Statistics for Biology and Health

For further volumes:
http://www.springer.com/series/2848

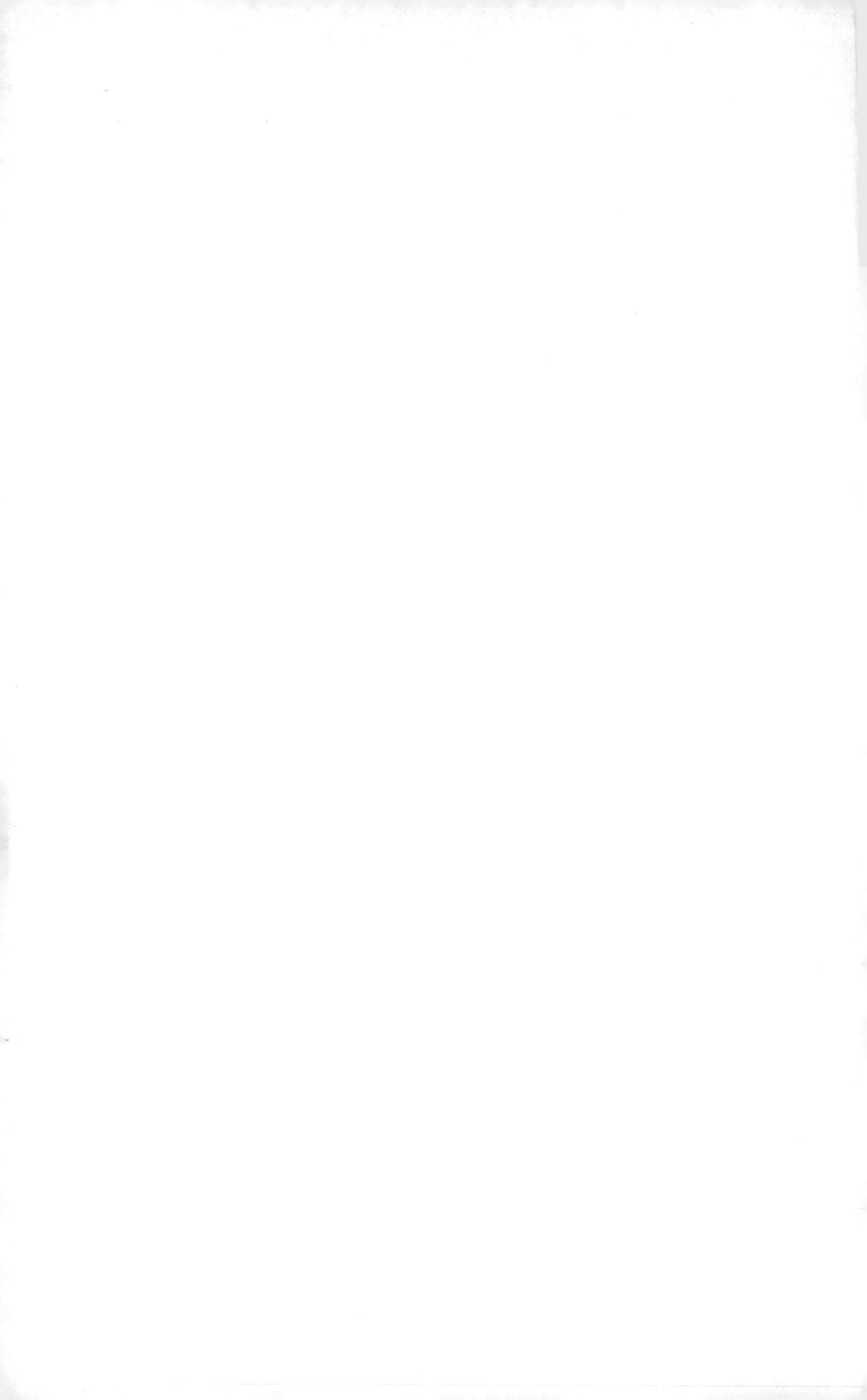

Bibhas Chakraborty • Erica E.M. Moodie

Statistical Methods for Dynamic Treatment Regimes

Reinforcement Learning, Causal Inference, and Personalized Medicine

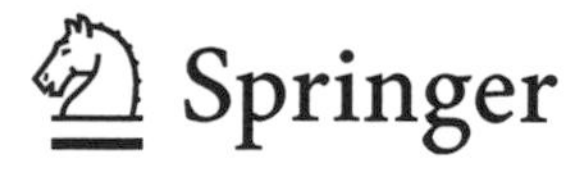

Bibhas Chakraborty
Department of Biostatistics
Columbia University
New York, USA

Erica E.M. Moodie
Department of Epidemiology, Biostatistics, and Occupational Health
McGill University
Montreal Québec
Canada

ISSN 1431-8776
ISBN 978-1-4899-9030-3 ISBN 978-1-4614-7428-9 (eBook)
DOI 10.1007/978-1-4614-7428-9
Springer New York Heidelberg Dordrecht London

Springer is part of Springer Science+Business Media (www.springer.com)

To my parents – Biman and Bani Chakraborty, and my wife Sanchalika: for all your love, support, and encouragement.

– Bibhas

To my family. Dave and my lovely boys, Gordie and Jamie: your unfailing encouragement and unconditional love keep me afloat. Mom and Dad: your guidance and support are invaluable. Zoe: you are my great listener and friend. I love you all.

– Erica

Preface

This book was written to summarize and describe the state of the art of statistical methods developed to address questions of estimation and inference for *dynamic treatment regimes*, a branch of personalized medicine. The study of dynamic treatment regimes is relatively young, and until now, no single source has aimed to provide an overview of the methodology and results which are dispersed in journals, proceedings, and technical reports so as to orient researchers to the field. Our primary focus is on description of the methods, clear communication of the conceptual underpinnings, and their illustration via analyses drawn from real applications as well as results from simulated data. The first chapter serves to set the context for the statistical reader in the landscape of personalized medicine; we assume a familiarity with elementary calculus, linear algebra, and basic large-sample theory. Important theoretical properties of the methods described will be stated when appropriate; however, the reader will, for the most part, be referred to the primary research articles for the proofs of the results. By doing so, we hope the book will be accessible to a wide audience of statisticians, epidemiologists, and medical researchers with some statistical training, as well as computer scientists (machine/reinforcement learning researchers) interested in medical applications.

Examples of data analyses from real applications are found throughout the book. From these, we hope to impart a sense of the power and versatility of the methods discussed to answer important problems in medical research. Where possible, we refer readers to available code or packages in different statistical languages to facilitate implementation; whether or not such code exists, we aim to describe all analytic approaches in sufficient detail that any researcher with a reasonable background in statistical programming could implement the methods from scratch.

We hope that the publication of this book will foster the genuine enthusiasm that we feel for this important area of research. Indeed, with the demographic shift of most Western populations to older age, the treatment of chronic conditions will bring increased pressure to develop evidence-based strategies for care that is tailored to individual changes in health status. The recently proposed methods have not yet reached a wide audience and consequently are underutilized. We hope that this text will serve as a useful handbook to those already active in the field of dynamic regimes and spark a new generation of researchers to turn their attention to this important and exciting area.

Acknowledgements

Bibhas Chakraborty would like to acknowledge support from the National Institutes of Health (NIH) grant R01 NS072127-01A1 and the Calderone Research Prize for Junior Faculty (2011) awarded by the Mailman School of Public Health of the Columbia University. Erica Moodie is supported by a Natural Sciences and Engineering Research Council (NSERC) University Faculty Award and by research grants from NSERC and the Canadian Institutes of Health Research (CIHR). Financial support for the writing of this book was provided by the Quebec Population Health Research Network (QPHRN).

We are indebted to numerous colleagues for lively and insightful discussions. Our research has been enriched by exchanges with Daniel Almirall, Ken Cheung, Nema Dean, Eric Laber, Bruce Levin, Susan Murphy, Min Qian, Thomas Richardson, Jamie Robins, Susan Shortreed, David Stephens, and Jonathan Wakefield. In particular, we wish to thank Ashkan Ertefaie, Eric Laber, Min Qian, Olli Saarela, and Michael Wallace for detailed comments on a first version of the text. Also, we would like to acknowledge help in software development and creation of some graphics for this book from Guqian Du, Tianxiao Huang, and Jingyi Xin – students in the Department of Biostatistics at Columbia University. Jonathan Weinberg, Benjamin Rich, and Yue Ru Sun, students in the Department of Mathematics & Statistics, the Department of Epidemiology, Biostatistics, & Occupational Health, and the school of Computer Science, respectively, at McGill University, also assisted in the preparation of some simulation results and graphics.

We wish to thank our many medical and epidemiological collaborators for thought-provoking discussions and/or the privilege of using their data: Dr. Michael Kramer (PROBIT), Drs. Merrick Moseley and Catherine Stewart (MOTAS), Dr. Augustus John Rush (STAR*D), and Dr. Victor J. Strecher (Project Quit – Forever Free). MOTAS was funded by the Guide Dogs for the Blind Association (UK); permission to analyze the data was granted by the MOTAS Cooperative. The follow-up of the PROBIT study was made possible by a grant from CIHR.

Data used in Sect. 5.2.4 were obtained from the limited access data sets distributed from the NIMH-supported "Clinical Antipsychotic Trials of Intervention Effectiveness in Schizophrenia" (CATIE-Sz). This is a multisite, clinical trial of persons with schizophrenia comparing the effectiveness of randomly assigned medication treatment. The study was supported by NIMH Contract #N01MH90001 to the University of North Carolina at Chapel Hill. The ClinicalTrials.gov identifier is NCT00014001. Analyses of the CATIE data presented in the book reflect the views of the authors and may not reflect the opinions or views of the CATIE-Sz Study Investigators or the NIH.

Data used in Sect. 8.9 were obtained from the limited access data sets distributed from the NIMH-supported "Sequenced Treatment Alternatives to Relieve Depression" (STAR*D) study. The study was supported by NIMH Contract # N01MH90003 to the University of Texas Southwestern Medical Center. The ClinicalTrials.gov identifier is NCT00021528. Analyses of the STAR*D data presented in the book reflect the views of the authors and may not reflect the opinions or views of the STAR*D Study Investigators or the NIH.

New York, USA — Bibhas Chakraborty
Montreal, Canada — Erica E.M. Moodie

Contents

Acronyms

AB	Adaptive bootstrap
ADHD	Attention deficit hyperactivity disorder
AFT	Accelerated failure time
ATT	Average treatment effect on the treated
BCAWS	Biased coin adaptive within-subject
BIC	Bayesian Information Criterion
BUP	Bupropion
BUS	Buspirone
CATIE	Clinical Antipsychotic Trials of Intervention Effectiveness
CBT	Cognitive behavioral therapy
CCM	Chronic care model
CCNIA	Characterizing Cognition in Nonverbal Individuals with Autism
CIT	Citalopram
CPB	Centered percentile bootstrap
CRAN	Comprehensive R Archive Network
CT	Cognitive psychotherapy
DAG	Directed acyclic graph
DB	Double bootstrap
DP	Dynamic programming
DTR	Dynamic treatment regime
EF	Estimating function
EM	Enhanced motivational program
GAM	Generalized additive model
GLM	Generalized linear model
HAART	Highly active antiretroviral therapy
HIV	Human immunodeficiency virus
HM	Hard-max
HT	Hard-threshold
IMOR	Iterative minimization of regrets
INR	International normalized ratio
IPTW	Inverse probability of treatment weighting

IPW	Inverse probability weighting
Li	Lithium
LQA	Local quadratic approximation
MC	Monte Carlo
MDP	Markov decision process
MIRT	Mirtazapine
MOTAS	Monitored Occlusion Treatment of Amblyopia Study
MSE	Mean Squared Error
MSM	Marginal structural model
NNR	Near-non-regular
NR	Non-regular
NTP	Nortriptyline
NTX	Naltrexone
NUC	No unmeasured confounding
OLS	Ordinary least squares
OWL	Outcome weighted learning
PANSS	Positive and Negative Syndrome Scale
PROBIT	Promotion of Breastfeeding Intervention Trial
PS	Propensity score
PSA	Prostate-specific antigen
QIDS	Quick Inventory of Depressive Symptomatology
RBT	Reinforcement-based treatment
RCT	Randomized controlled trial
RHS	Right-hand side
RL	Reinforcement learning
SER	Sertraline
SMART	Sequential multiple assignment randomized trial
SNMM	Structural nested mean model
SRA	Sequential randomization assumption
SSRI	Selective serotonin reuptake inhibitor
STAR*D	Sequenced Treatment Alternatives to Relieve Depression
ST	Soft-threshold
SUTVA	Stable unit treatment value assumption
SVR	Support vector regression
TCP	Tranylcypromine
THY	Thyroid hormone
TM	Telephone monitoring (only)
TMC	Telephone monitoring and counseling
VEN	Venlafaxine
WASI	Wechsler Abbreviated Scales of Intelligence
ZIPI	Zeroing instead of plugging in

Chapter 1
Introduction

1.1 Evidence-Based Personalized Medicine for Chronic Diseases

Personalized medicine is a medical paradigm that emphasizes systematic use of individual patient information to optimize that patient's health care. The primary motivation behind this paradigm is the well-established fact that patients often respond differently to a particular treatment, both in terms of the primary outcome and side-effects. This inherent heterogeneity across patients in response to any treatment prompted many health researchers to make an ideological transition from the *one-size-fits-all* approach of health care to the modern and more logical approach of personalized medicine. Benefits of personalized medicine include increased compliance or adherence to treatment, having the option of enhanced patient care by selecting the optimal treatment, and reduction of the overall cost of health care. While the increasing popularity of this paradigm within the medical community seems natural, it is less obvious why a statistician – or more generally a quantitative researcher – would be particularly interested in this topic. The primary reason is the growing interest in making the personalized treatments more *evidence-based* or *data-driven*, thus posing new methodological challenges that are often beyond the scope of traditional quantitative tools. As a natural consequence, there has been a recent surge of interest among statisticians, computer scientists and other quantitative researchers in this new arena of research leading to many exciting methodological developments.

This book focuses on personalized treatments for chronic diseases; we will describe various study designs as well as statistical analysis methods that aid in developing evidence-based personalized treatments for chronic diseases. Broadly speaking, chronic disorders constitute a considerable portion of today's pressing public health issues (WHO 1997; PFS 2004). For example, widely prevailing conditions like hypertension, obesity, diabetes, nicotine addiction, alcohol and drug abuse, cancer, HIV infection, and mental illnesses like depression and schizophrenia are all chronic. For effective long-term care of the patients, many of these chronic conditions require ongoing medical intervention, following the *chronic care model*

B. Chakraborty and E.E.M. Moodie, *Statistical Methods for Dynamic Treatment Regimes*,
Statistics for Biology and Health 76, DOI 10.1007/978-1-4614-7428-9_1,

(CCM) (Wagner et al. 2001) rather than the more traditional *acute care model*. Some of the key features of health care that the CCM emphasizes are as follows. First, clinicians following the CCM treat the patients by individualizing the treatment type, dosage and timing according to ongoing measures of patient response, adherence, burden, side effects, and preference; there is a strong emphasis on personalization of care according to patients' needs. Second, instead of deciding a treatment for once and all (*static* treatment), clinicians following CCM sequentially make decisions about what to do next to optimize patient outcome, given an individual patient's case history (*dynamic* treatment). The main motivations for considering sequences of treatments are high inter-patient variability in response to treatment, likely relapse, presence or emergence of co-morbidities, time-varying side effect severity, and reduction of costs and burden when intensive treatment is unnecessary (Collins et al. 2004). Third, while there exist traditional practice guidelines for clinicians that are primarily based on "expert opinions", the CCM advocates for making these regimes more objective and evidence-based. In fact, Wagner et al. (2001) described the CCM as "a synthesis of evidence-based system changes intended as a guide to quality improvement and disease management activities" (p. 69).

Since effective care for chronic disorders typically requires ongoing medical intervention, management of chronic disorders poses additional challenges for the paradigm of personalized medicine. This is because the personalization has to happen through multiple stages of intervention. In this context, *dynamic treatment regimes* (Murphy et al. 2001; Murphy 2003; Robins 2004; Lavori and Dawson 2004) offer a vehicle to operationalize the sequential decision making process involved in the personalized clinical practice consistent with the CCM, and thereby a potential way to improve it. In the following sections, we will develop key notions underlying dynamic treatment regimes.

1.2 Personalized Medicine and Medical Decision Making

Personalized treatments can be viewed as realizations of certain decision rules; these rules dictate what to do in a given state (e.g. demographics, case history, genetic information, etc.) of the patient. Thus, decision-theoretic notions, such as *utility*, can be employed in the development of these clinical decision rules. As argued by Parmigiani (2002), the main contribution of decision-theoretic ideas to medicine lies in providing a structure and formally defining a goal for the process of gathering, organizing, and integrating the quantitative information that is relevant to a decision. This justifies the role of decision-theoretic formalism in medical decision making despite the difficulties associated with its communication to the general public.

Use of decision-theoretic notions in medical and health care decision making has a long history. Early works in this domain include Lusted (1968), Weinstein et al. (1980), and Sox et al. (1988). More recent works include Chapman and Sonnenberg (2000), Clemen and Reilly (2001), and Parmigiani (2002). Specific discussion of the role of utility theory can be found in Pliskin et al. (1980) and Torrance (1986).

More statistically oriented works include Lindley (1985), French (1986), and Parmigiani (2002); in particular, Parmigiani (2002) provides an excellent account of the Bayesian approach to medical decision making. The type of decision problems studied in this book are, however, slightly different from the ones considered by the above authors. Below we briefly introduce the single-stage and multi-stage decision problems arising in personalized medicine that we will be considering in this book.

1.2.1 Single-stage Decision Problems in Personalized Medicine

For simplicity, first consider a single-stage decision problem, where the clinician has to decide on the optimal treatment for an individual patient. Suppose the clinician observes a certain characteristic (e.g. a demographic variable, a biomarker, or result of a diagnostic test) of the patient, say o, and based on that has to decide whether to prescribe treatment a or treatment a'. In this example, a decision rule could be: "give treatment a to the patient if his individual characteristic o is higher than a pre-specified threshold, and treatment a' otherwise". More formally, a decision rule is a mapping from currently available information, often succinctly referred to as the *state*, into the space of possible decisions.

Any decision, medical or otherwise, is statistically evaluated in terms of its *utility*, and the state in which the decision is made. For concreteness, let o denote the state (e.g. patient characteristic), a denote a possible decision (treatment), and $\mathscr{U}(o,a)$ denote the utility of taking the decision a while in the state o. Following Wald (1949), the current statistical decision problem can be formulated in terms of the opportunity *loss* (or *regret*) associated with each pair (o,a) by defining a loss function

$$\mathscr{L}(o,a) = \sup_{a} \mathscr{U}(o,a) - \mathscr{U}(o,a),$$

where the supremum is taken over all possible decisions for fixed o. The loss function is the difference between the utility of the optimal decision for state o, and the utility of the current decision a under that state. Clearly the goal is to find the decision that minimizes the loss function at the given state o; this is personalized decision making since the optimal decision depends on the state. Equivalently, the problem can be formulated directly in terms of the utility without defining the loss function; in that case the goal would be to choose a decision so as to maximize the utility for the given state o. The utility function can be specified in various ways, depending on the specific problem. One of the most common ways would be to set $\mathscr{U}(o,a) = E_a(Y|o)$, i.e. the conditional expectation of the primary outcome Y given the state, where the expectation is computed according to a probability distribution indexed by the decision a; we will make the underlying distributions precise in Chap. 3. Alternatively, one can define $\mathscr{U}(o,a) = E(Y(a)|o)$, where $Y(a)$ is the *potential outcome* of the decision a; see Chap. 2 for a precise description of the potential outcome framework.

In the econometrics literature, Manski (2000, 2002, 2004), Dehejia (2005), and Hirano and Porter (2009) use a similar decision-theoretic framework for the evaluation of social welfare programs, where the role of a clinician is replaced by a social planner, different welfare programs serve as different treatment choices, and the state again consists of individual characteristics. They use a slight variant of a loss or regret, and call it a *welfare contrast*. A welfare contrast is the difference between the utilities corresponding to two decisions, say a and a', under the same state o, i.e.

$$g(o,a,a') = \mathscr{U}(o,a) - \mathscr{U}(o,a').$$

Note that in the case where a is equal to the *optimal* decision, defined as the argument of the supremum of $\mathscr{U}(o,a)$, the welfare contrast coincides with the loss or regret associated with a'. Robins (2004) uses the term *blip* to denote a quantity similar to the welfare contrast in the multi-stage decision problems to be introduced next.

The focus of this book is multi-stage decision problems rather than the considerably simpler single-stage problems. However, we will use the single-stage decision framework at times to develop certain ideas to be ultimately used in the more complicated setting of multiple decisions. Theoretically oriented readers interested in the estimation of optimal single-stage decision rules and associated asymptotics may consult Hirano and Porter (2009) and Qian and Murphy (2011).

1.2.2 Multi-stage Decisions and Dynamic Treatment Regimes

Decision making problems arising not only in medicine but also in many other scientific domains like business, computer science, and social sciences often involve complex choices with multiple stages, where decisions made at one stage affect those to be made at another. In the context of multi-stage decisions, a *dynamic treatment regime* (DTR) is a sequence of decision rules, one per stage of intervention, for adapting a treatment plan to the time-varying state of an individual subject. Each decision rule takes a subject's individual characteristics and treatment history observed up to that stage as inputs, and outputs a recommended treatment at that stage; recommendations can include treatment type, dosage, and timing. DTRs are alternatively known as *treatment strategies* (Lavori and Dawson 2000; Thall et al. 2000, 2002, 2007a), *adaptive treatment strategies* (Murphy 2005a; Lavori and Dawson 2008), or *treatment policies* (Lunceford et al. 2002; Wahed and Tsiatis 2004, 2006). Conceptually, a DTR can be viewed as a *decision support system* of a clinician (or more generally, any decision maker), described as a key element of the CCM (Wagner et al. 2001). At a more basic level, it may be helpful to think of the regime as a rule-book and the specific treatment as the rules that apply to an individual case. The reason for considering a DTR as a whole instead of its individual stage-specific components is that the long-term effect of the current treatment may depend on the performance of future treatment choices. This issue will be discussed in greater detail in Chaps. 2 and 3.

In the current literature, a DTR is usually said to be *optimal* if it optimizes the mean long-term outcome (e.g. outcome observed at the end of the final stage of intervention). However, at least in principle, other utility functions (e.g. median or other quantiles, or some other feature of the outcome distribution) can be employed as optimization criteria. The main research goals in the arena of multi-stage decision making can be summarized as:

(a) To compare two or more preconceived DTRs in terms of their utility; and
(b) To identify the optimal DTR, i.e. to identify the sequence of treatments that result in the most favorable outcome possible (i.e. highest utility).

Thus, any attempt to achieve the above goals in a data-driven way essentially requires knowing or estimating the utility functions (or some variations). Key notions from the single-stage decision problems, as outlined above, can be extended to multi-stage decisions. For example, Murphy (2003) defines multiple stage-specific *regret* (loss) functions, and Robins (2004) defines stage-specific *blip* functions (welfare contrasts) in his framework of *structural nested mean models*. They provided methodologies to estimate the parameters of regret or blip functions, and thereby to identify the optimal DTR. Both of their approaches will be discussed in great detail in Chap. 4. On the other hand, *Q-learning*, a method originally developed in computer science but later adapted to statistics, targets estimating and maximizing the utility function (conditional expectation of the primary outcome), rather than minimizing the regret or any other blip; this method will be introduced in Chap. 3, and also will be used in some of the subsequent chapters in various contexts. All of these methods have their relative merits and demerits, which we will discuss as we go along. See also Dawid and Didelez (2010) for a decision-theoretic review of the DTRs from a causal inference perspective.

With the above broad picture of the multi-stage decision problems in mind, we provide a few concrete examples below.

Example 1: Treatment of HIV Infection

Patients with HIV infection are usually treated with *highly active antiretroviral therapy* (HAART). It is widely agreed that HAART should be initiated when CD4 cell count falls below 200 cells/μl, but a key question is whether to initiate HAART sooner in the course of the disease. In particular, it is of interest to know whether it is optimal to begin treatment when CD4 cell count first drops below a certain threshold, where that threshold may be as low as 200, or as high as 500, cells/μl (Sterne et al. 2009). Thus, the process of treating an HIV-infected patient is a multi-stage decision problem faced by the clinician who has to make treatment decisions based on the patient's CD4 count history (state) at a series of critical decision points (stages) (Cain et al. 2010).

Example 2: Treatment by Anticoagulation

Consider long-term anticoagulation treatment, as often given after events such as stroke, pulmonary embolism or deep vein thrombosis. The aim is to ensure that the patient's prothrombin time, measured by a quantity called the international normalized ratio (INR), is within a target range. Patients on this treatment are monitored regularly, and when their INR is outside the target range, the dose of anticoagulant is increased or decreased by the clinician so as to bring the INR level back within the target range. This is a multi-stage decision problem where the decisions are the doses and the previous INR observations and genetic markers comprise the state (Rosthøj et al. 2006).

Example 3: Treatment of Alcohol Addiction

Consider management of alcohol dependent subjects, with two clinical decisions: choosing the initial treatment and choosing the secondary treatment. Initially the clinician may prescribe either an opiate-antagonist called naltrexone (NTX) or cognitive behavioral therapy (CBT) to the alcohol dependent subjects. Subjects are classified as *responders* or *non-responders* based on their level of heavy drinking in the two months while they are on initial treatment. If at any time during this two-month period the subject experiences a third heavy drinking day, he is classified as a *non-responder* to the initial treatment. On the other hand, if the subject is able to avoid more than two heavy drinking days during the two-month period, he is considered a *responder*. If a subject is a non-responder to NTX, the clinician must decide whether to either switch to CBT or augment NTX with CBT and an enhanced motivational program (EM + CBT + NTX). If a subject is a non-responder to CBT, the clinician must decide whether to switch to NTX or augment CBT with NTX and an enhanced motivational program (EM + CBT + NTX). Responders to the initial treatment can be assigned either to telephone monitoring only (TM) or telephone monitoring and counseling (TMC) for an additional period of six months.

In this set-up, clinicians may want to use a DTR that maximizes the percent of days abstinent over a 12-month period (primary outcome). A DTR in this case consists of two decision rules: the first decision rule can use baseline level of addiction (e.g. number of heavy drinking days in a pre-specified period) to choose the initial treatment, and the second decision rule can utilize the intermediate outcome (responder/non-responder status) to choose the secondary treatment. One possible DTR can be: "as the initial treatment, prescribe NTX if the subject's baseline level of addiction is greater than a pre-specified threshold value, and prescribe CBT otherwise; as the secondary treatment, prescribe telephone monitoring if the subject is a responder to initial treatment, and prescribe a switch of treatment if the subject is a non-responder". Of course one can formulate many other DTRs in this set-up. Variations of this example have been discussed by Murphy (2005a), Chakraborty (2011), and Lei et al. (2012).

Example 4: Treatment of Cancer

Patients with cancer are often treated initially with a powerful chemotherapy, known as *induction therapy*, to induce remission of the disease. If the patient *responds* (e.g. shows sign of remission), the clinician tries to maintain remission for as long as possible before relapse by prescribing a *maintenance therapy* to intensify or augment the effects of the first-line induction therapy. If the patient *does not respond* (e.g. does not show sign of remission) to the first-line induction therapy, the clinician prescribes a second-line induction therapy to try to induce remission. Of course there exist many possible induction therapies and maintenance therapies. For treating a patient with cancer, a clinician may want to use a DTR that maximizes the disease-free survival time (primary outcome). One possible DTR can be: "initially prescribe the first-line induction therapy a; if the patient responds to a, prescribe maintenance therapy a', and if the patient does not respond to a, prescribe the second-line induction therapy a''". See, for example, Wahed and Tsiatis (2004) for further details on this two-stage clinical decision problem in the context of leukemia.

1.3 Outline of the Book

Constructing evidence-based (i.e. data-driven) dynamic treatment regimes comprises an emerging and important line of methodological research within the domain of personalized medicine, particularly in the context of chronic disorders. This book is an attempt to provide a comprehensive overview of this cutting-edge area of research. The methodologies emerged from at least two widely different academic disciplines, namely, reinforcement learning (within computer science) and causal inference (at the interface of statistics, epidemiology, economics and some other social sciences). Because of these very different origins, the methodologies are often described in different technical languages. In this book, we try to assimilate these into a coherent body of work.

In the present chapter, we have introduced the decision problems (both single- and multi-stage) arising in personalized medicine, and in particular, the concept of dynamic treatment regimes in the context of chronic diseases. Some concrete examples are provided to help readers appreciate the applications. In Chap. 2, we will describe different types of data sources and study designs relevant for constructing evidence-based DTRs. In this context, we will discuss both longitudinal observational studies and the sequential multiple assignment randomized trial designs that are tailor-made to produce high quality data for constructing dynamic treatment regimes. We will also review the potential outcome framework from causal inference in this chapter, while discussing observational studies.

The problem of estimating dynamic treatment regimes closely resembles reinforcement learning, and so we will review this area in Chap. 3, and develop a formal probabilistic framework in which we will work. In particular, we will introduce the Q-learning procedure, a simple yet powerful method for estimating optimal dynamic treatment regimes. In the following chapter, we will focus on methods from the statistical literature that hinge on direct modeling of contrasts of conditional mean outcomes under different regimes; this includes methods such as G-estimation of structural nested mean models and A-learning.

In Chap. 5, we turn to methods that model regimes directly. The chapter includes inverse probability of treatment weighted estimators such as marginal structural models as well as classification-based estimators. Chapter 6 takes a more model-based approach, and considers the likelihood-based method of G-computation.

The first six chapters focus on continuous outcome settings. In Chap. 7, we consider the literature to date on alternative outcome types: composite (multi-dimensional) outcomes, censored data, and discrete outcomes. A variety of methods from the previous chapters will be revisited.

Inference for optimal DTRs are discussed in Chap. 8. The issue of inference is particularly difficult in the DTR setting due to the phenomenon of *non-regularity*. Non-regularity and the ensuing complications arise because any method of estimating the optimal DTR involves non-smooth operations on the data. As a result, standard asymptotic theory or the usual bootstrap approach fail to produce valid confidence intervals for true treatment effect parameters. Various methods of avoiding this problem are discussed and compared in this chapter.

In Chap. 9, we will discuss some additional considerations, such as model building strategies and variable selection. In this chapter, we conclude the book with some overall discussion and remarks on the directions in which the field appears to be moving.

Chapter 2
The Data: Observational Studies and Sequentially Randomized Trials

The data for constructing (optimal) DTRs that we consider are obtained from either longitudinal observational studies or sequentially randomized trials. In this chapter we review these two types of data sources, their advantages and drawbacks, and the assumptions required to perform valid analyses in each, along with some examples. We also discuss a basic framework of causal inference in the context of observational studies, and power and sample size issues in the context of randomized studies.

2.1 Longitudinal Observational Studies

The goal of much of statistical inference is to quantify causal relationships, for instance to be able to assert that a specified treatment[1] improves patient outcomes rather than to state that treatment use or prescription of treatment is merely associated or correlated with better patient outcomes. Randomized trials are the "gold standard" in study design, as randomization coupled with compliance allows causal interpretations to be drawn from statistical association. Making causal inferences from observational data, however, can be tricky and relies critically on certain (unverifiable) assumptions which we will discuss in Sect. 2.1.3. The notion of causation is not new: it has been the subject matter of philosophers as far back as Aristotle, and more recently of econometricians and statisticians. Holland (1986) provides a nice overview of the philosophical views and definitions of causation as well as of the causal models frequently used in statistics. Neyman (1923) and later Rubin (1974) laid the foundations for the framework now used in modern causal inference. The textbook *Causal Inference* (Hernán and Robins 2013) provides a thorough description of basic definitions and most modern methods of causal inference for both

[1] In this book, we use the term *treatment* generically to denote either a medical treatment or an *exposure* (which is the preferred term in the causal inference literature and more generally in epidemiology).

B. Chakraborty and E.E.M. Moodie, *Statistical Methods for Dynamic Treatment Regimes*, Statistics for Biology and Health 76, DOI 10.1007/978-1-4614-7428-9_2,

point-source treatment (i.e. cross-sectional, or one-stage) settings as well as general longitudinal settings with time-varying treatments and the associated complexities.

2.1.1 The Potential Outcomes Framework

Much of the exposition of methods used when data are observational will rely on the notion of *potential outcomes* (also called *counterfactuals*), defined as a person's outcome had he followed a particular treatment regime, possibly different from the regime which he was actually observed to follow (hence, counter to fact). The individual-level causal effect of a regime may then be viewed as the difference in outcomes if a person had followed that regime as compared to a placebo regime or a standard care protocol. Consider, for example, a simple one-stage[2] randomized trial in which subjects can receive either a or a'. Suppose now that an individual was randomized to receive treatment a. This individual will have a single observed outcome Y which corresponds to the potential outcome "Y under treatment a", denoted by $Y(a)$, and one unobservable potential outcome, $Y(a')$, corresponding to the outcome under a'. An alternative notation to express counterfactual quantities is via subscripting: Y_a and $Y_{a'}$ (Hernán et al. 2000). Pearl (2009) uses an approach similar to that of the counterfactual framework, using what is called the "do" notation to express the idea that a treatment is administered rather than simply observed to have been given: in his notation, $E[Y|do(A = a)]$ is the expected value of the outcome variable Y under the intervention regime a, i.e. it is the population average were all subjects forced to take treatment a.

The so-called *fundamental problem of causal inference* lies in the definition of causal parameters at an individual level. Suppose we are interested in the causal effect of taking treatment a instead of treatment a'. An individual-level causal parameter that could be considered is a person's outcome under treatment a' subtracted from his outcome under treatment a, i.e. $Y(a) - Y(a')$. Clearly, it is not possible to observe the outcome under both treatments a and a' without further data and assumptions (e.g. in a cross-over trial with no carry-over effect) and so the individual-level causal effect can never be observed. However, population-level causal parameters or average causal effects can be identified under randomization with perfect compliance, or bounded under randomization with non-compliance. Without randomization, i.e. in observational studies or indeed randomized trials with imperfect compliance, further assumptions are required to estimate population-level causal effects, which we shall detail shortly.

Suppose now that rather than being a one-stage trial, subjects are treated over two stages, and can receive at each stage either a or a'. If an individual was randomized to receive treatment a first and then treatment a', this individual will have a single observed outcome Y which corresponds to the potential outcome "Y under regime

[2] While the term *stage* is commonly used in the randomized trial literature, the term *interval* is more popular in the causal inference literature. In this book, for consistency, we will use the term *stage* for both observational and randomized studies.

(a, a')", which we denote by $Y(a, a')$, and three unobservable potential outcomes: $Y(a, a)$, $Y(a', a)$, and $Y(a', a')$, corresponding to outcomes under each of the other three possible regimes. As is clear even in this very simple example, the number of potential outcomes and causal effects as represented by contrasts between the potential outcomes can be very large, even for a moderate number of stages. As shall be seen in Chap. 4, the optimal dynamic regime may be estimated while limiting the models specified to only a subset of all possible contrasts.

2.1.2 Time-Varying Confounding and Mediation

Longitudinal data are increasingly available to health researchers; this type of data presents challenges not observed in cross-sectional data, not the least of which is the presence of time-varying confounding variables and intermediate effects. A variable O is said to be a *mediating* or *intermediate* variable if it is caused by A and in turn causes changes in Y. For example, a prescription sleep-aid medication (A) may cause dizziness (O) which in turn causes fall-related injuries (Y). In contrast, a variable, O, is said to *confound* a relationship between a treatment A and an outcome Y if it is a common cause of both the treatment and the outcome. More generally, a variable is said to be a confounder (relative to a set of covariates X) if it is a pre-treatment covariate that removes some or all of the bias in a parameter estimate, when taken into account in addition to the variables X. It may be the case, then, that a variable is a confounder relative to one set of covariates X but not another, X'. If the effect of O on both A and Y is not accounted for, it may appear that there is a relationship between A and Y when in fact their pattern of association may be due entirely to changes in O. For example, consider a study of the dependence of the number of deaths by drowning (Y) on the use of sunscreen (A). A strong positive relationship is likely to be observed, however it is far more likely that this is due to the confounding variable air temperature (O). When air temperature is high, individuals may be more likely to require sunscreen and may also be more likely to swim, but there is no reason to believe that the use of sunscreen increases the risk of drowning. In cross-sectional data, eliminating the bias due to a confounding effect is typically achieved by adjusting for the variable in a regression model.

Directed Acyclic Graphs (DAGs), also called *causal graphs*, formalize the causal assumptions that a researcher may make regarding the variables he wishes to analyze. A graph is said to be *directed* if all inter-variable relationships are connected by arrows indicating that one variable causes changes in another and *acyclic* if it has no closed loops (no feedback between variables); see, for example, Greenland et al. (1999) or Pearl (2009) for further details. DAGs are becoming more common in epidemiology and related fields as researchers seek to clarify their assumptions about hypothesized relationships and thereby justify modeling choices (e.g. Bodnar et al. 2004; Brotman et al. 2008). In particular, confounding in its simplest form can be visualized in a DAG if there is an arrow from O into A, and another from O into Y. Similarly, mediation is said to occur if there is at least one directed path of arrows from A to Y that passes through O.

Let us now briefly turn to a two-stage setting where data are collected at three time-points: baseline (t_1=0), t_2, and t_3. Covariates are denoted O_1 and O_2, measured at baseline and t_2, respectively. Treatment at stages 1 and 2, received in the intervals $[0,t_2)$ and $[t_2,t_3)$, are denoted A_1 and A_2 respectively. Outcome, measured at t_3, is denoted Y. Suppose there is an additional variable, U, which is a cause of both O_2 and Y. See Fig. 2.1.

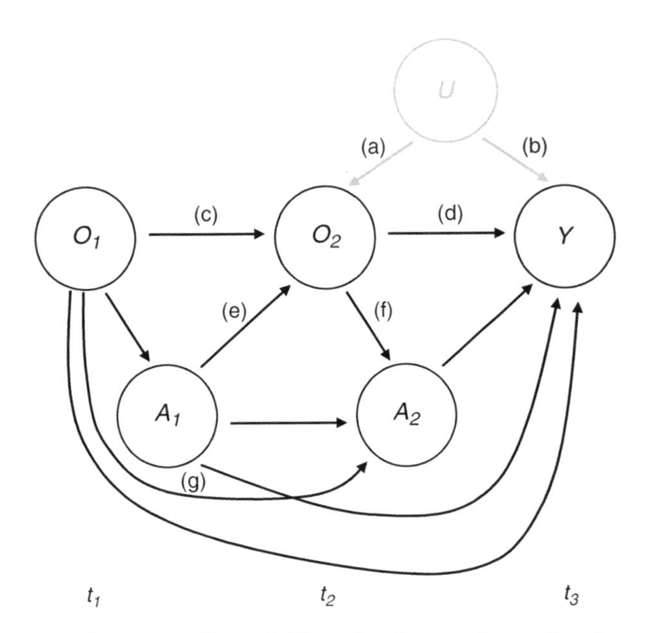

Fig. 2.1 A two-stage directed acyclic graph illustrating time-varying confounding and mediation

We first focus on the effect of A_1 on Y; A_1 acts directly on Y, but also acts indirectly through O_2 as indicated by arrows (e) and (d); O_2 is therefore a mediator. We now turn our attention to the effect of A_2 on Y; O_2 confounds this relationship, as can be observed by arrows (d) and (f). In this situation, adjustment for O_2 is essential to obtaining unbiased estimation of the effect of A_2 on Y. However, complications may arise if there are unmeasured factors that also act as confounders; in Fig. 2.1, U acts in this way. If one were to adjust for O_2 in a regression model, it would open what is called a "back-door" path from Y to A_2 via the path (b)→(a)→(c)→(g). This is known as *collider-stratification bias, selection bias, Berksonian bias, Berkson's paradox*, or, in some contexts, the *null paradox* (Robins and Wasserman 1997; Gail and Benichou 2000; Greenland 2003; Murphy 2005a); this problem will be considered in greater depth in Sect. 3.4.2 in the context of estimation. Collider-stratification bias can also occur when conditioning on or stratifying by variables that are caused by both the exposure and the outcome, and there has been a move in the epidemiology literature to use the term selection bias only for bias caused by conditioning on post-treatment variables, and the term confounding for bias caused by pre-treatment variables (Hernán et al. 2004).

Modeling choices become more complex when data are collected over time, particularly as a variable may act as both a confounder and a mediator. The use of a DAG forces the analyst to be explicit in his modeling assumptions, particularly as the absence of an arrow between two variables ("nodes") in a graph implies the assumption of (conditional) independence. Some forms of estimation are able to avoid the introduction of collider-stratification bias by eliminating conditioning (e.g. weighting techniques) while others rely on the assumption that no variables such as U exist. See Sect. 3.4.2 for a discussion on how *Q-learning*, a stage-wise regression based method of estimation, avoids this kind of bias by analyzing one stage at a time.

2.1.3 Necessary Assumptions

A fundamental requirement of the potential outcomes framework is the *axiom of consistency*, which states that the potential outcome under the observed treatment and the observed outcome agree: that is, the treatment must be defined in such a way that it must be possible for all treatment options to be assigned to all individuals in the population under consideration. Thus, the axiom of consistency requires that the outcome for a given treatment is the same, regardless of the manner in which treatments are 'assigned'. This is often plausible in studies of medical treatments where it is easy to conceive of how to manipulate the treatments given to the patients (this setting is relevant in the DTR context), but less obvious for exposures that are modifiable by a variety of means, such as body-mass index (Hernán and Taubman 2008), or that are better defined as (non-modifiable) characteristics, such as sex (Cole and Frangakis 2009).

Before stating the necessary assumptions for estimating DTRs, we introduce the following notations. Let $\bar{a}_K \equiv (a_1,\ldots,a_K)$ denote a K-stage sequence of treatments. Let $(d_1,\ldots,d_K)$ denote a treatment regime, i.e. a set of decision rules where d_j is a mapping from the history space to the treatment/action space for all j. Similarly let $\bar{O}_j \equiv (O_1,\ldots,O_j)$ denote the collection of covariates observed up to stage j and $\bar{A}_{j-1} \equiv (A_1,\ldots,A_{j-1})$ denote the collection of past treatments prior to stage j. We combine the treatment and covariate history up to the jth stage into a single *history* vector, $H_j \equiv (\bar{O}_j,\bar{A}_{j-1})$. To estimate a DTR from either randomized or observational data, two assumptions are required:

1. *Stable unit treatment value assumption (SUTVA)*: A subject's outcome is not influenced by other subjects' treatment allocation (Rubin 1980).
2. *No unmeasured confounders* (NUC): For any regime $\bar{a}_K$,

$$A_j \perp (O_{j+1}(\bar{a}_j),\ldots,O_K(\bar{a}_{K-1}),Y(\bar{a}_K))\Big| H_j \quad \forall j = 1,\ldots,K.$$

   That is, for any possible regime $\bar{a}_K$, treatment A_j received in the jth stage is independent of any future (potential) covariate or outcome, $O_{j+1}(\bar{a}_j),\ldots,O_K(\bar{a}_{K-1})$, $Y(\bar{a}_K)$, conditional on the history H_j (Robins 1997).

The first assumption – sometimes called *no interaction between units* or *no interference between units* (Cox 1958) – is often reasonable, particularly in the context of randomized trials where study participants are drawn from a large population. SUTVA may be violated in special cases such as vaccinations for contagious disease where the phenomenon of "herd immunity" may lead to protection of unvaccinated individuals or in the context of group therapy (e.g. a support group) where the inter-personal dynamics between group members could influence outcomes.

The NUC assumption always holds under either complete or sequential randomization, and is sometimes called the *sequential randomization assumption* (SRA), *sequential ignorability*, or *exchangeability*, which is closely linked to the concept of *stability* (Dawid and Didelez 2010; Berzuini et al. 2012). The assumption may also be (approximately) true in observational settings where all relevant confounders have been measured. No unmeasured confounding is a strong generalization of the usual concept of randomization in a single-stage trial, whereby it is assumed that, conditional on treatment and covariate history, *at each stage* the treatment actually received, A_j, is independent of future states and outcome under *any* sequence of future treatments, $\bar{a}_j$. That is, conditional on the past history, treatment received at stage j is independent of future potential covariates and outcome:

$$p(A_j|H_j, O_{j+1}(\bar{a}_j), \ldots, O_K(\bar{a}_{K-1}), Y(\bar{a}_K)) = p(A_j|H_j).$$

It is this assumption that allows us to effectively view each stage as a randomized trial, possibly with different randomization probabilities at stage j, given strata defined by the history H_j.

If subjects are censored (lost to follow-up or otherwise removed from the study), we must further assume that censoring is non-informative conditional on history, i.e. that the potential outcomes of those subjects who are censored follow the same distribution as that of those who are fully followed given measured covariates.

The optimal regime may only be estimated non-parametrically among the set of *feasible* regimes (Robins 1994). Let $p_j(a_j|H_j)$ denote the conditional probability of receiving treatment a_j given H_j, and let $f(H_K)$ denote the density function of H_K. Then for all histories h_K with $f(h_K) > 0$, a feasible regime $\bar{d}_K$ satisfies

$$\prod_{j=1}^{K} p_j(d_j(H_j)|H_j = h_j) > 0.$$

That is, feasibility requires some subjects to have followed regime $\bar{d}_K$ for the analyst to be able to estimate its performance non-parametrically. To express this in terms of decision trees, no non-parametric inference can be made about the effect of following a particular branch of a decision tree if no one in the sample followed that path.

Other terms have been used to describe feasible treatment regimes, including *viable* (Wang et al. 2012) and *realistic* (Petersen et al. 2012) rules. Feasibility is closely related to the *positivity*, or *experimental treatment assignment* (ETA), assumption. Positivity, like feasibility, requires that there are both treated and untreated individuals at every level of the treatment and covariate history. Positivity may be violated either *theoretically* or *practically*. A theoretical or structural violation occurs if the study design prohibits certain individuals from receiving a particular treatment, e.g. failure of one type of drug may preclude the prescription of other drugs in that class. A practical violation of the positivity assumption is said to occur when a particular stratum of subjects has a very low probability of receiving the treatment (Neugebauer and Van der Laan 2005; Cole and Hernán 2008). Visual and bootstrap-based approaches to diagnosing positivity violations have been proposed for one-stage settings (Wang et al. 2006; Petersen et al. 2012). Practical positivity violations may be more prevalent in longitudinal studies if there exists a large number of possible treatment paths; methods for handling such violations in multi-stage settings are less developed.

There is an additional assumption that is not required for estimation, but that is useful for understanding the counterfactual quantities and models that will be considered: the assumption of *additive local rank preservation*, which we shall elucidate in two steps. First, *local rank preservation* states that the ranking of subjects' outcomes under a particular treatment pattern $\overline{a}_K$ is the same as their ranking under any other pattern, say $\overline{d}_K$, given treatment and covariate history (see Table 2.1). In particular, if we consider two regimes $\overline{d}_K$ and $\overline{a}_K$, local rank preservation states that the ranking of patients' outcomes under regime $\overline{d}_K$ is the same as their ranking under regime $\overline{a}_K$ conditional on the history H_j. Local rank preservation is said to be *additive* when $Y(\overline{d}_K) = Y(\overline{a}_K) + \text{cons}$, where $\text{cons} = E[Y(\overline{d}_K) - Y(\overline{a}_K)]$, i.e., the individual causal effect equals the *average causal effect*. This is also called *unit treatment additivity*. Thus, rank preservation makes the assumption that the individuals who do best under one regime will also do so under another, and in fact the ranking of each individual's outcome will remain unchanged whatever the treatment pattern received. Additive local rank preservation makes the much stronger assumption that the difference between any two individuals' outcomes will be the same under all treatment patterns.

Table 2.1 Local rank preservation (LRP) and additive LRP, assuming all subjects have the same baseline covariates

			LRP		Additive LRP	
Subject	$Y(\overline{a}_K)$	Rank	$Y(\overline{d}_K)$	Rank	$Y(\overline{d}_K)$	Rank
1	12.8	3	15.8	3	13.9	3
2	10.9	1	14.0	1	13.0	1
3	13.1	4	16.0	4	14.2	4
4	12.7	2	14.5	2	13.8	2

2.2 Examples of Longitudinal Observational Studies

A variety of studies aimed at estimating optimal DTRs from observational data have been undertaken. Data sources include administrative (e.g. hospital) databases (Rosthøj et al. 2006; Cain et al. 2010; Cotton and Heagerty 2011), randomized encouragement trials (Moodie et al. 2009), and cohort studies (Van der Laan and Petersen 2007b). We shall briefly describe three here to demonstrate the variety of questions that can be addressed using observational data and DTR methodology. In particular, the data in the examples below have been addressed using regret-regression, G-estimation, and marginal structural models; these and related methods of estimation are presented in Chaps. 4 and 5.

2.2.1 Investigating Warfarin Dosing Using Hospital Data

Rosthøj et al. (2006) aimed to find a warfarin dosing strategy to control the risk of both clotting and excessive bleeding, by tailoring treatment using the international normalized ratio, a measure of clotting tendency of blood. Observational data were taken from hospital records over a five year period; recorded variables included age, sex, and diagnosis as well as a time-varying measure of INR. There exists a standard target range for INR, and so the vector-valued tailoring variable, O_j, was taken to be 0 if the most recent INR measurement lay within the target range and otherwise was taken to be the ratio of the difference between the INR measurement and the nearest boundary of the target range, and the width of that target range. Treatment at stage j, A_j, was taken to be the change in warfarin dose (with 0 being an acceptable option). The outcome of interest was taken to be the percentage of the time on study in which a subject's INR was within the target range.

Rosthøj et al. (2006) modeled the effect of taking the observed rather than the optimal dose of warfarin using parametric mean models that are quadratic in the dosing effect so that doses that are either too low or too high are penalized.

2.2.2 Investigating Epoetin Therapy Using the United States Renal Data System

Cotton and Heagerty (2011) performed an analysis of the United States Renal Data System, an administrative data set based on Medicare claims for hemodialysis with end-stage renal disease. Covariates included demographic variables as well as clinical and laboratory variables such as diabetes, HIV status, and creatinine clearance. Monthly information was also available on the number of dialysis sessions reported, the number of epoetin doses recorded, the total epoetin dosage, iron supplementation dose, the number of days hospitalized and the most recently recorded hematocrit measurement in the month.

Restricting their analysis to incident end-stage renal disease patients free from HIV/AIDS from 2003, Cotton and Heagerty (2011) considered treatment rules that adjust epoetin treatment at time j, A_j, multiplicatively based on the value of treatment in the previous month, A_{j-1}, and the most recent hematocrit measurement, O_j:

$$A_j \in \begin{cases} A_{j-1} \times (0,0.75) & \text{if } O_j \geq \psi - 3 \\ A_{j-1} \times (0.75,1.25) & \text{if } O_j \in (\psi - 3, \psi + 3) \\ A_{j-1} \times (1.25,\infty) & \text{if } O_j \leq \psi + 3 \end{cases}$$

where the target hematocrit range specified by the parameter ψ is varied to consider a range of different regimes. That is, O_j is the tailoring variable at each month, and the optimal regime is the treatment rule $d_j^{opt}(O_j, A_{j-1}; \psi)$ that maximizes survival time for $\psi \in \{31, 32, \ldots, 40\}$. Thus, in contrast to the strategy employed by Rosthøj et al. (2006), the decision rules considered in the analysis of Cotton and Heagerty (2011) did not attempt to estimate the optimal treatment changes/doses, but rather focused on estimating which target range of hematocrit should initiate a change in treatment dose from one month to the next. Note that the parameter ψ (the mid-value of the target hematocrit range) does not vary over time, but rather is common over all months; this is called *parameter sharing* (over time).

2.2.3 Estimating Optimal Breastfeeding Strategies Using Data from a Randomized Encouragement Trial

The Promotion of Breastfeeding Intervention Trial (PROBIT) (Kramer et al. 2001) has been used to explore several different dynamic regimes, with a view to optimizing growth (Moodie et al. 2009; Rich et al. 2010) and the vocabulary subtest of the Wechsler Abbreviated Scales of Intelligence (Moodie et al. 2012).

PROBIT randomized hospitals and affiliated polyclinics in the Republic of Belarus to a breastfeeding promotion intervention modeled on the WHO/UNICEF Baby-Friendly Hospital Initiative or standard care. Mother-infant pairs were enrolled during their postpartum stay, and follow-up visits were scheduled at 1, 2, 3, 6, 9, and 12 months of age for various measures of health and size, including weight, length, number of hospitalizations and gastrointestinal infections since the last scheduled visit. At each follow-up visit up to 12 months, it was established whether the infant was breastfeeding, as well as whether the infant was given other liquids or solid foods. In a later wave of PROBIT, follow-up interviews and examinations including the Wechsler test were performed on 13,889 (81.5 %) children at 6.5 years of age.

In analyses of these data, the treatment A_j was taken to be continued breastfeeding throughout the jth stage, and variables such as infant weight at the start of the stage or the number of gastrointestinal infections at the previous stage have been considered as potential tailoring variables, O_j.

2.3 Sequentially Randomized Studies

It is well known that estimates based on observational data are often subject to *confounding* and various hidden biases; hence randomized data, when available, are preferable for more accurate estimation and stronger statistical inference (Rubin 1974; Holland 1986; Rosenbaum 1991). This is especially important when dealing with DTRs since the hidden biases can compound over stages. One crucial point to note here is that developing DTRs is a developmental procedure rather than a confirmatory procedure. Usual randomized controlled trials are used as the "gold standard" for evaluating or confirming the efficacy of a newly developed treatment, not for developing the treatment *per se*. Thus, generating meaningful data for developing optimal DTRs is beyond the scope of the usual confirmatory randomized trials; special design considerations are required. A special class of designs called *sequential multiple assignment randomized trial* (SMART) designs, tailor-made for the purpose of developing optimal DTRs, is discussed below.

SMART designs involve an initial randomization of patients to possible treatment options, followed by re-randomizations at each subsequent stage of some or all of the patients to another treatment available at that stage. The re-randomizations at each subsequent stage may depend on information collected after previous treatments, but prior to assigning the new treatment, e.g. how well the patient responded to the previous treatment. Thus, even though a subject is randomized more than once, ethical constraints are not violated. This type of design was first introduced by Lavori and Dawson (2000) under the name *biased coin adaptive within-subject* (BCAWS) design, and practical considerations for designing such trials were discussed by Lavori and Dawson (2004). Building on these works, Murphy (2005a) proposed the general framework of the SMART design. These designs attempt to conform better to the way clinical practice for chronic disorders actually occurs, but still retain the well-known advantages of randomization over observational studies.

SMART-like trials, i.e. trials involving multiple randomizations had been used in various fields even before the exact framework was formally established; see for example, the CALGB Protocol 8923 for treating elderly patients with leukemia (Stone et al. 1995; Wahed and Tsiatis 2004, 2006), the CATIE trial for antipsychotic medications in patients with Alzheimer's disease (Schneider et al. 2001), the STAR*D trial for treatment of depression (Lavori et al. 2001; Rush et al. 2004; Fava et al. 2003), and some cancer trials conducted at the MD Anderson Cancer Center (Thall et al. 2000). Other examples include a smoking cessation study conducted by the Center for Health Communications Research at the University of Michigan (Strecher et al. 2008; Chakraborty et al. 2010), and a trial of neurobehavioral treatments for patients with metastatic malignant melanoma (Auyeung et al. 2009). More recently, Lei et al. (2012) discussed four additional examples of SMARTs: the Adaptive Characterizing Cognition in Nonverbal Individuals with Autism (CCNIA) Developmental and Augmented Intervention (Kasari 2009) for school-age, nonverbal children with autism spectrum disorders; the Adaptive Pharmacological and Behavioral Treatments for children with attention deficit hyperactivity disorder (ADHD) (see for example, Nahum-Shani et al. 2012a,b); the Adaptive Reinforcement-Based

Treatment for Pregnant Drug Abusers (RBT) (Jones 2010); and the ExTENd study for alcohol-dependent individuals (Oslin 2005). Lei et al. (2012) also discussed the subtle distinctions between different types of SMARTs in terms of the extent of multiple randomizations: (i) SMARTs in which only the non-responders to one of the initial treatments are re-randomized (e.g. CCNIA); (ii) SMARTs in which non-responders to all the initial treatments are re-randomized (e.g. the ADHD trial); and (iii) SMARTs in which both responders and non-responders to all the initial treatments are re-randomized (e.g. RBT, ExTENd).

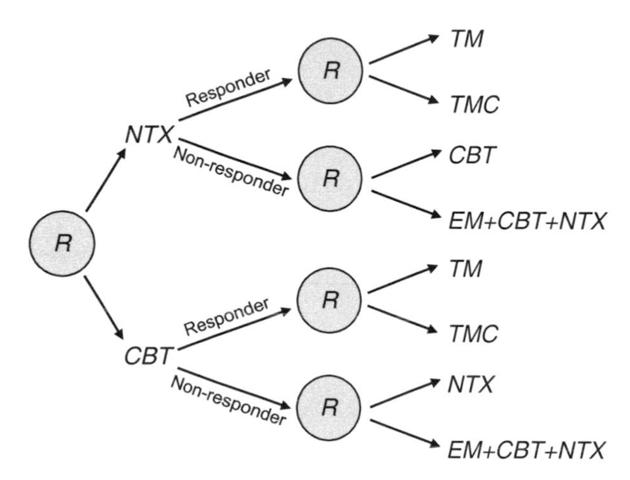

Fig. 2.2 Hypothetical SMART design schematic for the addiction management example (an "R" within a circle denotes randomization at a critical decision point)

In order to make the discussion more concrete, let us consider a hypothetical SMART design based on the addiction management example introduced in Chap. 1; see Fig. 2.2 for a schematic. In this trial, each subject is randomly assigned to one of two possible initial treatments: cognitive behavioral therapy (CBT) or naltrexone (NTX). A subject is classified as a *non-responder* or *responder* to the initial treatment according to whether he does or does not experience more than two heavy drinking days during the next two months. A non-responder to NTX is re-randomized to one of the two subsequent treatment options: either a switch to CBT, or an augmentation of NTX with CBT and an enhanced motivational program (EM + CBT + NTX). Similarly, a non-responder to CBT is re-randomized to either a switch to NTX or an augmentation (EM + CBT + NTX). Responders to the initial treatment are re-randomized to receive either telephone monitoring only (TM) or telephone monitoring and counseling (TMC) for an additional period of six months. The goal of the study is to maximize the number of non-heavy drinking days over a 12-month study period.

2.3.1 SMART Versus a Series of Single-stage Randomized Trials

Note that the goal of SMART design is to generate high quality data that would aid in the development and evaluation of optimal DTRs. A competing design approach could be to conduct separate randomized trials for each of the separate stages, to find the optimal treatment at each stage based on the trial data, and then combine these optimal treatments from individual stages to create a DTR. For example, instead of the SMART design for the addiction management study described above, the researcher may conduct two single-stage randomized trials. The first trial would involve a comparison of the initial treatments (CBT versus NTX). The researcher would then choose the best treatment based on the results of the first trial and move on to the second trial where all subjects would be initially treated with the chosen treatment and then responders would be randomized to one of the two possible options: TM or TMC, and non-responders would be randomized to one of the two possible options: switch of the initial treatment or a treatment augmentation (EM + CBT + NTX). However, when used to optimize DTRs, this approach suffers from several disadvantages as compared to a SMART design.

First, this design strategy is myopic, and may often fail to detect possible *delayed effects* of treatments, ultimately resulting in a suboptimal DTR (Lavori and Dawson 2000). Many treatments can have effects that do not occur until after the intermediate outcome (e.g. response to initial treatment) has been measured, such as improving the effect of a future treatment or long-term side effects that prevent a patient from being able to use an alternative useful treatment in future. SMART designs are capable of taking care of this issue while the competing approach is not. This point can be further elucidated using the addiction management example, following the original arguments of Murphy (2005a). Suppose counseling (TMC) is more effective than monitoring (TM) among responders to CBT; this is a realistic scenario since the subject can learn to use counseling during CBT at the initial stage and thus is able to take advantage of the counseling offered at the subsequent stage to responders. Individuals who received NTX during the initial treatment would not have learned to use counseling, and thus among responders to NTX the addition of counseling to the monitoring does not improve abstinence relative to monitoring alone. If an individual is a responder to CBT, it is best to offer TMC as the secondary treatment. But if the individual is a responder to NTX, it is best to offer the less expensive TM as the secondary treatment. In summary, even if CBT and NTX result in the same proportion of responders (or, even if CBT appears less effective at the initial stage), CBT may be the best initial treatment as part of the entire treatment sequence. This would be due to the enhanced effect of TMC when preceded by CBT. On the other hand, if the researcher employs two separate stage-specific trials, he would likely conduct the second trial with NTX (which is cheaper than CBT) as the initial treatment, unless CBT looks significantly better than NTX at the first trial. In that case, there would be no way for the researcher to discover the truly optimal regime.

Second, even though the results of the first trial may indicate that treatment a is initially less effective than treatment a', it is quite possible that treatment a may elicit valuable *diagnostic* information that would permit the researcher to better personalize the subsequent treatment to each subject, and thus improve the primary outcome. This issue can be better discussed using the ADHD study example (Nahum-Shani et al. 2012a,b), following the original discussion of Lei et al. (2012). In secondary analyses of the ADHD study, Nahum-Shani et al. (2012a,b) found evidence that children's adherence to the initial intervention could be used to better match the secondary intervention. More precisely, among non-responders to the initial intervention (either low-dose medication or low-dose behavioral modification), those with low adherence performed better when the initial intervention was augmented with the other type of intervention at the second stage, compared to increasing the dose or intensity of the initial treatment at the second stage. This phenomenon is sometimes called the *diagnostic effect* or *prescriptive effect*.

Third, subjects who enroll and remain in a single-stage trial may be inherently different from those who enroll and remain in a SMART. This is a type of *cohort effect* or *selection effect*, as discussed by Murphy et al. (2007a). Consider a single-stage randomized trial in which CBT is compared with NTX. First, in order to reduce variability in the treatment effect, investigators would tend to set very restrictive entry criteria (this is the case with most RCTs), which would result in a cohort that represents only a small subset of the treatable population. In contrast, researchers employing a SMART design would not try to reduce the variability in the treatment effect, since this design would allow varying treatment sequences for different types of patients. Hence SMARTs can recruit from a wider population of patients, and would likely result in greater *generalizability*. Furthermore, in a single-stage RCT, for subjects with no improvement in symptoms and for those experiencing severe side-effects, there is often no option but to drop out of the study or cease to comply with the study protocol. In contrast, non-responding subjects in a SMART would know that their treatments will be altered at some point. Thus it can be argued that non-responding subjects may be less likely to drop out from a SMART relative to a single-stage randomized trial. Consequently the choice of the best initial treatment obtained from a single-stage trial may be based on a sample less representative of the study population compared to the choice of the best initial treatment obtained from a SMART.

From the above discussion, it is clear that conducting separate stage-specific trials and combining best treatment options from these separate trials may fail to detect delayed effects and diagnostic effects, and may result in possible cohort effects, thereby rendering the developed sequence of treatment decisions potentially suboptimal. This has been the motivation to consider SMART designs.

2.3.2 Design Properties

For simplicity of exposition, let us focus on SMART designs with only two stages; however the ideas can be generalized to any finite number of stages. Denote the observable data trajectory for a subject in a SMART by (O_1, A_1, O_2, A_2, Y), where

O_1 and O_2 are the pretreatment information and intermediate outcomes, A_1 and A_2 are the randomly assigned initial and secondary treatments, and Y is the primary outcome, respectively. For example, in the addiction management study discussed earlier, O_1 may include addiction severity and co-morbid conditions, O_2 may include the subject's binary response status, side effects and adherence to the initial treatment, and Y may be the number of non-heavy drinking days over the 12-month study period. Under *the axiom of consistency* (see Sect. 2.1.3), the potential outcomes are connected to the observable data by $O_2 = O_2(A_1)$ and $Y = Y(A_1, A_2)$.

In a SMART, the randomization probabilities may depend on the available treatment and covariate *history*; more precisely, the randomization probabilities for A_1 and A_2 may depend on $H_1 \equiv O_1$ and $H_2 \equiv (O_1, A_1, O_2)$, respectively. Thus data from a SMART satisfy the *sequential ignorability* or *no unmeasured confounding* assumption (see Sect. 2.1.3). Under this assumption, the conditional distributions of the potential outcomes are the same as the corresponding conditional distributions of the observable data. That is,

$$P(O_2(a_1) \leq o_2 | O_1 = o_1) = P(O_2 \leq o_2 | O_1 = o_1, A_1 = a_1),$$

and

$$\begin{aligned} P(Y(a_1, a_2) \leq y | O_1 = o_1, O_2(a_1) = o_2) \\ = P(Y \leq y | O_1 = o_1, A_1 = a_1, O_2 = o_2, A_2 = a_2). \end{aligned}$$

This implies that the mean primary outcome of a DTR can be written as a function of the multivariate distribution of the observable data obtained from a SMART; see Murphy (2005a) for detailed derivation. This property ensures that data from SMARTs can be effectively used to evaluate pre-specified DTRs or to estimate the optimal DTR within a certain class. We defer our discussion of estimation of optimal DTRs to later chapters.

Power and Sample Size

As is the case with any other study, power and sample size calculations are crucial elements in designing a SMART. In a SMART, one can investigate multiple research questions, both concerning entire DTRs (e.g. comparing the effects of two DTRs) and concerning certain components thereof (e.g. testing the main effect of the first stage treatment, controlling for second stage treatment). To power a SMART, however, the investigator needs to choose a primary research question (primary hypothesis), and calculate the sample size based on that question. Additionally, one or more secondary questions (hypotheses) may be investigated in the study. While the SMART provides unbiased estimates (free from confounding) to these secondary questions by virtue of randomization, it is not necessarily powered to address these secondary hypotheses.

A good primary research question should be both scientifically important and helpful in developing a DTR. For example, in the addiction management study an interesting primary research question would be: "marginalizing over secondary treatments, what is the best initial treatment on average?". In other words, here the researcher wants to compare the mean primary outcome of the group of patients receiving NTX as the initial treatment with the mean primary outcome of those receiving CBT. Standard sample size formula for a large sample comparison of two means can be used in this case. Define the standardized effect size δ as the standardized difference in mean primary outcomes between two groups (Cohen 1988), i.e.

$$\delta = \frac{E(Y|A_1 = \text{NTX}) - E(Y|A_1 = \text{CBT})}{\sqrt{[Var(Y|A_1 = \text{NTX}) + Var(Y|A_1 = \text{CBT})]/2}}.$$

Suppose the randomization probability is $1/2$ for each treatment option at the first stage. Standard calculation yields a total sample size formula for the two sided test with power $(1-\beta)$ and size α:

$$n = 4(z_{\alpha/2} + z_{\beta})^2 \delta^{-2},$$

where $z_{\alpha/2}$ and z_{β} are the standard normal $(1-\alpha/2)$ percentile and $(1-\beta)$ percentile, respectively. To use the formula, one needs to postulate the effect size δ, as is the case in standard two-group randomized controlled trials (RCTs).

Another interesting primary question could be: "on average what is the best secondary treatment, TM or TMC, for responders to initial treatment?". In other words, the researcher wants to compare the mean primary outcomes of two groups of responders (those who get TM versus TMC as the secondary treatment). As before, standard formula can be used. Define the standardized effect size δ as the standardized difference in mean primary outcomes between two groups (Cohen 1988), i.e.

$$\delta = \frac{E(Y|Response, A_2 = \text{TM}) - E(Y|Response, A_2 = \text{TMC})}{\sqrt{[Var(Y|Response, A_2 = \text{TM}) + Var(Y|Response, A_2 = \text{TMC})]/2}}.$$

Let γ denote the overall response rate to initial treatment. Suppose the randomization probability is $1/2$ for each treatment option at the second stage. Standard calculation yields a total sample size formula for the two sided test with power $(1-\beta)$ and size α:

$$n = 4(z_{\alpha/2} + z_{\beta})^2 \delta^{-2} \gamma^{-1}.$$

To use the formula, one needs to postulate the overall initial response rate γ, in addition to postulating the effect size δ. A similar question could be a comparison of secondary treatments among non-responders; in this case the sample size formula would be a function of non-response rate to the initial treatment.

Alternatively researchers may be interested in primary research questions related to entire DTRs. In this case, Murphy (2005a) argued that the primary research questions should involve the comparison of two DTRs beginning with different initial treatments. Test statistics and sample size formulae for this type of research question have been derived by Murphy (2005a) and Oetting et al. (2011).

The comparison of two DTRs, say $\bar{d}$ and $\bar{d}'$, beginning with different initial treatments, can be obtained by comparing the subgroup of subjects in the trial whose treatment assignments are consistent with regime $\bar{d}$ with the subgroup of subjects in the trial whose treatment assignments are consistent with regime $\bar{d}'$. Note that there is no overlap between these two subgroups since a subject's initial treatment assignment can be consistent with only one of $\bar{d}$ or $\bar{d}'$. The standardized effect size in this context is defined as $\delta = (\mu_{\bar{d}} - \mu_{\bar{d}'})/\sqrt{(\sigma^2_{\bar{d}} + \sigma^2_{\bar{d}'})/2}$, where $\mu_{\bar{d}}$ is the mean primary outcome under the regime $\bar{d}$ and $\sigma^2_{\bar{d}}$ is its variance. Suppose the randomization probability for each treatment option is $1/2$ at each stage. In this case, using a large sample approximation, the required sample size for the two sided test with power $(1-\beta)$ and size α is

$$n = 8(z_{\alpha/2} + z_{\beta})^2 \delta^{-2}.$$

Oetting et al. (2011) discussed additional research questions and the corresponding test statistics and sample size formulae under different working assumptions. A web application that calculates the required sample size for sizing a study designed to discover the best DTR using a SMART design for continuous outcomes can be found at

http://methodologymedia.psu.edu/smart/samplesize.

Some alternative approaches to sample size calculations can be found in Dawson and Lavori (2010, 2012).

Furthermore, for time-to-event outcomes, sample size formulae can be found in Feng and Wahed (2009) and Li and Murphy (2011). A web application for sample size calculation in this case can be found at

http://methodologymedia.psu.edu/logranktest/samplesize.

Randomization Probabilities

Let $p_1(a_1|H_1)$ and $p_2(a_2|H_2)$ be the randomization probability at the first and second stage, respectively. Formulae for the randomization probabilities that would create equal sample sizes across all DTRs were derived by Murphy (2005a). This was motivated by the classical large sample comparison of means for which, given equal variances, the power of a test is maximized by equal sample sizes. Let $k_1(H_1)$ be the number of treatment options at the first stage with history H_1 and $k_2(H_2)$ be the number of treatment options at the second stage with history H_2, respectively. Then Murphy's calculations give the optimal values of randomization probabilities as

$$\begin{aligned} p_2(a_2|H_2) &= k_2(H_2)^{-1}, \text{ and} \\ p_1(a_1|H_1) &= \frac{E[k_2(H_2)^{-1}|O_1, A_1 = a_1]^{-1}}{\sum_{b=1}^{k_1(H_1)} E[k_2(H_2)^{-1}|O_1, A_1 = b]^{-1}}. \end{aligned} \quad (2.1)$$

If k_2 does not depend on H_2, the above formulae can be directly used at the start of the trial. Otherwise, working assumptions concerning the distribution of O_2 given (O_1, A_1) are needed in order to use the formulae. In the case of the addiction management example, $k_1(H_1) = 2$ and $k_2(H_2) = 2$ for all possible combinations of (H_1, H_2). Thus (2.1) yields an optimal randomization probability of $1/2$ for each treatment option at each stage. See Murphy (2005a) for derivations and further details.

2.3.3 Practical Considerations

Over the years, some principles and practical considerations have emerged mainly from the works of Lavori and Dawson (2004), Murphy (2005a) and Murphy et al. (2007a) which researchers should keep in mind as general guidelines when designing a SMART.

First, Murphy (2005a) recommended that the primary research question should consider simple DTRs, leading to tractable sample size calculations. For example, in the addiction management study, one can consider regimes where the initial decision rule does not depend on an individual's pre-treatment information and the secondary decision rule depends only on the individual's initial treatment and his response status (as opposed to depending on a large number of intermediate variables).

Second, when designing the trial, the class of treatment options at each stage should be restricted by ethical, scientific or feasibility considerations (Lavori and Dawson 2004; Murphy 2005a). It is better to use a low dimensional summary criterion (e.g. response status) instead of all intermediate outcomes (e.g. improvement of symptom severity, side-effects, adherence etc.) to restrict the class of possible treatments; in many contexts including mental health studies, feasibility considerations may often force researchers to use a patient's preference in this low dimensional summary. Lavori and Dawson (2004) demonstrated how to constrain treatment options (and thus decision rules) using the STAR*D study as an example (this study will be introduced later in this chapter). Yet, Murphy (2005a) warned against unnecessary restriction of the class of the decision rules. In our view, determining the "right class" of treatment options in any given study remains an art, and cannot be fully operationalized.

Third, a SMART should be viewed as one trial among a series of randomized trials intended to develop and/or refine a DTR (Collins et al. 2005). It should eventually be followed by a confirmatory randomized trial that compares the developed regime and an appropriate control (Murphy 2005a; Murphy et al. 2007a).

Fourth, like traditional randomized trials, SMARTs may involve usual problems such as dropout, non-compliance, incomplete assessments, etc. However, by virtue of the option to alter the non-functioning treatments at later stages, SMARTs should be more appealing to participants, which may result in greater recruitment success, greater compliance, and lower dropout compared to a standard RCT.

Finally, as in the context of any standard randomized trial, feasibility and acceptability considerations relating to a SMART can best be assessed via (external) *pilot studies* (see, e.g. Vogt 1993). Recently Almirall et al. (2012a) discussed how to effectively design a SMART pilot study that can precede, and thereby aid in fine-tuning, a full-blown SMART. They also presented a sample size calculation formula useful for designing a SMART pilot study.

2.3.4 SMART Versus Other Designs

The SMART design discussed above involves stages of treatment and/or experimentation. In this regard, it bears similarity with some other common designs, including what are known as *adaptive designs* (Berry 2001, 2004). Below we discuss the distinctions between SMART and some other multi-stage designs, to avoid any confusion.

SMART Design Versus Adaptive Designs

"Adaptive design" is an umbrella term used to denote a variety of trial designs that allow certain trial features to change from an initial specification based on accumulating data (evolving information) while maintaining statistical, scientific, and ethical integrity of the trial (Dragalin 2006; Chow and Chang 2008). Some common types of adaptive designs are as follows. A *response adaptive design* allows modification of the randomization schedules based on observed data at pre-set interim times in order to increase the probability of success for future subjects; Berry et al. (2001) discussed an example of this type of design. A *group sequential design* (Pocock 1977; Pampallona and Tsiatis 1994) allows premature stopping of a trial due to safety, futility and/or efficacy with options of additional adaptations based on the results of interim analyses. A *sample size re-estimation design* involves the re-calculation of sample size based on study parameters (e.g. revised effect size, conditional power, nuisance parameters) obtained from interim data; see Banerjee and Tsiatis (2006) for an example. An *adaptive dose-finding design* is used in early phase clinical development to identify the minimum effective dose and the maximum tolerable dose, which are then used to determine the dose level for the next phase clinical trials (see for example, Chen 2011). An *adaptive seamless phase II/III trial design* is a design that addresses within a single trial objectives that are normally achieved through separate trials in phase II and phase III of clinical development, by using data from patients enrolled before and after the adaptation in the final analysis; see Levin et al. (2011) for an example. In general, the aim of adaptive designs is to improve the quality, speed and efficiency of clinical development by modifying one or more aspects of a trial. Recent perspectives on adaptive designs can be found in Coffey et al. (2012).

Based on the above discussion, now we can identify the distinctions between the standard SMART design and adaptive designs. In a SMART design, each subject moves through multiple stages of treatment, while in most adaptive designs each stage involves different subjects. The goal of a SMART is to develop a good DTR that could benefit *future* patients. Many adaptive designs (e.g. response adaptive design) try to provide the most efficacious treatment to each patient *in the trial* based on the current knowledge available at the time that a subject is randomized. In a SMART, unlike in an adaptive design, the design elements such as the final sample size, randomization probabilities and treatment options are pre-specified. Thus, SMART designs involve *within-subject adaptation* of treatment, while adaptive designs involve *between-subject adaptation*.

Next comes the natural question of whether some adaptive features can be integrated into the SMART design framework. In some cases the answer is *yes*, at least in principle. For example, Thall et al. (2002) provided a statistical framework for an adaptive design in a multi-stage treatment setting involving two SMARTs. Thall and Wathen (2005) considered a similar but more flexible design where the randomization criteria for each subject at each stage depended on the data from all subjects previously enrolled. However, adaptation based on interim data is less feasible in settings where subjects' outcomes may only be observed after a long period of time has elapsed. How to optimally use adaptive design features within the SMART framework is an open question that warrants further research.

SMART Design Versus Crossover Trial Design

SMART designs have some operational similarity with classical crossover trial designs; however they are very different conceptually. First, treatment allocation at any stage after the initial stage of a SMART typically depends on a subject's intermediate outcome (response/non-response). However, in a crossover trial, subjects receive all the candidate treatments irrespective of their intermediate outcomes. Second, as the goal of a typical cross-over study is to determine the outcome of a one-off treatment, crossover trials consciously attempt to *wash out* the *carryover effects* (i.e. delayed effects), whereas SMARTs attempt to capture them and, where possible, take advantage of any interactions between treatments at different stages to optimize outcome following a sequence of treatments.

SMART Design Versus Multiphase Experimental Approach

As mentioned earlier, a SMART should be viewed as one trial among a series of randomized trials intended to develop and/or refine a DTR. It should eventually be followed by a confirmatory randomized trial that compares the developed regime and an appropriate control (Murphy 2005a; Murphy et al. 2007a). This purpose is shared by the *multiphase experimental approach* (with distinct phases for screening, refining, and confirming) involving factorial designs, originally developed in engineering

(Box et al. 1978), and recently used in the development of multicomponent behavioral interventions (Collins et al. 2005, 2009; Chakraborty et al. 2009). Note that DTRs are multicomponent treatments, and SMARTs are developmental trials to aid in the innovation of optimal DTRs. From this perspective, a SMART design can be viewed as one screening/refining experiment embedded in the entire multiphase experimental approach. In fact, Murphy and Bingham (2009) developed a framework to connect SMARTs with factorial designs. However, there remain many open questions in this context, and more research is needed to fully establish the connections.

2.4 Examples of Sequentially Randomized Studies

In this section, we consider two examples of SMARTs in great detail. An in-depth discussion of several other recently-conducted SMARTs can be found in Lei et al. (2012).

2.4.1 Project Quit – Forever Free: A Smoking Cessation Study

Here we briefly present a two-stage SMART design implemented in a study to develop/compare internet-based interventions (dynamic treatment regimes) for smoking cessation and relapse prevention. The study was conducted by the Center for Health Communications Research at the University of Michigan, and was funded by the National Cancer Institute (NCI). This study allowed the researchers to test cutting-edge web-based technology in a real-world environment that has the infrastructure for both evaluating and disseminating population-based cancer prevention and control programs. The first stage of this study, known as *Project Quit*, was conducted to find an optimal multi-factor behavioral intervention to help adult smokers quit smoking; and the second stage, known as *Forever Free*, was a follow-on study to help those (among the *Project Quit* participants) who had already quit remain non-smoking, and offer a second chance to those who failed to give up smoking at the previous stage. Details of the study design and primary analysis of the stage 1 data can be found in Strecher et al. (2008). Analysis of the data from the two stages considered together with a goal of finding an optimal DTR can be found in Chakraborty (2009) and Chakraborty et al. (2010).

At stage 1, although there were five two-level treatment factors in the original *fractional factorial* design, only two, `source` (of online behavioral counseling message) and `story` (of a hypothetical character who succeeded in quitting smoking) were significant in the primary analysis reported in Strecher et al. (2008). For simplicity of discussion, here we consider only these two treatment factors at stage 1, which would give a total of 4 treatment combinations at stage 1 corresponding to the 2×2 design. The treatment factor `source` was varied at two levels, e.g. high vs. low level of personalization; likewise the factor `story` was varied at two levels, e.g. high vs. low tailoring depth (degree to which the character in the story was tailored to the individual subject's baseline characteristics). Baseline variables at this stage included subjects' `motivation` to quit (on a 1–10 scale), `selfefficacy` (on a 1–10 scale) and `education` (binary, ≤high school vs.> high school). At stage 2, there were two treatment options: booster intervention and control. At the first stage, 1,848 subjects were randomized, out of which only 479 decided to continue to stage 2 and hence were subsequently randomized.

There was an outcome measured at the end of each stage in this study. The stage 1 outcome was binary quit status at 6 months from the date of initial randomization, called `PQ6Quitstatus` (1 = quit, 0 = not quit). The stage 2 outcome was binary quit status, called `FF6Quitstatus`, at 6 months from the date of stage 2 randomization (i.e., 12 months from the date of stage 1 randomization). We will re-visit this study in Sects. 3.4.3 and 8.3.3, in the context of estimating optimal DTRs and conducting inference about them.

*2.4.2 STAR*D: A Study of Depression*

Sequenced Treatment Alternatives to Relieve Depression (STAR*D) was a multi-site, multi-level randomized controlled trial designed to assess the comparative effectiveness of different treatment regimes for patients with major depressive disorder (MDD) (Fava et al. 2003; Rush et al. 2004). This study was funded by the National Institute of Mental Health (NIMH). The study enrolled a total of 4,041 patients, all of whom were treated with citalopram (CIT) at level 1. Clinic visits occurred several times during each treatment level, at 2- or 3-week intervals (weeks 0, 2, 4, 6, 9, 12). Severity of depression at any clinic visit was assessed using the clinician-rated and self-report versions of the *Quick Inventory of Depressive Symptomatology* (QIDS) scores (Rush et al. 2004). A schematic of the treatment assignment algorithm is given in Fig. 2.3. This study is more complex than the smoking cessation study in that there are more than two stages.

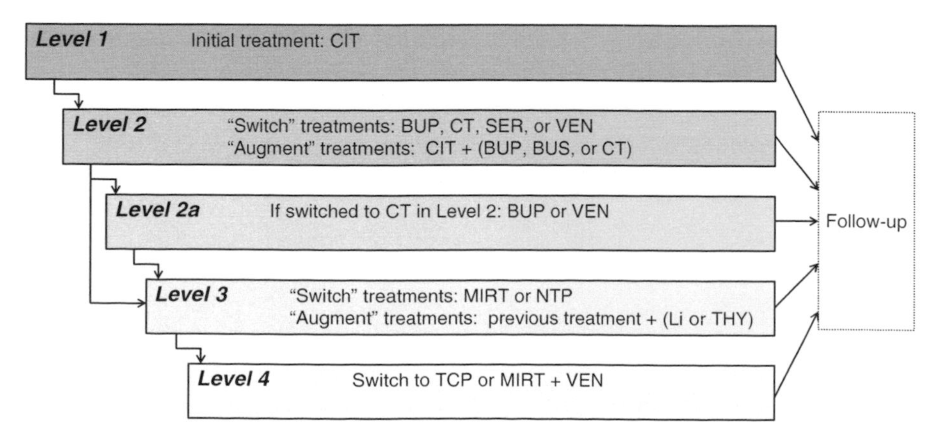

Fig. 2.3 A schematic of the algorithm for treatment assignment in the STAR*D study

Success was based on a total clinician-rated QIDS-score of ≤ 5 ("remission") during treatment with CIT. Those without remission were eligible to receive one of up to seven treatment options available at level 2, depending on their *preference* to switch or augment their level-1 treatment. Patients preferring a switch were randomly assigned to one of four treatment options: bupropion (BUP), cognitive psychotherapy (CT), sertraline (SER), or venlafaxine (VEN). Those preferring an augmentation were randomized to one of three options: CIT + BUP, CIT + buspirone (BUS), or CIT + CT. Only the patients assigned to CT or CIT + CT in level 2 were eligible, in the case of a non-satisfactory response, to move to a supplementary level of treatment (level 2A), to switch to either VEN or BUP. Patients not responding satisfactorily at level 2 (and level 2A, if applicable) would continue to level 3 treatment. Depending on the preference, patients at level 3 were randomly assigned to switch to either mirtazapine (MIRT) or nortriptyline (NTP), or randomly assigned to augment their previous treatment with lithium (Li) or thyroid hormone (THY). Patients without a satisfactory response at level 3 continued to level 4 treatments, which included two options: tranylcypromine (TCP) or MIRT + VEN. Patients achieving remission (QIDS ≤ 5) at any level entered a follow-up phase. Treatment assignment at each level took place via randomization within a patient's preference category. For a complete description of the STAR*D study design, see Fava et al. (2003) and Rush et al. (2004). We will re-visit this study in Chap. 8 in the context of making inference about the parameters indexing the optimal DTRs.

2.5 Discussion

In this chapter, we have described the two sources of data that are commonly used for estimating DTRs: observational follow-up studies and SMARTs. The use of observational data adds an element of complexity to the problem of estimation and requires careful handling and additional assumptions, due to the possibility of confounding. To assist in the careful formulation of causal contrasts in the presence of confounding, the potential outcomes framework was introduced. In contrast, SMARTs offer simpler analyses but often require significant investment to conduct a high quality trial with adequate power. We discussed conceptual underpinnings of and practical considerations for conducting a SMART, as well as its distinctions from other multiphase designs. We introduced several examples of observational and sequentially randomized studies, some of which we will investigate further in subsequent chapters.

Chapter 3
Statistical Reinforcement Learning

3.1 Multi-stage Decision Problems

Constructing optimal dynamic treatment regimes for chronic disorders based on patient data is a problem of multi-stage decision making about the best sequence of treatments. This problem bears strong resemblance to the problem of *reinforcement learning* (RL) in computer science. RL is a branch of machine learning that deals with the problem of multi-stage, sequential decision making by a *learning agent* (e.g. a robot). In this paradigm, a learning agent tries to optimize the total amount of reward it receives when interacting with an unknown environment. Unlike *supervised learning* (e.g. classification, regression) and *unsupervised learning* (e.g. clustering, density estimation), this branch of machine learning is relatively less known within the statistics community. However, there has been a recent surge of interest within the statistical and biomedical communities regarding the application of RL techniques to optimize DTRs. Recent efforts have targeted the development of DTRs for cancer (Zhao et al. 2009), epilepsy (Guez et al. 2008), depression (Murphy et al. 2007b; Pineau et al. 2007), schizophrenia (Shortreed et al. 2011), HIV infection (Ernst et al. 2006) and smoking cessation (Chakraborty et al. 2010), among others. In this chapter, we will review the necessary concepts of RL, connect them to the relevant statistical literature, and develop a mathematical framework that will enable us to treat the problem of estimating the optimal DTRs rigorously.

Historically, the first class of methods to solve multi-stage decision problems is *dynamic programming* (DP), which dates back to Bellman (1957). Classical DP algorithms are of limited practical utility in RL because of the following two reasons. First, they require a complete knowledge of the learning environment, often known as the *system dynamics*. In statistical terms, this means a complete knowledge about the multivariate distribution of the data. In many application areas, health-related or otherwise, it is often impractical to assume full distributional knowledge. Second, DP methods are computationally very expensive, and they become hard to manage in moderately high dimensional problems; in other words, they suffer from the *curse of dimensionality* (Sutton and Barto 1998). However, DP is still

B. Chakraborty and E.E.M. Moodie, *Statistical Methods for Dynamic Treatment Regimes*, Statistics for Biology and Health 76, DOI 10.1007/978-1-4614-7428-9_3,

important as a theoretical foundation for RL. The field of modern RL experienced a major breakthrough when Watkins (1989) developed *Q-learning*, a method to solve multi-stage decision problems based on sample data trajectories. This can be viewed as an *approximate dynamic programming* approach. In this book, we will focus on Q-learning as the main RL-based approach to estimating optimal DTRs; this will be implemented using primarily linear parametric models, although more flexible modeling is possible. A detailed introduction to the field of RL can be found in Sutton and Barto (1998), Bertsekas and Tsitsiklis (1996) and Kaelbling et al. (1996).

3.2 Reinforcement Learning: A Conceptual Overview

Reinforcement learning is characterized by a sequence of interactions between a *learning agent* and the *environment* it wants to learn about. At every decision point or *stage*, the agent observes a certain *state* of the environment, and chooses an *action* (makes a decision) from a set of possible actions. The environment responds to the action by making a transition to a new *state*. In addition to observing the new state, the agent observes a *reward*[1] that is meant to assess the immediate desirability of the action chosen by the agent. State, action and reward are the three basic elements of the RL framework. The most traditional (and perhaps the simplest) context in which RL is applied is called a *Markov decision process* (MDP). In an MDP setting, the probability of the environment making a transition to a new state, given the current state and action, does not depend on the distant past of the environment; more precisely, the state transition probabilities follow the well-known *Markov property* of memorylessness. In an MDP, the goal of RL is to learn how to map states to actions so as to maximize the total expected future reward (unless otherwise specified in a given problem, it is assumed that higher rewards are desirable). Note that the reward itself is usually a random variable, and hence the goal is formulated in terms of an expectation.

The number of stages in an RL problem can be either finite or infinite; accordingly it is called a *finite-horizon* or an *infinite-horizon* problem. In this book, we will only consider finite-horizon RL problems. In RL, a *policy* defines the agent's behavior (i.e. which action to take based on the current state) at any given stage. A *deterministic* policy is a vector of mappings, with as many components as the number of stages, where each component of the vector is a mapping from the *state space* (set of possible states) to the *action space* (set of possible actions) corresponding to a stage. More generally, a policy can be *stochastic*, in which case the mappings are from the stage-specific state spaces to the space of probability distributions over the stage-specific action spaces. Unless otherwise noted, by the term policy, we will generally mean deterministic policy throughout this book.

A useful quantity for assessing the merit of a policy is the *value function*, or simply, the *value*. While rewards reflect immediate desirability of an action, values represent what is good in the long run. Roughly speaking, the value of a given

[1] In some settings, there may only be a terminal reward for the entire sequence of agent-environment interactions.

state, with respect to a given policy, is the total expected future reward of an agent, starting with that state, and following the given policy to select actions thereafter. Thus the goal of RL, rephrased in terms of policy and value, is to estimate a policy that maximizes the value over a specified class of policies. Since the value is a function of two arguments, namely the state and the policy, the above-mentioned maximization of value over policy space can happen either for each state, or averaged over all the states. Unless otherwise specified, in this book, we will concentrate on maximization of value averaged over all the states.

Compare the above conceptual framework of traditional RL to the present problem of constructing DTRs for chronic disorders. The computerized *decision support system* of the clinician plays the role of the learning agent, while the population of subjects with the disorder of interest plays the role of the environment. Every time a patient visits the clinic defines a stage of potential clinical intervention. Pre-treatment observations on the patient constitute the state, and the treatment (type, dosage, timing etc.) serves as the action. A suitably-defined measure of the patient's well-being following the treatment can be conceptualized as the reward. For example, in the addiction management problem described in Chap. 1, reward can be the percentage of days abstinent in a given period of time following the treatment. However, it must be recognized that constructing good rewards in the medical setting is challenging, and how best to combine different outcomes of interest (e.g. efficacy and toxicity) into a single reward is an open question. Finally, policy is synonymous with dynamic treatment regime, and the value of a policy is the same as the expected primary outcome under a dynamic regime.

While the problem of constructing DTRs from patient data seems to be a special case of the classical RL, it has several unique features that distinguishes it from the classical RL problem. Below we list the major distinctions:

Unknown System Dynamics and the Presence of Unknown Causes: In many RL problems, the system dynamics (multivariate distribution of the data, including state transition probabilities) are known from the physical laws or other subject-matter knowledge. For example, in the case of a robot learning about its environment, the system dynamics are often known (Sutton and Barto 1998, p. 66). Unfortunately this is often not the case in the medical setting due to the presence of potentially many unknown causes of the outcome. Consider, for example, treatment of chronic depression. A patient's response to a treatment may depend on how well he adheres to the treatment assigned, his genetic composition, co-occurring family problems, etc. These unknown causes play an important role in treatment outcome, and in some cases interact with treatment to affect that outcome. Hence classical DP algorithms that use direct knowledge of the system dynamics are not suitable, and constructing DTRs in the medical setting using patient data is not a straightforward RL problem.

Furthermore, the unknown causes and system dynamics pose potential challenges to statistical methods for estimating treatment effects. In statistics, it is a common practice to collect data, whenever possible, on all potential risk factors and confounders and adjust for these by including them in regression models. However, it is not possible to collect data on a cause if it is unknown, and difficult to model a relationship (a component of the system dynamics) if it too is unknown or poorly understood. One might think to use nonparametric models to estimate the transition probabilities and then use DP methods to estimate the DTRs, provided the dimension of the problem is small relative to the sample size. When the state space and the action space are large, DP is a challenging computational problem. In most medical settings, particularly if the data arise from randomized trials (SMARTs), the number of subjects is typically not large compared to the size of the state space and the action space; hence nonparametric modeling of the system dynamics followed by DP has not become popular in the DTR literature.

Need to Pool over Subject-level Data: In some other classical RL problems, the system dynamics are not completely specified, rendering the DP methods unsuitable, however, good generative models are available from which one can simulate data on states, actions, and rewards – essentially as much data as one wants. In other words, data are often very cheap in these classical problems. The primary restrictive issue in this setting is the computational complexity. In the medical setting, however, data are extremely expensive in terms of both time and money. Furthermore, generative models from which to simulate patient data are rarely available due, in part, to the point noted above: that there may be unknown or poorly understood causes of the outcome in the medical setting. Thus, all that is typically available to the analyst is a sample consisting of treatment records (pre-treatment observations, treatments, and post-treatment outcomes) of n patients from a randomized or observational study. The sample size n is usually not very large compared to the size of the state space and the action space. Hence one is forced to use parametric or semi-parametric statistical models (called *function approximation* in computer science) to add some structure to the data and then pool over subjects' data to construct the decision rules. In computer science, a sample of data is often called a *batch*; hence a sub-class of RL algorithms that work with batch data are called *batch-mode* learning algorithms (Ernst et al. 2005; Murphy 2005b). In the medical setting, batch-mode RL algorithms with function approximation (as opposed to the more common *online* algorithms, which we will not discuss in this book) are suitable.

Non-Markovian Set-up: As mentioned earlier in this section, the most traditional setting in which the classical RL algorithms are applied is called an MDP, in which the state transition probabilities follow the Markov property. Roughly speaking, this means that the transition probabilities depend only on the immediate past as opposed to the entire history. In the medical setting, however, there is no reason to believe that the next state of the patient following a treatment depends on the immediately preceding state and treatment alone, and not on any distant history (there is no biological model indicating this). The main implication of this departure from the Markovian set-up is the need to introduce the notion of *history*; the history at any stage consists of all the present and past states, and also the past actions (treatments). Note that the space of history grows with the number of stages, and thus can quickly become high dimensional. Some of the previously defined terms need to be slightly re-defined in the non-MDP setting. For example, a policy is a mapping from the space of history (rather than just the immediate state space) to the action space at any stage. Also, in the non-MDP setting, one has to define the value of a certain history, rather than a state, with respect to a policy.

In spite of the above differences, one can think of RL algorithms as a good starting point for constructing DTRs. This book will focus largely on a particular RL algorithm named Q-learning, along with its variants. In the following, we will develop a probabilistic (statistical) framework to formalize the above concepts of RL.

3.3 A Probabilistic Framework

In a general RL problem, the agent and the environment interact at each of a possibly infinite number of stages. In the medical setting, we restrict ourselves to RL problems with a finite number of stages (say K). These are called *finite-horizon* problems. We do not assume Markov property here, since it is not appropriate in general.

At stage j ($1 \leq j \leq K$), the agent observes a state $O_j \in \mathscr{O}_j$ and executes an action $A_j \in \mathscr{A}_j$, where $\mathscr{O}_j$ is the state space and $\mathscr{A}_j$ is the action space. We will restrict ourselves to settings where the state O_j can be a vector consisting of discrete or continuous variables, but the action A_j can only be discrete. RL problems with a continuous action space are beyond the scope of this book, however exciting work on G-estimation of optimal strategies for dosing of continuous-valued treatments is being undertaken (Rich et al. 2010). Partly as a consequence of its action, the agent receives a real-valued reward $Y_j \in \mathscr{R}$, and moves on to the next stage with a new state $O_{j+1} \in \mathscr{O}_{j+1}$. As in Chap. 2, define $\bar{O}_j \equiv (O_1, \ldots, O_j)$ and $\bar{A}_j \equiv (A_1, \ldots, A_j)$. Also define the history H_j at stage j as the vector $(\bar{O}_j, \bar{A}_{j-1})$. At any stage j, the quantities O_j, A_j, Y_j and H_j are random variables, the observed values of which will be denoted respectively by o_j, a_j, y_j and h_j. The reward Y_j is conceptualized as a known function of the history H_j, the current action A_j, and the next state O_{j+1}. Thus,

$$Y_j = Y_j(H_j, A_j, O_{j+1}) = Y_j(\bar{O}_j, \bar{A}_j, O_{j+1}).$$

In some settings, there may be only one terminal reward Y_K; rewards at all previous stages are taken to be 0. In statistical terms, rewards may be taken to be synonymous with outcome.

Define a *deterministic policy* $d \equiv (d_1, \ldots, d_K)$ as a vector of decision rules, where for $1 \leq j \leq K$, $d_j : \mathscr{H}_j \to \mathscr{A}_j$ is a mapping from the history space $\mathscr{H}_j$ to the action space $\mathscr{A}_j$. A policy is called *stochastic* if the above mappings are from the history space $\mathscr{H}_j$ to the space of probability distributions over the action space $\mathscr{A}_j$ which, in a slight abuse of notation, we will denote $d_j(a_j|h_j)$. The collection of policies, depending on the history-space and action-space, defines a function space called *policy space* and is often denoted by $\mathscr{D}$.

A finite-horizon *trajectory* consists of the set $\{O_1, A_1, O_2, \ldots, A_K, O_{K+1}\}$. As mentioned earlier, the problem of constructing DTRs conforms to what is known as *batch-mode* RL in computer science. In a *batch-mode* RL problem, the data consist of a sample (*batch*) of n finite-horizon trajectories, each of the above form. That is, in the problem of constructing DTRs, the data consist of the treatment records of n subjects, i.e. n trajectories. We assume that the subjects are sampled at random according to a fixed distribution denoted by P_π. This distribution is composed of the unknown distribution of each O_j conditional on (H_{j-1}, A_{j-1}), and a fixed *exploration policy*[2] for generating the actions. Call the foregoing unknown conditional densities $\{f_1, \ldots, f_K\}$, and denote the exploration policy by $\pi = (\pi_1, \ldots, \pi_K)$, where the probability that action a_j is taken given history H_j is $\pi_j(a_j|H_j)$. We assume that $\pi_j(a_j|h_j) > 0$ for each action $a_j \in \mathscr{A}_j$ and for each possible value h_j; that is, all actions have a positive probability of being executed. Then the likelihood under P_π of the trajectory $\{o_1, a_1, o_2, \ldots, a_K, o_{K+1}\}$ is

$$f_1(o_1)\pi_1(a_1|o_1)\prod_{j=2}^{K} f_j(o_j|h_{j-1}, a_{j-1})\pi_j(a_j|h_j)f_{K+1}(o_{K+1}|h_K, a_K). \tag{3.1}$$

Denote the expectation with respect to the distribution P_π by E_π. As will be clear shortly, it is often useful to be able to write the likelihood of a trajectory under a policy different from the exploration policy that generated the observed data. Let P_d denote the distribution of a trajectory where an arbitrary policy $d = (d_1, \ldots, d_K)$ is used to generate the actions. If d is a deterministic policy, then the likelihood under P_d of the trajectory $\{o_1, a_1, o_2, \ldots, a_K, o_{K+1}\}$ is

$$f_1(o_1)\mathbb{I}[a_1 = d_1(o_1)]\prod_{j=2}^{K} f_j(o_j|h_{j-1}, a_{j-1})\mathbb{I}[a_j = d_j(h_j)]f_{K+1}(o_{K+1}|h_K, a_K). \tag{3.2}$$

For a stochastic policy d, the likelihood becomes

$$f_1(o_1)d_1(a_1|o_1)\prod_{j=2}^{K} f_j(o_j|h_{j-1}, a_{j-1})d_j(a_j|h_j)f_{K+1}(o_{K+1}|h_K, a_K). \tag{3.3}$$

Denote the expectation with respect to the distribution P_d by E_d. The primary goal in statistical RL is to estimate (learn) the optimal policy, say d^*, from the data on n finite-horizon trajectories, not necessarily generated by the optimal policy (hence the need for what are known as *off-policy* algorithms in RL). By optimal policy within a policy class, we mean the one with greatest possible *value* within that class. The precise definition of value follows.

The value function for a state o_1 with respect to an arbitrary policy d is

$$V^d(o_1) = E_d\Big[\sum_{j=1}^{K} Y_j(H_j, A_j, O_{j+1})\Big|O_1 = o_1\Big].$$

[2] In the case of a SMART, this policy consists of the randomization probabilities and is known by design, whereas for an observational study, this can be estimated by the propensity score (see Sect. 3.5 for definition).

This represents the total expected future reward starting at a particular state o_1 and thereafter choosing actions according to the policy d. Given a policy d, the stage j value function for a history h_j is the total expected future rewards from stage j onwards, and is given by

$$V_j^d(h_j) = E_d\Big[\sum_{k=j}^{K} Y_k(H_k, A_k, O_{k+1})\Big|H_j = h_j\Big], \quad 1 \le j \le K.$$

Note that, by definition, $V_1^d(\cdot) = V^d(\cdot)$. For convenience, set $V_{K+1}^d(\cdot) = 0$. Then the value functions can be expressed recursively as follows:

$$\begin{aligned}
V_j^d(h_j) &= E_d\Big[\sum_{k=j}^{K} Y_k(H_k, A_k, O_{k+1})\Big|H_j = h_j\Big] \\
&= E_d\Big[Y_j(H_j, A_j, O_{j+1})\Big|H_j = h_j\Big] + E_d\Big[\sum_{k=j+1}^{K} Y_k(H_k, A_k, O_{k+1})\Big|H_j = h_j\Big] \\
&= E_d\Big[Y_j(H_j, A_j, O_{j+1})\Big|H_j = h_j\Big] \\
&\qquad + E_d\Big[E_d\Big[\sum_{k=j+1}^{K} Y_k(H_k, A_k, O_{k+1})\Big|H_{j+1}\Big]\Big|H_j = h_j\Big] \\
&= E_d\Big[Y_j(H_j, A_j, O_{j+1})\Big|H_j = h_j\Big] + E_d\Big[V_{j+1}^d(H_{j+1})\Big|H_j = h_j\Big] \\
&= E_d\Big[Y_j(H_j, A_j, O_{j+1}) + V_{j+1}^d(H_{j+1})\Big|H_j = h_j\Big], \quad 1 \le j \le K. \qquad (3.4)
\end{aligned}$$

The optimal stage j value function for a history h_j is

$$V_j^{opt}(h_j) = \max_{d \in \mathscr{D}} V_j^d(h_j).$$

The optimal value functions satisfy the Bellman equation (Bellman 1957),

$$V_j^{opt}(h_j) = \max_{a_j \in \mathscr{A}_j} E\Big[Y_j(H_j, A_j, O_{j+1}) + V_{j+1}^{opt}(H_{j+1})\Big|H_j = h_j, A_j = a_j\Big], \qquad (3.5)$$

when all observations and actions are discrete (see Sutton and Barto, 1998, pp. 76, for details). The Bellman equation also holds for more general scenarios, but with additional assumptions.

Finally, the (*marginal*) value of a policy d, written V^d, is the average value function under that policy, averaged over possible initial observations, i.e.,

$$V^d = E_{O_1}[V^d(O_1)] = E_d\Big[\sum_{k=1}^{K} Y_k(H_k, A_k, O_{k+1})\Big]. \qquad (3.6)$$

Note that the above expectation is taken with respect to entire likelihood of the data, as given by (3.2) or (3.3), for the case of deterministic or stochastic policy respectively. Thus the value of a policy is simply the marginal mean outcome under that policy.

Given a policy, the primary statistical goal is to estimate its value. A related problem would be to compare the values of two or more pre-specified policies; this is, in fact, an extension of the problem of comparing mean outcomes of two or more (static) treatments. Note that this is often the primary analysis of a SMART. In Sect. 5.1, we will consider some methods for estimating the value of a pre-specified policy developed in the statistics literature.

In many classical RL as well as medical domains, researchers often seek to estimate a policy that maximizes the value (i.e. the *optimal* policy). One approach is to first specify a policy space, and then employ some method to estimate the value of each policy in that space to find the best one. An alternative approach is to work with what is known as *action-value function* or simply the *Q-function* (where "Q" stands for the "quality of action") instead of the value function V^d defined above. Q-functions are defined as follows.

The stage j *Q-function* for policy d is the total expected future reward starting from a history h_j at stage j, taking an action a_j, and following the policy d thereafter. Thus,

$$Q_j^d(h_j, a_j) = E[Y_j(H_j, A_j, O_{j+1}) + V_{j+1}^d(H_{j+1})|H_j = h_j, A_j = a_j].$$

The optimal stage j Q-function is

$$Q_j^{opt}(h_j, a_j) = E[Y_j(H_j, A_j, O_{j+1}) + V_{j+1}^{opt}(H_{j+1})|H_j = h_j, A_j = a_j].$$

In the medical decision making paradigm (also in many classical RL domains), a major interest lies in estimating Q_j^{opt}, since this can directly lead to the optimal policy; see Sect. 3.4 for further details.

3.4 Estimation of Optimal DTRs by Modeling Conditional Means

The primary goal in statistical RL is to estimate the optimal policy. As briefly mentioned in Sect. 3.3, one approach to achieve this goal is to first specify a policy space $\mathscr{D}$, and then employ any suitable method to estimate the value of each candidate policy $d \in \mathscr{D}$ to estimate the best one, say $\hat{d}^{opt}$. More precisely,

$$\hat{d}^{opt} = \arg\max_{d \in \mathscr{D}} \hat{V}^d.$$

This class of methods is known as the *policy search methods* in the RL literature (Ng and Jordan 2000). Methods like *inverse probability weighting* and *marginal structural models* developed in the causal inference literature also fall in this category; we will discuss these approaches in considerable detail in Chap. 5. While the policy search approach is typically non-parametric or semi-parametric, requiring only mild assumptions about the data, the main issue is the high variability of the value function estimates, and the resulting high variability in the estimated optimal policies.

With reference to estimating the optimal policy, one can conceive of methods that lie at the other end of the parametric spectrum, in the sense that they model the entire multivariate distribution of the data, and then apply *dynamic programming* methods to learn the optimal policy. Likelihood-based methods, including G-computation and Bayesian methods, fall in that category; we will briefly discuss them in Chap. 9. One downside of this class of methods is that the entire likelihood of the data may not be relevant for choosing optimal actions, and hence these methods run the risk of providing a biased estimator of the value function (and hence the optimal policy) if the model specification is incorrect. Since there is more modeling involved in this approach, there are more chances to get it wrong.

In between these two extremes, there exist attractive methods that model only part of the entire likelihood, e.g. the conditional expectation of the reward given history and action. In other words, these methods model the Q-functions (*Q-learning*) or even only parts of the Q-functions relevant for decision making (e.g. *A-learning*, *G-estimation*, etc.). In the present chapter and Chap. 4, we will be focusing on this class of methods. Modeling the conditional expectation can be done via regression. Below we introduce a simple version of Q-learning that estimates the optimal policy in two steps: (1) estimate the stage-specific Q-functions by using parametric models (e.g. linear models), and (2) recommend the actions that maximize the estimated Q-functions. In its simplest incarnation (using linear models for the Q-functions), Q-learning[3] can be viewed as an extension of least squares regression to multi-stage decision problems. However, one can use more flexible models (e.g. splines, neural networks, trees etc.) for the Q-functions.

3.4.1 Q-learning with Linear Models

For clarity of exposition, we will first describe Q-learning for studies with two stages, and then generalize to $K (\geq 2)$ stages. In a two-stage study, longitudinal data on a single subject are given by the trajectory $(O_1, A_1, O_2, A_2, O_3)$, where notations are defined in Sect. 3.3. The histories at each stage are given by $H_1 \equiv O_1$ and $H_2 \equiv (O_1, A_1, O_2)$. The data available for estimation consist of a random sample of n subjects. For simplicity, assume that the data arise from a SMART with two possible treatments at each stage, $A_j \in \{-1, 1\}$ and that they are randomized (conditionally on history) with known randomization probabilities. The study can have either a single terminal reward (primary outcome), Y, observed at the end of stage

[3] The version of Q-learning we will be using in this book is similar to the *fitted Q-iteration* algorithm in the RL literature. This version is an adaptation of Watkins' classical Q-learning to batch data, involving function approximation.

2, or two rewards (intermediate and final outcomes), Y_1 and Y_2, observed at the end of each stage. The case of a single terminal outcome Y is viewed as a special case with $Y_1 \equiv 0$ and $Y_2 = Y$. A two-stage policy (DTR) consists of two decision rules, say (d_1, d_2), with $d_j(H_j) \in \{-1, 1\}$.

One simple method to construct the optimal DTR $d^{opt} = (d_1^{opt}, d_2^{opt})$ is Q-learning (Watkins 1989; Sutton and Barto 1998; Murphy 2005b). First define the optimal Q-functions for the two stages as follows:

$$Q_2^{opt}(H_2, A_2) = E\left[Y_2 | H_2, A_2\right],$$
$$Q_1^{opt}(H_1, A_1) = E\left[Y_1 + \max_{a_2} Q_2^{opt}(H_2, a_2) | H_1, A_1\right].$$

If the above two Q-functions were known, the optimal DTR (d_1^{opt}, d_2^{opt}), using a backwards induction argument (as in dynamic programming), would be

$$d_j^{opt}(h_j) = \arg\max_{a_j} Q_j^{opt}(h_j, a_j), \quad j = 1, 2. \tag{3.7}$$

In practice, the true Q-functions are not known and hence must be estimated from the data. Note that Q-functions are conditional expectations, and hence a natural approach to model them is via regression models. Consider linear regression models for the Q-functions. Let the stage j ($j = 1, 2$) Q-function be modeled as

$$Q_j^{opt}(H_j, A_j; \beta_j, \psi_j) = \beta_j^T H_{j0} + (\psi_j^T H_{j1}) A_j, \tag{3.8}$$

where H_{j0} and H_{j1} are two (possibly different) vector summaries (or, features) of the history H_j, with H_{j0} denoting the "main effect of history" (H_{j0} includes the intercept term) and H_{j1} denoting the "treatment effect of history" (the vector H_{j1} also includes an intercept-like term that corresponds to the main effect of treatment). The collections of variables H_{j0} are often termed *predictive*, while H_{j1} is said to contain *prescriptive* or *tailoring* variables. The Q-learning algorithm involves the following steps:

1. Stage 2 regression: $(\hat{\beta}_2, \hat{\psi}_2) = \arg\min_{\beta_2, \psi_2} \frac{1}{n} \sum_{i=1}^n \left(Y_{2i} - Q_2^{opt}(H_{2i}, A_{2i}; \beta_2, \psi_2)\right)^2$.
2. Stage 1 pseudo-outcome: $\hat{Y}_{1i} = Y_{1i} + \max_{a_2} Q_2^{opt}(H_{2i}, a_2; \hat{\beta}_2, \hat{\psi}_2)$, $i = 1, \ldots, n$.
3. Stage 1 regression: $(\hat{\beta}_1, \hat{\psi}_1) = \arg\min_{\beta_1, \psi_1} \frac{1}{n} \sum_{i=1}^n \left(\hat{Y}_{1i} - Q_1^{opt}(H_{1i}, A_{1i}; \beta_1, \psi_1)\right)^2$.

Note that in step 2 above, the quantity $\hat{Y}_{1i}$ is a predictor of the unobserved random variable $Y_{1i} + \max_{a_2} Q_2^{opt}(H_{2i}, a_2)$, $i = 1, \ldots, n$. Once the Q-functions have been estimated, finding the optimal DTR is easy. The estimated optimal DTR using Q-learning is given by $(\hat{d}_1^{opt}, \hat{d}_2^{opt})$, where the stage j optimal rule is specified as

$$\hat{d}_j^{opt}(h_j) = \arg\max_{a_j} Q_j^{opt}(h_j, a_j; \hat{\beta}_j, \hat{\psi}_j), \; j = 1, 2.$$

The above procedure can be easily generalized to $K > 2$ stages. Define $Q_{K+1}^{opt} \equiv 0$, and

$$Q_j^{opt}(H_j, A_j) = E\left[Y_j + \max_{a_{j+1}} Q_{j+1}^{opt}(H_{j+1}, a_{j+1}) | H_j, A_j\right], \quad j = 1, \ldots, K.$$

Stage specific Q-functions can be parameterized as before, e.g.

$$Q_j^{opt}(H_j, A_j; \beta_j, \psi_j) = \beta_j^T H_{j0} + (\psi_j^T H_{j1}) A_j, \quad j = 1, \ldots, K.$$

Finally, for $j = K, K-1, \ldots, 1$, moving backward through stages, the regression parameters can be estimated as

$$(\hat{\beta}_j, \hat{\psi}_j) = \arg\min_{\beta_j, \psi_j} \frac{1}{n} \sum_{i=1}^{n} \Big(\underbrace{Y_{ji} + \max_{a_{j+1}} Q_{j+1}^{opt}(H_{j+1}, a_{j+1}; \hat{\beta}_{j+1}, \hat{\psi}_{j+1})}_{\text{stage } j \text{ pseudo-outcome}} - Q_j^{opt}(H_{ji}, A_{ji}; \beta_j, \psi_j) \Big)^2.$$

As before, the estimated optimal DTR is given by $(\hat{d}_1^{opt}, \ldots, \hat{d}_K^{opt})$, where

$$\hat{d}_j^{opt}(h_j) = \arg\max_{a_j} Q_j^{opt}(h_j, a_j; \hat{\beta}_j, \hat{\psi}_j), \; j = 1, \ldots, K.$$

Q-learning with linear models and $K = 2$ stages has been implemented in the R package `qLearn` that is freely available from the Comprehensive R Archive Network (CRAN):

`http://cran.r-project.org/web/packages/qLearn/index.html.`

3.4.2 *Why Move Through Stages?*

Some readers, especially those unfamiliar with causal inference, may find the indirect, two-step procedure of Q-learning a bit strange, at least on the surface. To them, the following one-step procedure for estimating the optimal DTR might seem more natural. In this approach, one would model the conditional mean outcome $E(Y|O_1, A_1, O_2, A_2)$ and run an all-at-once regression analysis; the estimated optimal policy would be given by

$$\left(\hat{d}_1^{opt}, \hat{d}_2^{opt}\right) = \arg\max_{(a_1, a_2)} E(Y|o_1, a_1, o_2, a_2).$$

Unfortunately, this is not a good idea because of the possibility of bias in the estimation of stage 1 treatment effect; this arises as a consequence of what is known as *collider-stratification bias* or *Berkson's paradox* (Gail and Benichou 2000; Greenland 2003; Murphy 2005a; Chakraborty 2011). This phenomenon was first described in the context of a retrospective study examining a risk factor for a disease in a sample from a hospital in-patient population by Berkson (1946). The phenomenon can be explained with the help of the addiction management example (see Sect. 2.3). Suppose there is an unobserved variable U that affects a patient's ability to respond to treatment. For simplicity, let us conceptualize U as the stability in one's life ($U = 1$ if stable, and 0 otherwise). One can expect that U is positively correlated with the intermediate outcome responder/non-responder status (O_2), and also U is positively correlated with Y, percent days abstinent. Suppose that the initial treatments have differing effects on responder/non-responder status (O_2). Since the initial treatment assignment is randomized, U and A_1 should be uncorrelated. However, there will be a conditional correlation between U and A_1, given non-response to initial treatment (i.e. given O_2). Intuitively, a non-responder who received the better initial treatment is more likely to have an unstable life ($U = 0$).

To make the above concept more concrete, consider the following example described by Murphy and Bingham (2009). Suppose $U \sim Bernoulli(\frac{1}{2})$ and $Y = \delta_0 + \delta_1 U + \varepsilon$, where ε has zero mean, finite variance, and is independent of O_1, A_1, O_2, A_2, U. Thus in truth, there is no effect of A_1 or A_2 on Y. Next suppose that

$$P(O_2 = 1|O_1, U, A_1) = U\left[\frac{q_1+q_2}{2} + \frac{q_1-q_2}{2}A_1\right] + (1-U)\left[\frac{q_3+q_4}{2} + \frac{q_3-q_4}{2}A_1\right],$$

where each $q_j \in [0,1]$. That is, the binary intermediate outcome O_2 (responder/non-responder status to initial treatment) depends on U and also on the treatment A_1 (when $q_1 - q_2 \neq 0$ and $q_3 - q_4 \neq 0$). By applying Bayes' theorem and some algebra, one can see that

$$\begin{aligned} E(Y|O_1, A_1, O_2 = 0, A_2) &= \delta_0 + \delta_1 E(U|O_1, A_1, O_2 = 0) \\ &= \delta_0 + \delta_1 P(U = 1|O_1, A_1, O_2 = 0) \\ &= \delta_0 + \frac{\delta_1}{2}\left(\frac{1-q_1}{2-q_1-q_3} + \frac{1-q_2}{2-q_2-q_4}\right) \\ &\quad + \frac{\delta_1}{2}\left(\frac{1-q_1}{2-q_1-q_3} + \frac{1-q_2}{2-q_2-q_4}\right)A_1. \end{aligned}$$

Thus, conditional on the intermediate outcome O_2, the effect of A_1 on Y can be non-zero, which is different from the true effect. Note that when one runs a regression of Y on (O_1, A_1, O_2, A_2), among other things, one conditions on O_2. Conditionally on O_2, the unobserved variable U and A_1 will be correlated. This correlation, coupled with the correlation between U and Y, will induce a spurious (non-causal) correlation between A_1 and Y (even though A_1 is randomized). As a consequence, the stage 1 treatment effect will be estimated with bias.

Figure 3.1 (where O_1 and A_2 are excluded to simplify the diagram) may help to demonstrate the situation visually. The direct arrow (solid) from A_1 to Y is the true stage 1 treatment effect we want to estimate. However since U is unobserved and thus not included in the regression, the spurious effect arising out of Berkson's paradox, represented by the dotted path from A_1 to Y via O_2 and U, contaminates the true effect of A_1. Thus, including both the stage 1 and stage 2 variables in one

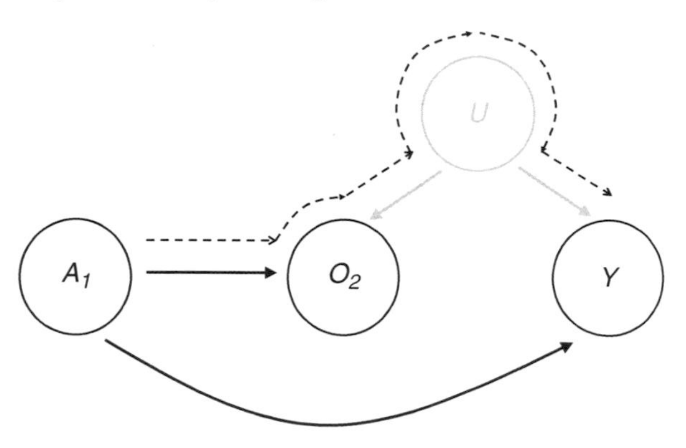

Fig. 3.1 A diagram displaying the spurious effect between A_1 and Y, as a consequence of Berkson's paradox

regression is potentially problematic. However, any method that moves stage by stage does not suffer from this problem since stage-wise methods do not condition on any covariate that occurs after the treatment of interest in that stage. Q-learning, as outlined above, is one such stage-wise method that avoids this unwanted bias.

3.4.3 Analysis of Smoking Cessation Data: An Illustration

To demonstrate the use of Q-learning in a health application, here we present the analysis of a data set from a randomized, two-stage, internet-based smoking cessation study, introduced in Sect. 2.4.1.

As described in Sect. 2.4.1, there were two treatment components, `source` (of online behavioral counseling message) and `story` (of a hypothetical character who succeeded in quitting smoking) at stage 1 of the study. The treatment component `source` was varied at two levels, high vs. low level of personalization, coded 1 and -1; also the treatment component `story` was varied at two levels, high vs. low tailoring depth (degree to which the character in the story was tailored to the individual subject's baseline characteristics), coded 1 and -1. Baseline variables included subjects' `motivation` to quit (on a 1–10 scale), `selfefficacy` (on a 1–10 scale) and `education` (binary, $\leq$high school vs.$>$ high school, coded 1 and -1). At stage 2, the treatment variable was called `FFarm`, coded 1 and -1 ($1 =$ booster intervention, $-1 =$ control). There were two outcomes at the two stages: the binary quit status at 6 months from the date of initial randomization, called `PQ6Quitstatus` ($1 =$quit, $0 =$not quit), and the binary quit status, called `FF6Quitstatus`, at 6 months from the date of stage 2 randomization (i.e., 12 months from the date of stage 1 randomization).

Having reviewed the study, let us now identify the setup for a dynamic treatment regime. Here O_1 consists of baseline variables (e.g., motivation, self-efficacy, education), O_2 consists of several stage 1 outcomes (e.g., quit status, reduction in the average number of cigarettes smoked per day, number of months not smoked during the study period, all measured at 6 months from the baseline), and O_3 consists of the same outcome variables measured at stage 2 (12 months from the baseline). A_1 and A_2 represent the behavioral interventions given at stages 1 and 2 respectively. The outcome Y could be the quit status at the end of the study. An example DTR can have the following form: "At stage 1, if a subject's baseline `selfefficacy` is greater than a threshold (say 7, on a 1–10 scale), then provide the highly-personalized level of the treatment component `source`; and if the subject is willing to continue treatment, then at stage 2 provide booster intervention if he continues to be a smoker at the end of stage 1 and control otherwise". Of course characteristics other than `selfefficacy` or a combination of more than one characteristic can be used to specify a DTR. To find the optimal DTR, we applied the two-stage Q-learning procedure involving the following steps.

1. Fit stage 2 regression ($n = 281$) of `FF6Quitstatus` using the model:

$$\begin{aligned}\texttt{FF6Quitstatus} = {} & \beta_{20} + \beta_{21} \times \texttt{motivation} + \beta_{22} \times \texttt{source} \\ & + \beta_{23} \times \texttt{selfefficacy} + \beta_{24} \times \texttt{story} \\ & + \beta_{25} \times \texttt{education} + \beta_{26} \times \texttt{PQ6Quitstatus} \\ & + \beta_{27} \times \texttt{source} \times \texttt{selfefficacy} \\ & + \beta_{28} \times \texttt{story} \times \texttt{education} \\ & + \left(\psi_{20} + \psi_{21} \times \texttt{PQ6Quitstatus}\right) \times \texttt{FFarm} + \texttt{error}.\end{aligned}$$

2. Construct the pseudo-outcome ($\hat{Y}_1$) for the stage 1 regression by plugging in the stage 2 estimates:

$$\begin{aligned}\hat{Y}_1 = {} & \texttt{PQ6Quitstatus} + \hat{\beta}_{20} + \hat{\beta}_{21} \times \texttt{motivation} + \hat{\beta}_{22} \times \texttt{source} \\ & + \hat{\beta}_{23} \times \texttt{selfefficacy} + \hat{\beta}_{24} \times \texttt{story} \\ & + \hat{\beta}_{25} \times \texttt{education} + \hat{\beta}_{26} \times \texttt{PQ6Quitstatus} \\ & + \hat{\beta}_{27} \times \texttt{source} \times \texttt{selfefficacy} + \hat{\beta}_{28} \times \texttt{story} \times \texttt{education} \\ & + \left|\hat{\psi}_{20} + \hat{\psi}_{21} \times \texttt{PQ6Quitstatus}\right|.\end{aligned}$$

   Note that in this case one can construct the pseudo-outcome for everyone who participated at stage 1, since there are no variables from post-stage 1 required to do so.

3. Fit stage 1 regression ($n = 1{,}401$) of the pseudo-outcome using a model of the form:

$$\begin{aligned}\hat{Y}_1 = {} & \beta_{10} + \beta_{11} \times \texttt{motivation} + \beta_{12} \times \texttt{selfefficacy} + \beta_{13} \times \texttt{education} \\ & + \left(\psi_{10}^{(1)} + \psi_{11}^{(1)} \times \texttt{selfefficacy}\right) \times \texttt{source} \\ & + \left(\psi_{10}^{(2)} + \psi_{11}^{(2)} \times \texttt{education}\right) \times \texttt{story} + \texttt{error}.\end{aligned}$$

Table 3.1 Regression coefficients and 95 % bootstrap confidence intervals at stage 1 (significant effects are in bold)

Variable	Coefficient	95 % CI
motivation	0.04	(−0.00, 0.08)
selfefficacy	**0.03**	(0.00, 0.06)
education	−0.01	(−0.07, 0.06)
source	−0.15	(−0.35, 0.06)
source × selfefficacy	**0.03**	(0.00, 0.06)
story	0.05	(−0.01, 0.11)
story × education	**−0.07**	(−0.13, −0.01)

Note that the sample sizes at the two stages differ because only 281 subjects were willing to continue treatment into stage 2 (as allowed by the study protocol). No significant treatment effect was found in the regression analysis at stage 2. The stage 1 analysis summary, including the regression coefficients and 95 % bootstrap confidence intervals[4] (using 1,000 replications) is presented in Table 3.1.

The conclusions from the present data analysis can be summarized as follows. Since no significant stage 2 treatment effect was found, this analysis suggests that the stage 2 behavioral intervention need not be adapted to the smoker's individual characteristics, interventions previously received, or stage 1 outcome. More interesting results are found at stage 1. It is found that subjects with higher levels of `selfefficacy` are more likely to quit. The highly personalized level of `source` is more effective for subjects with a higher `selfefficacy` ($\geq$7), and deeply tailored level of `story` is more effective for subjects with lower `education` ($\leq$high school); these two conclusions can be drawn from the interaction plots (with confidence intervals) presented in Fig. 3.2. Thus, according to this data analysis, to maximize each individual's chance of quitting over the two stages, the web-based smoking cessation intervention should be designed in future such that: (1) smokers with high `selfefficacy` ($\geq$7) are assigned to highly personalized level of `source`, and (2) smokers with lower `education` are assigned to deeply tailored level of `story`.

3.5 Q-learning Using Observational Data

Until recently, Q-learning had only been studied and implemented in settings where the exposure was randomized. However, as the development of DTRs is often exploratory, the power granted by the large samples often available using observational data may be a good means of discovering potentially optimal DTRs which may later be assessed in a confirmatory randomized trial. It has long been believed that Q-learning could easily be adapted to observational (non-randomized) treatment

[4] Inference for stage 1 parameters in Q-learning is problematic due to an underlying lack of smoothness, so usual bootstrap inference is not theoretically valid. Nevertheless, we use it here for illustrative purposes only. Valid inference procedures will be discussed in Chap. 8.

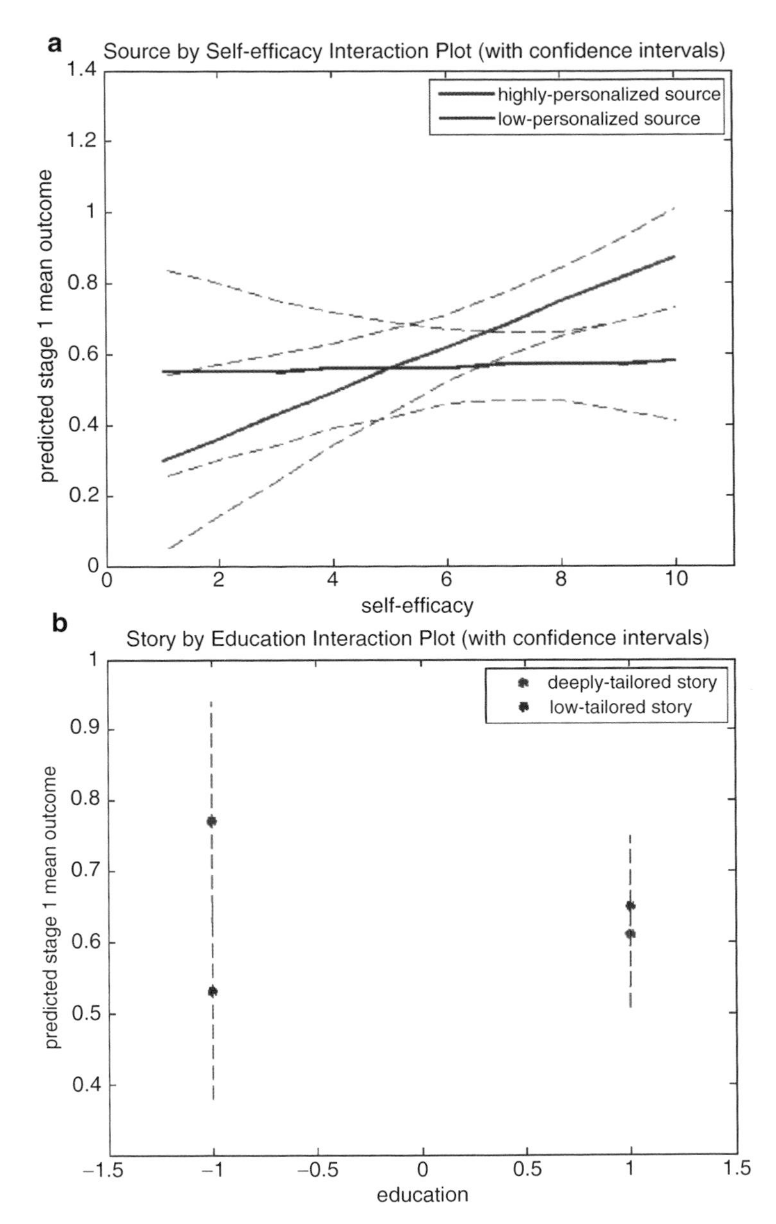

Fig. 3.2 Interaction plots: (**a**) source by self-efficacy (*upper panel*), (**b**) story by education (*lower panel*), along with confidence intervals for predicted stage 1 pseudo-outcome

settings, provided all confounding covariates are measured, using covariate adjustment or so-called causal methods, i.e. propensity score approaches, including regression, matching, and inverse probability of treatment weighting.

The propensity score (PS) is defined to be

$$\pi(o) = P(A = 1|O = o)$$

where A is a binary treatment and O is a collection of measured covariates (Rosenbaum and Rubin 1983). The PS is a balancing score such that, given the propensity score, treatment received is independent of known covariates O used to construct the PS. This property is used to obtain unbiased estimates of the treatment effect based on conditional expectation modeling of the outcome and conditioning on some form of the PS or based on simple comparisons of the treated and untreated using a PS-matched subsample of the full sample data. When using the PS for adjustment, quintiles of the propensity score are often included as covariates (D'Agostino 1998; Rosenbaum and Rubin 1983, 1984) as a means of providing a substantial reduction in bias without making strict assumptions about the functional form of the relationship between the outcome and the propensity score that is made when including the PS as a linear term, or without the loss of power associated with the reduction in sample size incurred when matching.

Unbiasedness can be achieved if the PS conditions on all confounding variables, i.e. all confounding variables are measured and included in the PS model (Ertefaie et al. 2012). In an inverse probability of treatment weighted (IPW) analysis, weighting is used to achieve a pseudo-sample in which covariates do not predict treatment (Robins et al. 2000). As with the PS adjustment methods, we require no unmeasured confounding, and that the PS is neither 0 nor 1 to ensure the resulting weights are well-defined (this is the positivity assumption).

We briefly present a basic no-adjustment implementation of Q-learning with five approaches to confounder adjustment, and examine their performance in a small simulation study. In this section, we shall distinguish between the components O_j that are tailoring variables, and those that are predictive variables including potential confounders, denoted C_j, $j = 1,2$. Three of the adjustment methods adapt Q-learning by redefining the history vectors, H_1 and H_2. The fourth approach uses a caliper-matched sample of the data (Rosenbaum and Rubin 1985), while the fifth relies on inverse probability weighting. If we denote the interval-specific propensity scores by $PS_1 = P(A_1 = 1|C_1)$, $PS_2 = P(A_2 = 1|C_1,C_2)$, then we will compare Q-learning using the following implementations:

1. Including only tailoring variables in the Q-function: $H_1 = O_1; H_2 = O_2$.
2. Including all covariates as linear terms in the Q-function: $H_1 = (C_1,O_1)$, $H_2 = (C_1,C_2,O_1,A_1,O_2)$,
3. Including the propensity score as a linear term in the Q-function: $H_1 = (PS_1,O_1)$, $H_2 = (PS_2,O_1,A_1,O_2)$,
4. Including quintiles of PS_j as covariates in the j-th stage Q-function,
5. Caliper matching on the propensity score with $H_1 = O_1; H_2 = O_2$,
6. Inverse probability of treatment weighting with $H_1 = O_1; H_2 = O_2$.

Caliper matching with replacement into pairs was accomplished using the Matching package in R (Sekhon 2011). For simplicity, we focus on the IPW estimator which uses unstabilized weights, defined as $w_1 = \mathbb{I}[A_1 = 1]/PS_1 + (1 - \mathbb{I}[A_1 = 1])/(1 - PS_1)$

at the first interval and $w_2 = w_1 * \{\mathbb{I}[A_2 = 1]/PS_2 + (1 - \mathbb{I}[A_2 = 1])/(1 - PS_2)\}$ at the second interval, although the conclusions of the simulations which follow are unaltered by the use of the more efficient, stabilized weights.

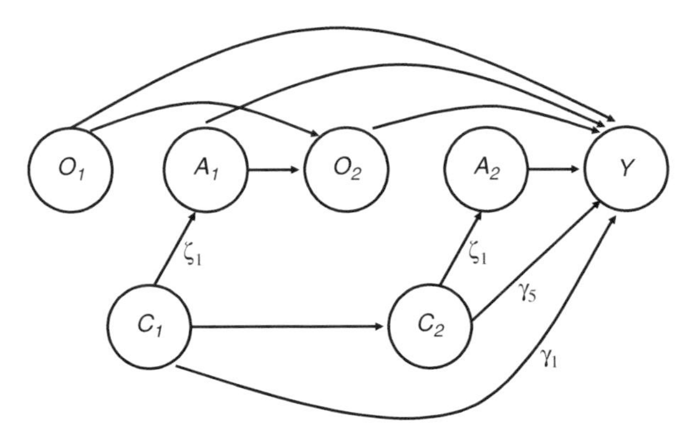

Fig. 3.3 Causal diagram for generative model for simulations in Sect. 3.5

We consider five scenarios:

Scenario A: Consider a single continuous confounder, C_j, at each interval, where $C_1 \sim \mathcal{N}(0,1)$ and $C_2 \sim \mathcal{N}(\eta_0 + \eta_1 C_1, 1)$ for $\eta_0 = -0.5$, $\eta_1 = 0.5$. Treatment assignment is dependent on the value of the confounding variable: $P[A_j = 1|C_j] = 1 - P[A_j = -1|C_j] = \text{expit}(\zeta_0 + \zeta_1 C_j)$, $j = 1,2$. The binary covariates which interact with treatment to produce a personalized rule are generated via

$$P[O_1 = 1] = P[O_1 = -1] = \frac{1}{2},$$
$$P[O_2 = 1|O_1, A_1] = 1 - P[O_2 = -1|O_1, A_1] = \text{expit}(\delta_1 O_1 + \delta_2 A_1).$$

Let $\mu = E[Y|C_1, O_1, A_1, C_2, O_2, A_2]$, and $\varepsilon \sim N(0,1)$ be the error term. Then $Y = \mu + \varepsilon$, with

$$\mu = \gamma_0 + \gamma_1 C_1 + \gamma_2 O_1 + \gamma_3 A_1 + \gamma_4 O_1 A_1 + \gamma_5 C_2 + \gamma_6 A_2 + \gamma_7 O_2 A_2 + \gamma_8 A_1 A_2.$$

See Fig. 3.3 for the causal diagram corresponding to the data generating models. Parameters were chosen to produce regular settings (see Chap. 8 for consideration of non-regularity): $\gamma = (0, \gamma_1, 0, -0.5, 0, \gamma_5, 0.25, 0.5, 0.5)$ and $\delta = (0.1, 0.1)$. We begin with a randomized treatment setting, $\zeta_0 = \zeta_1 = 0$ and $\gamma_1 = \gamma_5 = 0$. This is the reference scenario.

Scenario B: This setting is the same as Scenario A, except that $\gamma_1 = \gamma_5 = 1$. Note that this is again a randomized treatment setting.

Scenario C: This setting is the same as Scenario A, except that $\gamma_1 = \gamma_5 = 1$ and $\zeta_0 = -0.8$, $\zeta_1 = 1.25$. Treatment is now confounded by C_1 and C_2.

Scenario D: Here, we made the confounders C_1 and C_2 binary rather than continuous: $P[C_1 = 1] = 1 - P[C_1 = -1] = 1/3$ and $P[C_2 = 1] = 1 - P[C_2 = -1] = \text{expit}(0.6C_1)$. We set $\gamma_1 = \gamma_5 = 1$.

Scenario E: This setting is the same as Scenario D, except that $\gamma_1 = 0$ so that C_2 is a predictor of Y, but C_1 is not.

We focus our attention on the parameter ψ_{10}, the parameter in the analytic model for the first-stage Q-function which corresponds to the main effect of A_1. Performance of the six different Q-learning approaches under are given in Table 3.2 for a sample size of 250. Note that when the confounders are binary, PS matching and partitioning of the PS into quintiles are not feasible strategies.

All methods perform well when treatment is randomly allocated, with better performance when C_j does not predict the outcome. This would suggest that correct specification of the Q-function is not essential in the RCT setting.

In settings where treatment is confounded by the continuous confounders C_1 and C_2, only covariate adjustment provides unbiased estimates. The same general pattern holds when confounders are binary, with one exception: if there exists a single confounder at each interval, and only C_2 but not C_1 affects Y then including the PS in the Q-function model performs as well as including C_2 in the model, since the PS acts as a re-scaled version of C_2. Although the PS regression-based methods yield unbiased estimates of the parameters associated with treatment A_2 (i.e. the variables contained in H_{21}), the methods do not yield a good prediction of the stage 1 pseudo-outcome itself, since the model mis-specifies the functional form of the dependence of that pseudo-outcome on important predictors C_1 and C_2. This leads to bias in the stage 1 parameter estimates. Furthermore, we note that the PS matching estimator targets the average treatment effect on the treated (ATT), and has increased variability due the re-use of data in matching with replacement.

In the simulations above, the data were generated in such a way that a model that includes the confounding variables as linear terms in the Q-function was correctly specified. We therefore pursue an alternative approach to generating data that will allow us to examine the performance of the adjustment methods without the additional complication of incorrect model specification by generating data in which confounding is introduced by allowing the choice of treatment received to depend on the counterfactual outcomes.

In particular, the data are created by generating the outcome under each of the four potential treatment paths $(-1,-1)$, $(-1,1)$, $(1,-1)$, and $(1,1)$:

1. Generate the first-stage tailoring variable, O_1, using $P[O_1 = 1] = P[O_1 = -1] = \frac{1}{2}$.
2. Generate the potential value of the second-stage tailoring variable, $O_2(A_1)$, using $P[O_2 = 1|O_1,A_1] = 1 - P[O_2 = -1|O_1,A_1] = \text{expit}(\delta_1 O_1 + \delta_2 A_1)$ for each possible value of A_1, thereby generating the potential second-stage value that would occur under each of $A_1 = -1$ and $A_1 = 1$.
3. Generate the vector of potential outcomes, $\mathbf{Y} = \mu + \varepsilon$, where ε is a multivariate normal error term with mean $(0,0,0,0)^T$ and a covariance matrix that takes the value 1 on its diagonal and 0.5 on all off-diagonals, and

Table 3.2 Performance of Q-learning adjustment methods: Bias, Monte Carlo Variance (MC var), and Mean Squared Error (MSE)

Method	Bias	MC var	MSE
Scenario A			
None	−0.0004	0.0080	0.0080
Linear	−0.0005	0.0079	0.0079
PS (linear)	−0.0006	0.0079	0.0079
PS (quintiles)	−0.0007	0.0080	0.0080
PS (matching)	−0.0066	0.0164	0.0164
IPW	−0.0006	0.0080	0.0080
Scenario B			
None	0.0073	0.0297	0.0298
Linear	0.0088	0.0121	0.0122
PS (linear)	0.0054	0.0188	0.0188
PS (quintiles)	0.0056	0.0204	0.0204
PS (matching)	−0.0109	0.0431	0.0432
IPW	0.0080	0.0224	0.0224
Scenario C			
None	−0.7201	0.0256	0.5441
Linear	−0.0027	0.0116	0.0116
PS (linear)	−0.2534	0.0233	0.0875
PS (quintiles)	−0.3151	0.0213	0.1206
PS (matching)	−0.2547	0.0681	0.1330
IPW	−0.4304	0.0189	0.2042
Scenario D			
None	−0.5972	0.0211	0.3777
Linear	0.0075	0.0120	0.0121
PS (linear)	−0.2599	0.0227	0.0902
IPW	−0.3274	0.0159	0.1231
Scenario E			
None	−0.2475	0.0114	0.0727
Linear	0.0075	0.0120	0.0121
PS (linear)	0.0050	0.0141	0.0141
IPW	−0.1381	0.0116	0.0306

$$\mu = \gamma_0^* + \gamma_1^*\mathbf{O}_1 + \gamma_2^*\mathbf{A}_1 + \gamma_3^*\mathbf{O}_1\mathbf{A}_1 + \gamma_4^*\mathbf{A}_2 + \gamma_5^*\mathbf{O}_2\mathbf{A}_2 + \gamma_6^*\mathbf{A}_1\mathbf{A}_2 \tag{3.9}$$

where $\mathbf{O}_1$ is the 4×1 vectors consisting of O_1 from step (1) repeated four times, $\mathbf{A}_1 = (-1,-1,1,1)$, $\mathbf{O}_2 = (O_2(-1), O_2(-1), O_2(1), O_2(1))$ using the potential values generated in step (2), and $\mathbf{A}_2 = (-1,1,-1,1)$.

4. Set the confounders to be $C_1 = \overline{\mathbf{Y}}$ and $C_2 = \max(\mathbf{Y})$.
5. From among the four possible treatment paths and corresponding potential outcomes, select the "observed" data using $P[A_j = 1|C_j] = 1 - P[A_j = -1|C_j] = \text{expit}(\zeta_0 + \zeta_1 C_j)$, $j = 1,2$.

The vector of δs was set to $(0.1, 0.1)$, while the vector of γ^*s was taken to be $(0, 0, -0.5, 0, 0.25, 0.5, 0.5)$, indicating a regular (large effect) scenario. In simulations where treatment was randomly allocated, $\zeta_0 = \zeta_1 = 0$, while for confounded treatment, $\zeta_0 = 0.2$, $\zeta_1 = 1$. As can be observed from Eq. (3.9), the Q-functions will not depend on the values of C_1 and C_2 so that any model for the Q-function that includes O_1, A_1, O_2, A_2 and the appropriate interactions will be correctly specified. However the observed or selected treatment depends on C_1 and C_2, which are functions of the potential outcomes, hence the treatment-outcome relationship is confounded by these variables.

Under this data-generating approach, we observe that all methods of adjusting for confounding provide considerably improved estimates in terms of bias for small samples, but in large samples, only inverse probability weighting or directly adjusting for covariates by including them as linear terms in the model for the Q-function provide the required bias-removal (Table 3.3). While these simulations provide a useful demonstration of the methods of adjustment in principle, it is not clear whether these results generalize to real-data scenarios as it is difficult to conceive of a situation in which counterfactual outcomes could be measured and used as covariates. Rather, the results of these simulations should serve to provide a cautionary note on the importance of adequately modeling the Q-function, particularly in observational data settings.

Table 3.3 Performance of Q-learning adjustment methods under the confounding by counterfactuals simulations: Bias, Monte Carlo Variance (MC var), Mean Squared Error (MSE) and coverage of 95 % bootstrap confidence intervals

Adjustment method	Randomized treatment				Confounded treatment			
	Bias	MC var	MSE	Cover	Bias	MC var	MSE	Cover
$n = 250$								
None	0.0020	0.0082	0.0082	94.0	0.2293	0.0080	0.0605	26.4
Linear	0.0011	0.0032	0.0032	95.1	0.0051	0.0039	0.0039	93.8
PS (linear)	0.0010	0.0052	0.0052	96.2	0.0548	0.0060	0.0090	89.4
PS (quintiles)	0.0008	0.0056	0.0056	96.1	0.0779	0.0061	0.0121	83.2
PS (matching)	0.0027	0.0099	0.0099	98.0	0.1375	0.0107	0.0295	75.9
IPW	0.0004	0.0046	0.0046	93.9	0.0108	0.0075	0.0076	92.8
$n = 1{,}000$								
None	−0.0012	0.0022	0.0022	93.4	0.2246	0.0021	0.0525	0.5
Linear	0.0001	0.0009	0.0009	93.5	0.0037	0.0010	0.0010	93.5
PS (linear)	−0.0002	0.0014	0.0014	95.5	0.0446	0.0015	0.0035	77.0
PS (quintiles)	−0.0004	0.0015	0.0015	95.7	0.0699	0.0015	0.0064	55.0
PS (matching)	−0.0015	0.0026	0.0026	97.5	0.1256	0.0027	0.0184	31.0
IPW	−0.0008	0.0012	0.0012	93.6	0.0018	0.0018	0.0018	93.6

3.6 Discussion

In this chapter, we have delved into the mathematical complexities of multi-stage decision problems, and placed them in context in both the statistical and computer sciences literature. In particular, the terminology of the two fields has been brought together to assist researchers in each field understand that a policy is a treatment regime or set of decision rules, a state space is a set of covariates, and an action space is the set of treatments under consideration.

In Sect. 3.3, the longitudinal data structure was described. In Sect. 3.4, Q-learning was introduced. This is a semi-parametric approach to estimation that we will return to throughout the remainder of the text. In its typical implementation, it employs a sequence of regressions, initially aiming to determine the optimal treatment strategy at the last stage, then at each previous stage assuming the optimal DTR is followed in later stages. The method is appealing for its computational and conceptual simplicity, and as we will see in the next chapter, it ties closely with other methods of estimation from the statistical literature. However, Q-learning may depend heavily on being able to correctly specify the model for the Q-function, as we observed in Sect. 3.5. The approach must therefore be undertaken with particular caution when non-randomized data are used.

Chapter 4
Semi-parametric Estimation of Optimal DTRs by Modeling Contrasts of Conditional Mean Outcomes

In this chapter, we will focus on semi-parametric estimation of optimal DTRs by modeling contrasts of conditional mean outcomes, as opposed to modeling the conditional means themselves (e.g. Q-learning). Within the statistics (causal inference) literature, Robins has been a pioneer in the domain of time-varying treatment regimes (Robins 1986, 1994, 1997), while Murphy (2003) produced one of the first methods to estimate optimal dynamic regimes semi-parametrically using regret functions. Robins produced a number of estimating equation-based methods for finding optimal regimes relying on *structural nested mean models* (SNMM); a review of SNMMs can be found in Vansteelandt and Goetghebeur (2003). The term *structural* is used to indicate that the model is for a counterfactual quantity and therefore is meant to capture a *causal* rather than merely associational relationship. SNMMs are used to model the function of an exposure (treatment) at stage j as a function of the state history up to that stage; the approach therefore requires a model for each stage, and these models are said to be *nested* within stages.

As we shall see in Sect. 4.1.1, the regret is a special case of SNMMs. A SNMM parameterizes the causal effect that is the *difference* between the conditional expectation of an outcome in the observed data and the conditional expectation of an outcome under some potential outcome scenario. To return to the two-treatment, two-stage example of previous chapters, a model specifying the form of $E[Y(a,a) - Y(a,a')|\text{Covariates}]$ is a SNMM; a key notion is that only differences in outcomes under different treatment regimes must be parameterized, rather than the full outcome distribution. This chapter focuses attention on situations where the outcome of interest is a continuous measure; other outcome types are considered briefly in Chap. 7.

4.1 Structural Nested Mean Models

Define an *optimal blip-to-reference function*, $\gamma_j(h_j, a_j)$, at any stage j to be the expected difference in outcome when using a reference regime d_j^{ref} instead of a_j at

B. Chakraborty and E.E.M. Moodie, *Statistical Methods for Dynamic Treatment Regimes*, Statistics for Biology and Health 76, DOI 10.1007/978-1-4614-7428-9_4,

stage j, in persons with treatment and covariate history h_j who subsequently receive the optimal regime $\underline{d}^{opt}_{j+1}$:

$$\gamma_j(h_j,a_j) = E[Y(\bar{a}_j,\underline{d}^{opt}_{j+1}) - Y(\bar{a}_{j-1},d^{ref}_j,\underline{d}^{opt}_{j+1})|H_j = h_j],$$

where "optimal" refers to treatment subsequent to stage j and "blip" refers to the single-stage change in treatment at stage j, i.e., a "blip" of treatment given at stage j. Note that at least one of $Y(\bar{a}_j,\underline{d}^{opt}_{j+1})$, $Y(\bar{a}_{j-1},d^{ref}_j,\underline{d}^{opt}_{j+1})$ is a counterfactual outcome unless the reference regime is optimal in stage j and the patient was treated optimally at stage j and thereafter, in which case $\gamma_j(h_j,a_j) = 0$.

As noted previously, a dynamic treatment regime $\bar{d}^{opt}_K$ is optimal if it maximizes the expectation of the outcome Y; define components of the optimal regime recursively starting at K as

$$d^{opt}_j(h_j) = \underset{a_j}{\text{argmax}}\, E[Y(\bar{a}_{j-1},a_j,\underline{d}^{opt}_{j+1})|H_j = h_j].$$

In general, $d^{opt}_j(h_j)$ depends on $\bar{o}_j$ and $\bar{a}_{j-1}$, however as in previous chapters, we will sometimes suppress the argument of the treatment regime function and simply write d^{opt}_j. Note that both of the counterfactual outcomes $Y(\bar{a}_j,\underline{d}^{opt}_{j+1})$ and $Y(\bar{a}_{j-1},d^{ref}_j,\underline{d}^{opt}_{j+1})$ in the optimal blip-to-reference assume that the optimal regime is followed from stage $j+1$ to the end of treatment. However, the actual treatments prescribed by the optimal regime may differ because the treatments which maximize outcome given treatment history $\bar{a}_j$ may not correspond to those that maximize outcome given treatment history $(\bar{a}_{j-1},d^{ref}_j)$. Thus, we must keep in mind the subtle distinction between the optimal regime and the specific optimal treatment prescribed by that regime given an individual's particular history.

Optimal regimes are defined for any sequence of treatment and covariate history, even a sequence h_j that might not be possible to observe had the optimal regime been followed by all participants from the first stage. Thus, an optimal regime provides information not only on the best treatment choices from "time zero", but also on the treatment choices that would maximize outcome from some other time or stage, even if a sub-optimal regime had been followed up to that point. The *sequential randomization* or *no unmeasured confounding assumption* discussed in Chap. 2 is important as it allows us to infer that the average counterfactual outcome of people who received treatments $\bar{a}_K$ had they instead received $\underline{d}_j$ from stage j onwards is the same as the average outcome in those people who *actually received* treatments $(\bar{a}_{j-1},\underline{d}_j)$ conditional on history, and thus identify the parameters of the blip function.

The assumption of rank preservation, introduced in Chap. 2, provides a simplistic situation in which the parameters of a SNMM may be interpreted at the individual level. That is, *additive local rank preservation* gives that the difference in the outcome that would be observed for each particular person (who has history $H_j = h_j$) should he be treated with regime $(\bar{a}_{j-1},d^{ref}_j,\underline{d}^{opt}_{j+1})$ instead of regime $(\bar{a}_j,\underline{d}^{opt}_{j+1})$ is equal to $\gamma_j(h_j,a_j)$ given some treatment a_j at stage j. However, SNMMs may be used without making such assumptions, relying instead on an arguably more useful population-level interpretation of average causal effects.

4.1.1 Special Cases of Optimal SNMMs

There are two special cases of optimal blip-to-reference functions that are commonly used in the dynamic regimes literature and applications. We focus here on binary treatment, i.e. $A_j \in \{-1,1\}$,[1] however the two SNMMs discussed below are mathematically equivalent under more general treatment types (Robins 2004, pp. 243–245).

The first of these, suggested by Robins (2004), takes the reference regime to be the zero regime, where by "zero regime" we mean some substantively meaningful treatment such as placebo or standard care. Of course, like the optimal regime, what is considered to be standard care may be different for participants with different covariates or in different stages of treatment. Call this the *optimal blip-to-zero* function.

A second special case of the optimal blip-to-reference function, called the regret function, takes the negative of the optimal blip-to-reference that uses optimal treatment at stage j as the reference regime. Denote this by

$$\mu_j(h_j,a_j) = E[Y(\bar{a}_{j-1},\underline{d}_j^{opt}) - Y(\bar{a}_j,\underline{d}_{j+1}^{opt})|H_j = h_j]$$

for $j = 1,\ldots,K$. Thus the regret at stage j is the expected difference in the outcome that would have been observed had the participant taken the optimal treatment in stage j instead of treatment regime a_j in participants who followed $\bar{a}_j$ up to stage j and the optimal regime from stage $j+1$ onwards; note that this is identical in spirit the loss-function $\mathscr{L}(o,a)$ introduced in Chap. 1.

For binary treatment and continuous outcome, the correspondence between the optimal blip-to-reference functions and regrets is:

$$\mu_j(h_j,a_j) = \max_{a_j} \gamma_j(h_j,a_j) - \gamma_j(h_j,a_j), \text{ or}$$

$$\gamma_j(h_j,a_j) = \mu_j(h_j,d_j^{ref}) - \mu_j(h_j,a_j).$$

It is evident from these identities that if the regret is smooth in its arguments, the optimal blip-to-zero will also be smooth. The converse does not hold: a smooth optimal blip-to-zero may imply a discontinuous regret function. We shall henceforth assume that d_j^{ref} equals the zero regime (coded -1), and simply refer to the optimal blip-to-zero function as the optimal blip.

[1] While the 0/1 coding of treatment is widely used in the causal inference literature, the $-1/1$ coding is more common in Q-learning and SMART design literature, and hence we will adopt it in this chapter as in the rest of the book.

4.1.2 Standard SNMMs

Another class of SNMM is the *standard* blip-to-reference functions, which consider the expected difference in outcome when using a reference regime d_j^{ref} instead of a_j at stage j, in persons with treatment and covariate history h_j who subsequently receive the zero regime rather than subsequently being treated optimally as in optimal SNMM.

These models require knowledge of the longitudinal distribution of states and outcome to be able to specify the optimal regime. To see this, consider a two-stage example where we take the reference regime to be the zero (placebo/standard care) regime. Leave the distribution of O_1 unspecified and assume

$$O_2 = \beta_{10} + \beta_{11}O_1 + (\psi_{10} + \psi_{11}O_1)(A_1+1)/2 + \varepsilon_1$$

$$Y(A_1,A_2) = \beta_{20} + \beta_{21}O_2 + (\psi_{20} + \psi_{21}O_2 + \psi_{22}(A_1+1)/2)(A_2+1)/2 + \varepsilon_2,$$

where ε_1, ε_2 are mean zero random variables.

At the final stage, the standard blip function and the optimal blip function are equal:

$$E[Y(A_1,A_2) - Y(A_1,-1)|H_2] = (\psi_{20} + \psi_{21}O_2 + \psi_{23}(A_1+1)/2)(A_2+1)/2$$

giving $d_2^{opt} = sign(\psi_{20} + \psi_{21}O_2 + \psi_{23}(A_1+1)/2)$. However at previous stages (in this example, there is only one prior stage: the first), the standard blip:

$$E[Y(A_1,-1) - Y(-1,-1)|H_1] = (A_1+1)/2(\beta_{21}\psi_{10} + \beta_{21}\psi_{11}O_1),$$

differs from the optimal blip:

$$\begin{aligned} E[Y(A_1,A_2^{opt}(\bar{O}_2,A_1)) - Y(-1,A_2^{opt}(\bar{O}_2,-1))|H_1] = \\ E\Big[(\beta_{21}\psi_{10} + \beta_{21}\psi_{11}O_1)(A_1+1)/2 + \\ (\varepsilon' + c_1 + c_2)(sign(\varepsilon' + c_1 + c_2) + 1)/2 - \\ (\varepsilon' + c_1)(sign(\varepsilon' + c_1) + 1)/2|H_1\Big], \end{aligned}$$

where

$$\begin{aligned} \varepsilon' &= \psi_{21}\varepsilon_1 \\ c_1 &= c_1(O_1) = \psi_{20} + \psi_{21}\beta_{10} + \psi_{21}\beta_{11}O_1 \\ c_2 &= c_2(O_1,A_1) = (\psi_{22} + \psi_{21}\psi_{10} + \psi_{21}\psi_{11}O_1)(A_1+1)/2. \end{aligned}$$

This gives

$$d_1^{opt} = \underset{A_1 \in \{-1,1\}}{\text{argmax}}\ E\left[(\beta_{21}\psi_{10} + \beta_{21}\psi_{11}O_1)(A_1+1)/2 + \right.$$
$$\left. (\varepsilon' + c_1 + c_2)(sign(\varepsilon' + c_1 + c_2) + 1)/2 | H_1\right]. \quad (4.1)$$

The presence of ε_1 in non-linear functions within the expectations requires a model for its distribution in order to estimate the optimal rule. More concretely, suppose $\varepsilon' \sim \mathcal{N}(0,\sigma^2)$. Then the optimal rule is given by

$$d_1^{opt} = \underset{A_1 \in \{-1,1\}}{\text{argmax}} \left\{ (\beta_{21}\psi_{10} + \beta_{21}\psi_{11}O_1)(A_1+1)/2 + \sigma\phi\left(\frac{c_1+c_2}{\sigma}\right) + \right.$$
$$\left. (c_1+c_2)\Phi\left(\frac{c_1+c_2}{\sigma}\right)\right\}.$$

The optimal rule contains both the probability and cumulative density functions of the normal distribution. Specific parametric knowledge of the distribution of the state variable is required to estimate the optimal rule – but of course this is precisely what we wish to avoid when using semi-parametric methods such as G-estimation, which will be presented shortly, in Sect. 4.3. The study of standard SNMMs will not be pursued further in this chapter, as, for the present, our interest lies in estimating optimal dynamic regimes *without* explicitly modeling all aspects of the longitudinal distribution of the data.

4.2 Model Parameterizations and Optimal Rules

Let ψ be parameters for the SNMM, $\gamma_j(h_j,a_j;\psi)$ or $\mu_j(h_j,a_j;\psi)$. If the true form of the SNMM and the true values of ψ were known then the optimal regime is

$$d_j^{opt}(h_j;\psi) = \arg\max_{a_j} \gamma_j(h_j,a_j;\psi) \qquad \text{or}$$

$$d_j^{opt}(h_j;\psi) = \{a_j \text{ such that } \mu_j(h_j,a_j;\psi) = 0\}$$

for $j = 1,2,\ldots,K$. Sections 4.3 and 4.4 discuss in greater detail methods of finding estimators $\hat{\psi}$ of ψ so that the optimal rules may be estimated to be the treatment a_j which maximizes $\gamma_j(h_j,a_j;\hat{\psi})$ over all possible treatments at stage j. A number of estimators for ψ have been proposed. For example, in some cases solutions can be found in closed form while in others, an objective function must be minimized or iteration is required (Murphy 2003). Once $\hat{\psi}$ has been found by an appropriate method, the optimal treatments are found by maximizing the regret or the optimal blip function over all treatments where $\hat{\psi}$ is used in place of ψ.

There is a variety of parameterizations that may be chosen to describe the optimal blip function at each stage. For instance, we may suppose that the blips are time-dependent (non-stationary), so that $\gamma_j(h_j,a_j;\psi_j)$ is such that $\psi_j \neq \psi_k$ whenever

$j \neq k$. On the other hand, when the state variable, O_j, measures the same quantity at each stage, for example CD4 cell count in an HIV setting or white blood cell count in a cancer trial, it may be more reasonable to assume that parameters are shared across stages: $\psi_j = \psi_k$ for all j,k. We consider the shared parameters case in more detail in Chap. 9.

Define $\mathscr{D}_j(\gamma)$ to be the set of rules, d_j^{opt}, that are optimal under the optimal blip function model $\gamma_j(h_j, a_j; \psi)$ as ψ is varied:

$$\mathscr{D}_j(\gamma) = \{d_j^{opt}(\cdot;\psi) | d_j^{opt}(h_j;\psi) = \underset{a_j}{\text{argmax}} \;\; \gamma_j(h_j, a_j; \psi) \text{ for some } \psi\}.$$

Similarly, let $\mathscr{D}_j(\mu)$ be the set of optimal rules that are compatible with regret model $\mu_j(h_j, a_j; \psi)$:

$$\mathscr{D}_j(\mu) = \{d_j^{opt}(\cdot;\psi) | \mu_j(h_j, d_j^{opt}(h_j;\psi);\psi) = 0 \text{ for some } \psi\}.$$

Murphy (2003) proposes modeling regrets using a known link function, $f(u)$, that relates the regret and the decision rule. For a scale parameter $\eta_j(h_j) \geq 0$, set

$$\mu_j^f(h_j, a_j) = \eta_j(h_j) \times f(a_j - d_j^{opt}(h_j;\psi)),$$

where $f(\cdot)$ is required to be non-negative and the superscript f is used to remind the reader of the parametric form assumed. When there is an effect of treatment, the regret is zero if and only if a_j is optimal. Consequently, $f(0) = 0$ if and only if $d_j^{opt}(h_j;\psi)$ is the optimal rule. Note that when treatment has no effect, every regime is equally optimal (or sub-optimal), and the regret and blip functions equal zero for all treatments. The form of the optimal decision rule must be postulated to specify $f(\cdot)$ (see below). The parameters in $d_j^{opt}(h_j;\psi)$ are not defined when the scale parameter, η_j, equals zero.

Murphy (2003) models discrete decisions via a smooth approximation in order to facilitate estimation. For example, if using a 0/1 coding of treatment, the analyst may choose to approximate an indicator function for the binary decision rule with the inverse logit function expit$(x) = e^x(e^x+1)^{-1}$; equivalently, one could use $2[e^x(e^x+1)^{-1} - 0.5]$ for treatment coded $-1/1$. When the decision in the regret model is approximated as is the case when using the inverse logit in place of an indicator function, use $\breve{\mu}_j(h_j, a_j)$ to denote the *approximation* of regret $\mu_j(h_j, a_j)$, and let

$$\mathscr{D}_j(\breve{\mu}_j) = \{d_j^{opt}(\cdot;\psi) | d_j^{opt}(h_j;\psi) = \arg\min_{a_j} \breve{\mu}_j(h_j, a_j;\psi) \text{ for some } \psi\}$$

denote the set of optimal rules that are compatible with the approximation $\breve{\mu}_j(h_j, a_j)$ of $\mu_j(h_j, a_j)$. The approximate regret may not equal zero at the optimal regime. In particular, using the expit function gives $\breve{\mu}_j(h_j, a_j) = 0.5$ at the optimal regime for individuals whose covariates values lie exactly on the optimal decision rule threshold (i.e., people for whom the optimal rule is not unique).

Suppose $\gamma_j(h_j, a_j) = c'(o_j;\psi)(a_j+1)/2$ is monotonic and increasing in o_j so that treatment is beneficial if a subject is above a threshold value of the random variable O_j. If treatment is binary, the corresponding regret is

$$\mu_j(h_j,a_j) = |c'(o_j;\psi)| \times [a_j - sign(c'(o_j;\psi))]^2/4,$$

and $\mathscr{D}_j(\gamma) = \mathscr{D}_j(\mu) = \{sign(c'(o_j;\psi))\}$. This holds true since whenever the optimal blip is positive, the outcome is being maximized by taking treatment ($A = 1$) rather than not ($A = -1$), while when the optimal blip is negative, the best one could do is to have an expected difference in potential outcomes of zero, which is achieved by not being treated (Fig. 4.1).

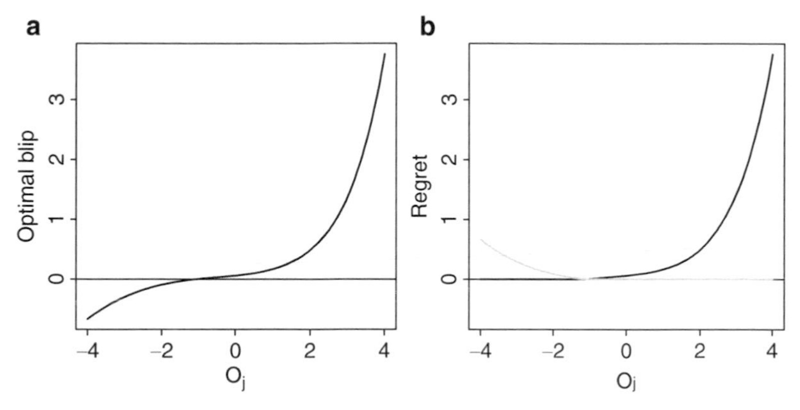

Fig. 4.1 (**a**) Monotonic, increasing optimal blip and (**b**) corresponding regret functions. The regret in *black* is for $A = -1$, and in *grey*, for $A = 1$. Note that the regrets, where non-zero, are a reflection of the optimal blip above the x-axis

The parameterization of the underlying data generating procedure by the analyst is key to obtaining good estimates of the DTR (Robins 2004, p. 243). For example, suppose the optimal blip, $\gamma_j(h_j,a_j;\psi) = c'(o_j;\psi)(a_j+1)/2$, is such that $c'(o_j;\psi) = \psi_0 + \psi_1 o_j$ and treatment a_j is binary. The corresponding regret is $\mu_j(h_j,a_j) = |\psi_0 + \psi_1 o_j| \times (a_j - sign(\psi_0 + \psi_1 o_j))^2/4$ and $\mathscr{D}_j(\gamma) = \mathscr{D}_j(\mu) = \{sign(\psi_0 + \psi_1 o_j)\}$. If in fact $\psi_1 > 0$ so that treatment is beneficial when O_j is above the threshold $\beta = -\psi_0/\psi_1$, we may re-parameterize the regret to obtain the threshold, β: $\mu_j^*(h_j,a_j) = |o_j - \beta| \times (a_j - sign(o_j - \beta))^2/4$, which gives $\mathscr{D}_j(\mu^*) = \{sign(o_j - \beta)\}$. However, if $\psi_1 < 0$ so that now subjects should be treated when $O_j < \beta$, $\mu_j^*(h_j,a_j) = |o_j - \beta| \times (a_j + sign(o_j - \beta))^2/4$ and so $\mathscr{D}_j(\mu^*) = \{-sign(o_j - \beta)\}$. Thus, one consequence of using the re-parameterized regret is that the analyst must know in advance whether it is optimal to treat patients for low or high values of O_j. Incorrectly specifying for whom treatment will be beneficial can lead to false conclusions such as failure to detect a treatment effect, however this can be overcome simply by using a richer class of models for the regret, such as the two-parameter model in this example (see the reply to the discussion of (Murphy 2003)).

4.3 G-estimation

Robins (2004) proposed finding the parameters ψ of the optimal blip function or regret function via G-estimation. This method is a generalization of estimating equations designed to account for time-varying covariates and general treatment regimes. There are close ties between G-estimation and instrumental variables methods. To use an instrumental variable analysis to estimate a causal effect requires a variable (the instrument) that is associated with the outcome only through its effect on the treatment received and possibly also through measured confounders (Angrist et al. 1996). All that is required to define an unbiased estimating equation is that the model residual is conditionally uncorrelated with the instrument. Viewing the expected counterfactual outcome ($G_j(\psi)$, defined below) as the model and a centered function of treatment as the instrument, we may think of G-estimation as an instrumental variables analysis (Joffe 2000); by the assumption of no unmeasured confounding, treatment allocation at stage j is independent of outcome and state in any future stage, conditional on treatment and state history. See Joffe and Brensinger (2003) for a detailed one-stage explanation and implementation. Instrumental variables analysis and G-estimation fall under the wider umbrella of the Generalized Methods of Moments approach, thoroughly treated by Newey and McFadden (1994).

Define

$$\begin{aligned}
G_j(\psi) &= Y + \sum_{k=j}^{K} \left[\gamma_k(h_k, d_k^{opt}; \psi) - \gamma_k(h_k, a_k; \psi)\right] \\
&= Y + \sum_{k=j}^{K} E\Big[\{Y(\bar{a}_{k-1}, \underline{d}_k^{opt}) - Y(\bar{a}_{k-1}, 0_k, \underline{d}_{k+1}^{opt})\} - \\
&\qquad \{Y(\bar{a}_k, \underline{d}_{k+1}^{opt}) - Y(\bar{a}_{k-1}, 0_k, \underline{d}_{k+1}^{opt})\} \,|H_k = h_k\Big] \\
&= Y + \sum_{k=j}^{K} E\left[Y(\bar{a}_{k-1}, \underline{d}_k^{opt}) - Y(\bar{a}_k, \underline{d}_{k+1}^{opt})|H_k = h_k\right].
\end{aligned}$$

In the two-stage case, this gives

$$\begin{aligned}
G_2(\psi) &= Y + E\left[Y(a_1, d_2^{opt}) - Y(\bar{a}_2)|H_2 = h_2\right] \\
&= Y - E[Y(\bar{a}_2)|H_2 = h_2] + E[Y(a_1, d_2^{opt})|H_2 = h_2]
\end{aligned}$$

at the second stage, which is the observed outcome minus the expected counterfactual outcome under the observed treatment (given the observed covariate history) plus the expected counterfactual outcome under the observed treatment at the first stage and the optimal treatment at the second stage (given the observed covariate history). In expectation, the first of two terms cancel out, leaving only the expected counterfactual outcome under the observed treatment at the first stage and the optimal treatment at the second stage. Similarly, for the first stage in a two-stage setting, we have

$$G_1(\psi) = Y + E\Big[Y(\underline{d}_1^{opt}) - Y(a_1, d_2^{opt})|H_1 = h_1\Big] + E\Big[Y(a_1, d_2^{opt}) - Y(\bar{a}_2)|H_2 = h_2\Big].$$

The third and fourth terms, $-E\Big[Y(a_1, d_2^{opt})|H_1 = h_1\Big] + E\Big[Y(a_1, d_2^{opt})|H_2 = h_2\Big]$ cancel in expectation, as do the first and last, leaving only the expected counterfactual outcome under optimal treatment at both stages.

Therefore, $G_j(\psi)$ is a person's outcome adjusted by the expected difference between the average outcome for someone who received a_j and someone who was given the optimal treatment at the start of stage j, where both had the same treatment and covariate history to the start of stage $j-1$ and were subsequently treated optimally. Under the assumption of additive local rank preservation, $G_j(\psi)$ *equals* the counterfactual outcome, not simply its expectation (Robins 2004); i.e., $G_j(\psi) = Y(\bar{a}_{j-1}, \underline{d}_j^{opt})$. Now, let $S_j(A_j) = s_j(H_j, A_j)$ be a vector-valued function that is chosen by the analyst to contain the variables thought to interact with treatment to effect a difference in the outcome; the range of the function is in $\mathbb{R}^{dim(\psi_j)}$. For example, if $K = 2$, we may choose $S_1(A_1) = (A_1 + 1)/2 \cdot (1, O_1)^T$ and $S_2(A_2) = (A_2 + 1)/2 \cdot (1, O_1, A_1, O_1 A_1)^T$, which is simply the derivative of the stage j blip function with respect to ψ.

Model the probability of receiving treatment a_j by $p_j(A_j = 1|H_j; \alpha)$, where α may be vector-valued; for binary treatment, this model is the propensity score which was first introduced in Sect. 3.5. A common parametric model used to describe the treatment allocation probabilities is the logistic model when treatment is binary, however non-parametric models may also be used. Let

$$U(\psi, \alpha) = \sum_{j=1}^{K} G_j(\psi)\{S_j(A_j) - E[S_j(A_j)|H_j; \alpha]\}. \tag{4.2}$$

Then $E[U(\psi, \alpha)] = 0$ is an unbiased estimating equation from which consistent, asymptotically normal estimators $\hat{\psi}$ of ψ may be found under standard regularity conditions provided the treatment allocation probabilities, $p_j(A_j = 1|H_j)$, are known or modeled correctly with respect to confounding variables (using estimates $\hat{\alpha}$) and there are no distributions of the data for which more than one treatment is optimal. This latter condition, also known as requiring no *exceptional laws*, will be considered in greater detail in Chap. 8; when this condition is violated, estimators may be non-regular. Even when the treatment model and its parameters are known, it is more efficient to estimate the treatment model parameters than to substitute in known values (Robins 2004, p. 211); this is analogous to the gains in efficiency observed by adjusting for covariates in a randomized trial to account for chance imbalance between treatment groups. The unbiasedness of Eq. (4.2) is due to the fact that counterfactual outcomes under different treatment regimes at stage j are independent of any function of actual treatment conditional on prior treatment and covariates (by the assumption of no unmeasured confounding). These estimators are not semi-parametric efficient. Note that semi-parametric efficiency is a concept similar to efficiency in a simple parametric case; semi-parametric analogs to the Cramer-Rao lower bound on the variability of an estimator can be derived.

4.3.1 More Efficient G-estimation

Robins refined the estimating equation in (4.2) to gain efficiency by making an additional modeling assumption for the form of $E[G_j(\psi_j)|H_j]$. For example, we may use ordinary least squares to model $E[G_j(\psi_j)|H_j;\varsigma]$ with (possibly vector-valued) parameters ς. Let

$$U(\psi,\varsigma(\psi),\alpha) = \sum_{j}^{K}(G_j(\psi) - E[G_j(\psi)|H_j;\varsigma])\{S_j(A_j) - E[S_j(A_j)|H_j;\alpha]\}. \quad (4.3)$$

Robins (2004) proved that the estimator $\hat{\psi}$ of ψ using Eq. (4.3) is consistent provided that *either* $E[G_j(\psi)|H_j;\varsigma]$ *or* $p_j(A_j = 1|H_j;\alpha)$ is correctly modeled, and thus the estimate is said to be *doubly-robust*. In fact, the propensity score model $p_j(A_j = 2|H_j;\alpha)$ need not be correctly specified in the sense of capturing the data-generating mechanism, but rather it must include and correctly model the impact of all confounding variables on the choice of treatment. To use Eq. (4.3), typically estimates $\hat{\varsigma}$ and $\hat{\alpha}$ of the nuisance parameters ς and α are substituted into the estimating equation. Estimates from Eq. (4.3) may be considerably less variable than those from Eq. (4.2), but they are still not efficient. As with Eq. (4.2), if the treatment model and its parameters are known (as they would be, for instance, in a randomized trial with perfect compliance), estimates from (4.3) are more efficient using estimated treatment probabilities than the known values (Robins 2004).

Efficient estimates can be found with judicious choice of the function $S_j(A_j)$. Unfortunately, the form of $S_j(A_j)$ that leads to efficient estimates is typically complex except in the special case where

$$\text{Var}[G_j(\psi)|H_j,A_j] = \text{Var}[G_j(\psi)|H_j]$$

for all j (Robins 1994). In the particular situation where this variance assumption holds, setting

$$S_j(A_j;\psi) = E\left[\frac{\partial}{\partial\psi}G_j(\psi)\right](\text{Var}[G_j(\psi)|H_j])^{-1}$$

yields estimators that are semi-parametric efficient provided each of $E[G_j(\psi)|H_j]$, $p_j(A_j = 1|H_j;\alpha)$, $E[\frac{\partial}{\partial\psi}G_j(\psi)]$, and $\text{Var}[G_j(\psi)|H_j]$ is correctly specified. Note, however, that "correct" specification of the treatment model does not in fact require complete knowledge of the treatment assignment mechanism, but only that the model $p_j(A_j = 1|H_j;\alpha)$ conditions on all variables that confound the relationship between treatment in the jth stage, A_j, and the outcome; Ertefaie et al. (2012) prove this in the context of propensity score adjustment and inverse probability weighting.

4.3.2 Recursive G-estimation

When optimal blips are linear in ψ and parameters are not assumed to be shared across stages, we can solve for $\hat{\psi}$ explicitly. In general, for instance when blips are not linear or parameters are shared across stages, search algorithms may be required. Use the modification

$$G_{\text{mod},j}(\psi) = Y - \gamma_j(h_j, a_j; \psi) + \sum_{k=j+1}^{K} \left[\gamma_k(h_k, d_k^{opt}; \psi) - \gamma_k(h_k, a_k; \psi)\right],$$

which is a person's outcome adjusted by the expected difference between the average outcome for someone who received a_j and someone who was given the zero regime at stage j, where both had the same treatment and covariate history to stage $j-1$ and were treated optimally from stage $j+1$ onwards. Under additive local rank preservation, $G_{\text{mod},j}(\psi) = Y(\bar{a}_{j-1}, -1, d_{j+1}^{opt})$.

This modification allows recursive estimation using Eqs. (4.2) or (4.3). At the last stage, we first estimate the nuisance parameter (ς_K, α_K) and note that $G_{\text{mod},K}(\psi)$ and consequently $U_K(\psi)$ now has only a single (possibly vector) unknown parameter as well as ψ_K. Solve for $\hat{\psi}_K$. Now estimate $(\varsigma_{K-1}, \alpha_{K-1})$ at the second-to-last stage, $K-1$. Substitution of these estimates $\hat{\psi}_K$ leaves us with only the parameter ψ_{K-1} unknown in $U_{K-1}(\psi)$, and so $\hat{\psi}_{K-1}$ may be found. Continuing in this manner yields recursive G-estimates for all optimal regime parameters, ψ_j, $j = 1, \ldots, K$.

Recursive G-estimation is particularly useful when parameters are not shared across stages (i.e., not stationary or common to different stages). An example of blip functions for two stages which are linear in ψ but *do* have common parameters between stages are $\gamma_1(h_1, a_1) = (\psi_0 + \psi_1 o_1)(a_1 + 1)/2$ and $\gamma_2(h_2, a_2) = (\psi_0 + \psi_1 o_2 + \psi_2 a_1)(a_2 + 1)/2$, since ψ_0 and ψ_1 appear in the blip functions at both stages. In fact, recursive G-estimation may still be used when parameters are shared by first assuming no sharing and then taking, for instance, the inverse-covariance weighted average or even the simple average of the stage-specific estimates. Note that $G_{\text{mod},j}(\psi)$ could also be used in G-estimation (Eqs. (4.2) or (4.3)) without recursion.

To accomplish G-estimation (using either the standard or the recursive approach) requires estimates of the nuisance parameters ς and α. Thus, we can perform G-estimation in two steps: find $\varsigma(\psi)$ analytically by ordinary least squares and α by some possibly non-parametric method of estimation (step 1), then plug these estimates into Eqs. (4.2) or (4.3) and solve to find ψ (step 2). For recursive G-estimation, we in fact have two steps of estimation at each stage for a total of $2K$ steps. The impact of this two-step approach on estimation of standard errors will be considered in Chap. 8.

4.3.3 G-estimation Versus OLS Regression for a One-Stage Problem

In the one-stage case with univariate O and binary A, a linear (optimal) blip function gives

$$E[Y|O=o,A=a]-E[Y|O=o,A=-1]=(\psi_0+\psi_1 o)(a+1)/2$$

so that $E[Y|O=o,A=a]=(\psi_0+\psi_1 o)(a+1)/2+b(o)$ where the form of $b(o)$ is not specified. In this simple context, we may model $b(o)$ non-parametrically and use ordinary least squares to model the optimal blip as an alternative to G-estimation (Robins 2004); in fact, the ordinary least squares (OLS) approach is a simplified implementation of Q-learning. We consider two examples; in both, we generate the state and treatment data such that $O\sim$ Uniform$(-0.5,3)$ and A takes the value 1 with probability expit$(-2+1.8O)$. In the first example,

$$Y(A)=-1.4+0.8+(5+2O)(A+1)/2+\varepsilon,$$

and in the second,

$$Y(A)=-1.4O^3+e^O+(5+2O)(A+1)/2+\varepsilon,$$

with $\varepsilon\sim\mathcal{N}(0,1)$ for each. For both G-estimation approaches based on (4.2) and (4.3), take $S(A)=(A+1)/2\cdot(1,O)^T$. To perform G-estimation more efficiently, model $E[H(\psi)|O]$ as a linear function of O. Recall that the estimator is doubly-robust, so that it is consistent even when $E[H(\psi)|O]$ is incorrectly specified provided treatment allocation probabilities are correctly modeled with respect to the confounding variables. For the regression method, model $b(o)$ in two ways: non-parametrically with a smoothing spline and parametrically via a linear model.

Table 4.1 shows results from 1,000 simulations in which G-estimation is compared to modeling outcome, Y, among those who were not treated with a straight line and with a smoothing spline, and the regressing observed outcome minus the predicted value from the initial regression on the state variable. When $Y(A=-1)$ depends linearly on O, all four methods exhibit little bias, with the smallest variability exhibited by the regression method which models $b(o)$ linearly, followed closely by the G-estimation using Eq. (4.3).

In the second example, where the dependence of Y on O is highly non-linear, G-estimation using (4.2) demonstrates the least bias of the three approaches, however it is also the most highly variable. Using the more efficient G-estimating Eq. (4.3) reduces the standard error considerably, at the cost of an introduction of some bias at small sample sizes. The regression method that models $b(o)$ linearly exhibits a low variance but considerable bias even at large sample sizes.

Table 4.1 Comparison of G-estimation and OLS regression for a one-stage case

		G-estimation				Linear regression			
		Eq. (4.2)		Eq. (4.3)		Linear $b(o)$		Smooth $b(o)$	
n	ψ	$\hat{\psi}$	SE	$\hat{\psi}$	SE	$\hat{\psi}$	SE	$\hat{\psi}$	SE
$Y=-1.4+0.8O+A(5+2O)+\varepsilon$									
50	$\psi_0=5$	5.183	1.071	5.020	0.777	5.029	0.599	5.062	1.004
	$\psi_1=2$	1.864	0.823	1.978	0.563	1.975	0.412	1.938	0.778
100	$\psi_0=5$	5.040	0.602	4.984	0.476	4.976	0.381	4.996	0.598
	$\psi_1=2$	1.963	0.464	2.000	0.355	2.007	0.263	1.993	0.480
1,000	$\psi_0=5$	5.008	0.176	5.001	0.150	5.000	0.123	4.998	0.172
	$\psi_1=2$	1.993	0.136	1.998	0.111	1.999	0.084	2.001	0.130
$Y=-1.4O^3+e^O+A(5+2O)+\varepsilon$									
50	$\psi_0=5$	4.626	3.846	5.655	1.917	11.358	2.389	7.449	2.018
	$\psi_1=2$	2.167	3.494	1.452	1.501	−3.134	1.585	−0.018	1.695
100	$\psi_0=5$	4.940	1.893	5.318	1.187	10.982	1.541	6.817	1.208
	$\psi_1=2$	1.944	1.980	1.680	0.990	−2.907	1.098	0.523	1.086
1,000	$\psi_0=5$	4.981	0.481	5.011	0.355	10.726	0.476	6.319	0.286
	$\psi_1=2$	2.011	0.550	1.990	0.295	−2.654	0.337	1.001	0.244

4.3.4 Q-learning and G-estimation

Under the following sufficient conditions, it has been shown that Q-learning and G-estimation are algebraically equivalent when linear models are used for the Q-functions (Chakraborty et al. 2010):

(i) The parameters in Q_1^{opt} and Q_2^{opt} are distinct;
(ii) A_j has zero conditional mean given the history $H_j=(\bar{O}_j,\bar{A}_{j-1})$, $j=1,2$; and
(iii) The covariates used in the model for Q_1^{opt} are nested within the covariates used in the model for Q_2^{opt}, i.e., $(H_{10}^T,H_{11}^TA_1)\subset H_{20}^T$ where H_{j0} and H_{j1} are two vector summaries of the history H_j, denoting the main effect of history and the part of history that interacts with treatment.

Recall that with binary treatments A_j coded $-1/1$, the random variable A_j may in fact have a zero mean conditional on covariate history.

Recall that the regret is given by $\mu_j(h_j,a_j)=E[Y(\bar{a}_{j-1},\underline{d}_j^{opt})-Y(\bar{a}_j,\underline{d}_{j+1}^{opt})|H_j=h_j]$, which can also be expressed as

$$-\mu_j(h_j,a_j)=Q_j^{opt}(h_j,a_j)-\max_{a_j}Q_j^{opt}(h_j,a_j)$$

for $j=1,2$. Using linear models parameterized by β,ψ of the form $Q_j^{opt}(H_j,A_j;\beta_j,\psi_j)=\beta_j^TH_{j0}+(\psi_j^TH_{j1})A_j$ for the Q-functions, this gives

$$-\mu_j(H_j,A_j;\psi_j)=\psi_j^TH_{j1}a_j-|\psi_j^TH_{j1}|,\ j=1,2.$$

Define $m_2(H_2)=E[Q_2^{opt}(H_2,A_2)|H_2]$. Since we assume no parameter sharing, we can perform the estimation recursively, beginning at the last stage.

The recursive form of G-estimation using Eq. (4.3) first solves

$$\mathbb{P}_n\left[(Y_2+\mu_2(H_2,A_2;\psi_2)-E[Y_2+\mu_2(H_2,A_2;\psi_2)|H_2])\,(H_{21}A_2-E[H_{21}A_2|H_2])\right]=0,$$

where $\mathbb{P}_n$ denotes the empirical average function, thereby finding estimates of $\theta_2^T=(\beta_2^T,\psi_2^T)$. By assumption (ii), the left-hand side reduces to

$$\begin{aligned}
&\mathbb{P}_n\left[H_{21}A_2\,(Y_2+\mu_2(H_2,A_2;\psi_2)-E[Y_2+\mu_2(H_2,A_2;\psi_2)|H_2])\right]\\
&\quad=\mathbb{P}_n\left[H_{21}A_2\left(Y_2-\psi_j^T H_{j1}A_j+|\psi_j^T H_{j1}|-(m_2(H_2)+|\psi_j^T H_{j1}|)\right)\right]\\
&\quad=\mathbb{P}_n\left[H_{21}A_2\left(Y_2-m_2(H_2)-\psi_j^T H_{j1}A_j\right)\right]
\end{aligned}$$

since $-\mu_2(H_2,A_2;\psi_2)=\psi_j^T H_{j1}A_j-|\psi_j^T H_{j1}|$ and so $E[\mu_2(H_2,A_2;\psi_2)|H_2]=|\psi_j^T H_{j1}|$. Then, taking $m_2(H_2)=H_{j0}^T\hat{\beta}_2$ where

$$\hat{\beta}_2=\left[\mathbb{P}_n(H_{20}H_{20}^T)\right]^{-1}\left[\mathbb{P}_n(H_{20}Y_2)-\mathbb{P}_n(H_{20}H_{21}^T A_2\psi_2)\right],$$

we have shown that the G-estimating equation is identical to the second-stage least squares regression performed in Q-learning. The proof for the first stage estimation follows in a similar fashion.

In the case of shared parameters, the G-estimating functions are stacked and solved simultaneously. Approximate solutions to the G-estimation functions and Q-learning functions have been considered by taking the outer product of the estimation functions and searching for values of ψ that minimize the resulting quadratic function (Chakraborty and Moodie 2013). In such circumstances, assuming conditions (ii) and (iii) above, it can again be shown that Q-learning and G-estimation are equivalent.

As noted previously, even in randomized trial settings where treatment probabilities are fixed and known, it is more efficient to use estimates of the propensity score rather than known randomization probabilities; as this expectation does not involve parameters ψ_j, it is typically estimated at the outset of a G-estimation analysis and substituted into the G-estimating functions for the DTR parameters. Thus, while Q-learning and G-estimation are in some instances equivalent, the typical implementation of these methods leads to estimates which are not identical.

4.4 Regret-Based Methods of Estimation

Advantage learning, or *A-learning*, is a method of identifying optimal dynamic regimes by focusing on modeling the advantage, the regret, or a similar quantity such as the difference between the Q-function and the untreated outcome:

$$\tilde{\mu}_j=Q_j^{opt}(H_j,A_j)-Q_j^{opt}(H_j,-1)$$

where −1 is used to indicate a standard or zero treatment, such as placebo or usual care. Since the Q-function can be written as the sum of the advantage function and the value function, we can see that A-learning requires a model for only part of the Q-function, namely the interaction terms specific to the decision making or tailoring part of the Q-function.

4.4.1 Iterative Minimization of Regrets

Murphy (2003) developed a method that estimates the parameters of the optimal regime, ψ, by searching for $(\hat{\psi}, \hat{c})$ which satisfy

$$\sum_{j=1}^{K} \mathbb{P}_n \Big[Y + \hat{c} + \sum_{k=1}^{K} \mu_k(H_k, A_k; \hat{\psi}) - \sum_a \mu_j(H_j, a; \hat{\psi}) p_j(a|H_j; \hat{\alpha}) \Big]^2$$

$$\leq \sum_{j=1}^{K} \mathbb{P}_n \Big[Y + c + \sum_{k \neq j} \mu_k(H_k, A_k; \hat{\psi}) + \mu_j(H_j, A_j; \psi)$$

$$- \sum_a \mu_j(H_j, a; \psi) p_j(a|H_j; \hat{\alpha}) \Big]^2 \quad (4.4)$$

for all c and all ψ. Treatment probabilities – i.e., parameters α of the propensity score – can be estimated in the same fashion as for G-estimation. The scalar quantity c is not easily interpreted, except in the special case of no effect of treatment, when $\hat{c} = -\mathbb{P}_n(Y)$ i.e. it is the negative of the sample mean of the outcomes. In fact, c $(\hat{c})$ may be omitted from (4.4); it is not required for estimation but greatly improves the stability of the procedure (Murphy 2003). The estimator $\hat{\psi}$ is consistent for ψ provided the treatment allocation probabilities, $p_j(A_j = 1|H_j; \alpha)$, are correctly specified with respect to confounding variables.

Murphy (2003) described an iterative method of finding solutions to (4.4), which begins by selecting an initial value of $\hat{\psi}$, say $\hat{\psi}^{(1)}$, then minimizing the right-hand side (RHS) of the equation over (ψ, c) to obtain a new value of $\hat{\psi}$, $\hat{\psi}^{(2)}$, and repeating this until convergence. This *iterative minimization of regrets* (IMOR) method may not produce a monotonically decreasing sequence of RHS values of Eq. (4.4). Furthermore, this iterative procedure may not converge to a minimum; use of several starting seeds and profile plots of the RHS of (4.4) for each parameter in a stage about its estimate may reassure the analyst that a minimum was reached. Rosthøj et al. (2006) provided an empirical demonstration of the method applied to estimate the optimal dose of anticoagulation medication, and investigated convergence properties through extensive simulations. The simulation study suggested that IMOR may not converge when samples are small (e.g. 300), there is considerable noise in the data, or the researcher cannot posit good initial values for the search algorithm; mis-specification of the treatment model can lead to serious convergence problems, indicating that IMOR is not a doubly-robust procedure.

In the following section, we will see that IMOR is closely connected to, but not in general the same as, Robins' more efficient estimation (Eq. (4.3)) and that these are equivalent under the null hypothesis of no treatment effect for particular model choices in Eq. (4.3). Note that the term "more efficient G-estimation" is used to distinguish between the two G-estimating Eqs. (4.2) and (4.3), and is not meant to imply that G-estimation is more efficient than IMOR.

4.4.1.1 Connections to G-estimation: The One-Stage Case

Consider the one-stage case with observed variables O, A, and Y where A is binary and O and Y are both univariate. We shall demonstrate that G-estimation and IMOR are equivalent, given specific choices of models. Robins (2004, Theorem 9.1) proves that for

$$\gamma(o,a;\psi) = E[Y|O=o,A=a] - E[Y|O=o,A=-1],$$

which equals $E[Y(a)-Y(-1)|O=o]$ under the no unmeasured confounding assumption, $\gamma(o,a)$ is the unique function $g(o,a)$ minimizing

$$E\left[\{Y-g(o,a)-E[Y-g(o,a)|O=o]\}^2\right] \tag{4.5}$$

subject to $g(o,-1)=0$. This constraint on $g()$ is required to restrict the function to be in the class of blip functions. In G-estimation, minimization occurs when the derivative of Eq. (4.5),

$$\frac{\partial}{\partial\psi}E\left[\{Y-g(o,a)-E[Y-g(o,a)|O=o]\}^2\right] \propto$$
$$E\left[\{Y-g(o,a)-E[Y-g(o,a)|O=o]\}\times\left\{-\frac{\partial}{\partial\psi}g(o,a)+E[\frac{\partial}{\partial\psi}g(o,a)|O=o]\right\}\right],$$

equals zero. At the minimum, $g(o,a)=\gamma(o,a)$, which gives $Y-g(o,a)=G(\psi)=G_{\text{mod}}(\psi)$. Taking $S(A)$ equal to $-\frac{\partial}{\partial\psi}g(O,A)$, Eq. (4.5) equals Eq. (4.3), the more efficient G-estimating equation.

For a one-stage problem, IMOR proceeds directly by minimizing the left-hand side of Eq. (4.4). At the minimum we have:

$$\begin{aligned}
E&\left[\left\{Y-g(o,a)-E[Y-g(o,a)|O]\right\}^2\right]\\
&=E\left[\left\{Y-\gamma(o,a)-E[Y-\gamma(o,a)|O=o]\right\}^2\right]\\
&=E\left[\left\{Y-(\mu(o,-1)-\mu(o,a))-E[Y-(\mu(o,-1)-\mu(o,a))|O=o]\right\}^2\right]\\
&=E\left[\left\{Y+\hat{c}+\mu(o,a)-E[\mu(o,a)|O=o]\right\}^2\right]
\end{aligned}$$

with $\hat{c}=-\mu(o,-1)+E[\mu(o,-1)-Y|O=o]$, which can be re-expressed as

$$-\hat{c} = E[G_{\text{mod}}(\psi)|O = o] + \mu(o,-1) - E[\mu(o,a)|O = o].$$

One critical difference exists: IMOR does not model $E[G_{\text{mod}}(\psi)|O = o]$ explicitly, but rather does so through the regrets and $\hat{c}$. This expression for $\hat{c}$ makes clear that, under the null hypothesis of no treatment effect, $\hat{c} = E[G_{\text{mod}}(\psi)] = E[Y]$, and IMOR is equivalent to G-estimation using Eq. (4.3) with $E[G_{\text{mod}}(\psi)|O = o]$ modeled by a constant.

4.4.1.2 Connections to G-estimation: *K* Stages

Suppose now that we have K stages and we observe $\bar{O}_K$, $\bar{A}_K$, and Y where A_j is binary and O_j, Y are univariate for all j. Suppose also that parameters are not shared across stages, so that $\psi_j \neq \psi_k$ for $j \neq k$. Robins (2004, Corollary 9.2) extended Eq. (4.5), proving that for an optimal blip $\gamma_j(h_j, a_j)$ with parameters ψ_j, the unique function $g(h_j, a_j)$ minimizing

$$E\left[\left\{Y - g(h_j,a_j) + \sum_{k=j+1}^{K} \left[\gamma_k(h_k, d_k^{opt}; \psi_k) - \gamma_k(h_k, a_k; \psi_k)\right]\right.\right.$$
$$\left.\left. - E\left[Y - g(h_j,a_j) + \sum_{k=j+1}^{K} \left[\gamma_k(h_k, d_k^{opt}; \psi_k) - \gamma_k(h_k, a_k; \psi_k)\right] |H_k = h_k\right]\right\}^2\right] \quad (4.6)$$

subject to $g(h_j, a_j) = 0$ for $a_j = -1$ is $\gamma_j(h_j, a_j)$. For this to be of any use in estimating ψ_j, ψ_k for $k = j+1, \ldots, K$ must have been estimated already. For any arbitrary function $q_j(\cdot)$, it is not possible to minimize

$$E\left[\left\{Y - q_j(h_j,a_j) + \sum_{k=j+1}^{K} \left[q_k(h_k, d_k^{opt}) - q_k(h_k, a_k)\right]\right.\right.$$
$$\left.\left. - E\left[Y - q_j(h_j,a_j) + \sum_{k=j+1}^{K} \left[q_k(h_k, d_k^{opt}) - q_k(h_k, a_k)\right] |H_k = h_k\right]\right\}^2\right]$$

simultaneously over $q_j(\cdot)$ (Robins 2004). In G-estimation, simultaneous minimization is avoided by proceeding recursively, estimating first ψ_K, then ψ_{K-1} and so on until all parameters have been estimated. As observed in the case of a single stage, G-estimation for several stages is equivalent to minimizing Eq. (4.6) at each stage by setting its derivative to zero. At the minimum, $g(h_j, a_j) = \gamma_j(h_j, a_j)$ and so

$$Y - g(h_j,a_j) + \sum_{k=j+1}^{K} \left[\gamma(h_k, d_k^{opt}; \psi_k) - \gamma(h_j, a_j; \psi_k)\right] = G_{\text{mod},j}(\psi_j).$$

When $S(A_j) = -\frac{\partial}{\partial \psi_j} g(H_j, A_j)$, Eq. (4.6) equals a G-estimating equation of the same form as Eq. (4.3) using the modified version of the counterfactual quantity $G_j(\psi)$.

IMOR is another method of recursive minimization. At any stage j, taking $g(h_j, a_j) = \gamma_j(h_j, a_j; \psi_j) = \mu_j(h_j, -1; \psi_j) - \mu_j(h_j, a_j; \psi_j)$ in Eq. (4.6) leads to the RHS of (4.4) for a single stage with

$$\begin{aligned}
-\hat{c} &= \mu_j(h_j, -1; \psi_j) + \sum_{k=1}^{j-1} \mu_k(h_k, a_k; \hat{\psi}_k) \\
&\quad - E\left[\mu_j(h_j, -1; \psi_j) + \sum_{k=j+1}^{K} \mu_k(h_k, a_k; \hat{\psi}_k) - Y \middle| H_j = h_j\right] \\
&= E\left[G_{\text{mod},j}(\psi) | H_j = h_j\right] + \mu_j(h_j, -1; \psi_j) \\
&\quad + \sum_{k=1}^{j-1} \mu_k(h_k, a_k; \hat{\psi}_k) - E\left[\mu_j(h_j, a_j; \psi_j) | H_j = h_j\right].
\end{aligned}$$

However, the parameter c in Eq. (4.4) is *not* stage-specific and IMOR and G-estimation are not in general equivalent. As in the one-stage instance, there is the important difference between the way the methods achieve their solutions that is due to whether or not $E[G_{\text{mod},j}(\psi)|H_j = h_j]$ is modeled explicitly or through the regrets and $\hat{c}$. As in the case of a single stage, under the null hypothesis of no treatment effect, $\hat{c} = E[G_{\text{mod},j}(\psi)] = E[Y]$, so there is equivalence between IMOR and G-estimation (4.3) when $E[G_{\text{mod},j}(\psi)|H_j = h_j]$ is modeled with a constant (which is stationary across all stages) and $S(A_j) = -\frac{\partial}{\partial \psi_j} g(H_j, A_j)$.

Regarding the relative efficiency, we can make the following points:

(i) Under the null hypothesis of no treatment effect, IMOR is a special case of G-estimation using Eq. (4.3) in which $E[G_{\text{mod},j}(\psi_j)|H_j]$ is assumed to be constant.
(ii) Under regularity conditions, estimates from Eq. (4.3) are the most efficient among the class of G-estimates using a given function $S(A_j)$ when both the propensity score (w.r.t. confounders) and expected counterfactual models are correctly specified (Robins 2004, Theorems 3.3(ii), 3.4).
(iii) Equation (4.3) does not satisfy the regularity conditions under the null hypothesis due to non-differentiability of the estimating equation in a neighborhood of $\psi = 0$. However, the conditions hold for constant blip functions, $\gamma_j(h_j, a_j) = a_j \psi_j$ (which may depend on j but not h_j) which posit no treatment interactions. (See Chap. 8 for a thorough consideration of the problem of non-regularity and solutions.)

Therefore, we may say that if the null hypothesis holds and we estimate a constant blip model (which trivially is correctly specified under the null hypothesis of no treatment effect), then G-estimation is more efficient than IMOR when $E[G_{\text{mod},j}(\psi)|H_j = h_j] = E[Y|H_j = h_j]$ depends on H_j and is correctly specified in G-estimating Eq. (4.3). If $E[G_{\text{mod},j}(\psi)|H_j = h_j]$ is constant, IMOR and Eq. (4.3) yield efficient estimators.

4.4.2 A-Learning

Recall that a regret is a difference in Q-functions. *A-learning* is an approach to DTR estimation that focuses on modeling only Q-function contrasts, rather than the full Q-function, since it is only the contrast which is required to identify the optimal DTR. By reducing the dependence of the estimation procedure on the full data-distribution, robustness to model mis-specification is won.

The A-learning procedure solves, at each stage j, the equation

$$\{Y - C(H_j,A_j;\psi_j) - \theta(H_K)\}\{S_j(A_j) - E[S_j(A_j)|H_j;\alpha]\} = 0$$

where $C(H_j,A_j;\psi_j)$ is a contrast of Q-functions. For linear Q-functions of the form $\beta_j^T H_{j0} + (\psi_j^T H_{j1})(A_j+1)/2$, $C(H_j,A_j;\psi_j) = (\psi_j^T H_{j1})(A_j+1)/2$, the same form as the optimal blip function. Like the more efficient G-estimation, A-learning using the above estimating equation is doubly-robust: it suffices for either $S_j(A_j) - E[S_j(A_j)|H_j;\alpha]$ or $Y - C(H_j,A_j;\psi_j) - \theta(H_K)$ to have mean zero (and thus, it suffices to adequately model either the treatment or the outcome) to obtain a consistent estimator of the DTR parameters, ψ. Indeed, for certain choices of $\theta(H_k)$, A-learning and G-estimation are identical.

Schulte et al. (2012) have provided a detailed and self-contained comparison of A-learning and Q-learning, in which they performed several simulations aimed at identifying regions in which one method is superior to the other. In a two-stage problem, they found that when all models were correctly specified, Q-learning was nearly twice as efficient in estimating the second stage parameters relative to A-learning, while gains at the first stage were much more modest. Q-learning was also more efficient than A-learning when the treatment model was mis-specified. However, if the Q-function was mis-specified, there were values of the parameters for which gains in efficiency exhibited by Q-learning were clearly outweighed by the bias incurred, making A-learning preferable in terms of mean squared error.

4.4.3 Regret-Regression

Two very similar methods have been proposed to model blip or regret function parameters using *regret-regression*. The first, proposed by Almirall et al. (2010), relies on the observation that, in a two-stage setting, the marginal mean of the counterfactual outcome $Y(a_1,a_2)$ can be expressed as

$$\begin{aligned}
E[Y(a_1,a_2)|H_j,A_j] &= E[Y(-1,-1)] + E\Big[Y(\bar{a}_2) - Y(a_1,-1)|H_2 = h_2\Big] + \\
&\qquad E\Big[Y(a_1,-1) - Y(-1,-1)|H_1 = h_1\Big] + \sum_{j=1}^{2} \varepsilon_j(H_j) \\
&= \beta_0 + \sum_{j=1}^{2} \gamma_j^0(H_j,A_j;\psi_j) + \sum_{j=1}^{2} \varepsilon_j(H_j)
\end{aligned}$$

where $\beta_0 = E[Y(-1,-1)]$ and γ_j^0 are zero blip-to-zero functions, i.e. blip functions that consider the zero treatment regime to be the reference at stage j and assume zero treatment at all subsequent stages. The functions $\varepsilon_j(H_j)$ are nuisance functions which must have mean zero for equality of the above equation to hold. In particular, $\varepsilon_1(H_1) = E[Y(-1,-1)|H_1] - E[Y(-1,-1)]$ and $\varepsilon_2(H_2) = E[Y(a_1,-1)|H_2] - E[Y(a_1,-1)|H_1]$. One modeling possibility is to set the functions equal to a linear function of the residual obtained after subtracting O_j from its estimated conditional mean: $\varepsilon_j(H_j) = \beta_j(O_j - \hat{E}[O_j|H_{j-1},A_{j-1}])$. A linear model implementation of the algorithm can thus be described in brief as following the steps:

1. At each stage, regress O_j on the history H_{j-1} and A_{j-1} and set $Z_j = O_j - \hat{E}[O_j|H_{j-1},A_{j-1}]$.
2. Estimate the parameters of

$$E[Y|H_j,A_j;\beta_j,\psi_j] = \beta_0 + \sum_{j=2}^{K} \beta_j^T Z_j - \sum_{j=1}^{K} \gamma^0(H_j,A_j;\psi_j)$$

   using a standard linear regression of Y on a column of 1s, the nuisance functions Z_j and all covariate-interaction terms $H_{j1}A_j$.

Henderson et al. (2010) propose a very similar method, which they term regret-regression. The algorithm for estimation proceeds as follows:

1. At each stage, regress O_j on H_{j-1},A_{j-1} and set $Z_j = O_j - \hat{E}[O_j|H_{j-1},A_{j-1}]$.
2. Assuming

$$E[Y|H_j,A_j;\beta_j,\psi_j] = \beta_0(O_1) + \sum_{j=2}^{K} \beta_j^T Z_j - \sum_{j=1}^{K} \mu(H_j,A_j;\psi_j)$$

   is a correct specification for the conditional mean of Y, estimate the parameters β and ψ of this function by minimizing

$$\sum_{i=1}^{n} \left(Y - \beta_0(H_1) - \sum_{j=2}^{K} \beta_j^T(H_{j-1})Z_j + \sum_{j=1}^{K} \mu(H_j,A_j;\psi_j) \right)^2 .$$

In simulation, this method appeared to perform better than IMOR in terms of both bias and variability.

The regret-regression methods described above require estimation of the components of the full data-likelihood that involve the time-varying covariates O_j, but not the treatment decisions, A_j. In contrast, G-estimation and IMOR do not require estimating the components of the data relating to state variables. It has been argued that it may be easier to model the treatment mechanism than the covariate mechanism. This is undoubtedly the case in sequentially randomized trials, but may be subject to debate in observational studies. Finally, as noted in Sect. 4.3.1, G-estimation enjoys the property of double-robustness, which is not a feature of the regret-based methods described in this section. However, under correct model-specification, the regression-based estimators appear to enjoy lower variability than G-estimators and it is reasonable to conjecture that the regret-regression estimator will as well. Furthermore, as the above methods are regression-based, the usual linear-regression residual diagnostic techniques may be used to guide the choice of the regret-function. See Sect. 9.2 for further discussion of model-checking in DTR estimation.

4.4.4 Occlusion Therapy for Amblyopia: An Illustration

To demonstrate the use of G-estimation and IMOR, we consider a simplified analysis using data from the Monitored Occlusion Treatment of Amblyopia Study (MOTAS). Amblyopia is the most common visual problem among children in Western societies, resulting from an interruption of development during a susceptible period of childhood. It causes visual impairment and is usually treated by occlusion (eye patching) of the dominant eye. MOTAS was conducted in 87 children aged 3–8 years in the United Kingdom, and was the first to describe the dose-response relationship of occlusion to improvement in visual acuity (Stewart et al. 2002). Briefly, MOTAS followed a three-phase design: (1) children were assessed and monitored to ensure baseline vision was stable, (2) children needing glasses received them and were monitored until vision was stable, and (3) all children were prescribed 6 hours of occlusion per day and followed until visual acuity ceased to improve. All children who entered the third phase of the study, regardless of age, were prescribed 6 hours of occlusion daily. We consider the first 12 weeks of the occlusion phase as a single stage in order to demonstrate G-estimation and IMOR in the simplest context; the purpose of this example is purely illustrative.

Patch use data were obtained from a dose monitor built into the eye patch and visual acuity was measured on the logMAR scale (a scale in which smaller numbers are indicative of better visual acuity). Of the 80 children eligible for the occlusion phase of the trial, eight dropped out before any dose was given and three dropped out after less than 15 min of occlusion. These 11 participants were excluded, leaving 69 subjects for analysis. Thirty-one children missed their week 12 visit. Missing values were imputed by using a child's linear prediction plus a randomly selected residual term (taken from any child). The vision of 15 children ceased to improve with occlusion before 12 weeks. For these children, their last measurement was carried forward and a randomly selected residual from the linear regressions was added.

Age is the state variable, O. Take Y to be a utility defined as the *negative* of week 12 visual acuity, so that high values of Y are desirable. It has been postulated that 200 hours of occlusion are sufficient to achieve improvement in visual acuity of at least 0.2 on the logMAR scale (Stewart et al. 2004). Thus, we consider a child to have been treated if he received at least 200 hours of occlusion in the first 12 weeks; 25 (36.2 %) children were treated under this definition. Treatment allocation probabilities were estimated via logistic regression, so that the probability of being treated is $E(A=1|O) = \text{expit}(\hat{\alpha}_0 + \hat{\alpha}_1 O)$.

4.4.4.1 Analysis Using G-estimation

To implement G-estimation for one stage, we modeled the optimal blip function with a simple linear model,

$$\begin{aligned}\gamma(o,a;\psi) &= E[Y|O=o,A=a;\psi] - E[Y|O=o,A=-1;\psi]\\ &= \frac{1}{2}(a+1)\cdot(\psi_0+\psi_1 o).\end{aligned} \tag{4.7}$$

For $S(O,A) = \frac{1}{2}(A+1)\cdot(1,O)^T$, $E[S(A)|O] = (P(A=1|O), O\cdot P(A=1|O))^T$ when A is binary and so the resulting G-estimation function for Eq. (4.2) is

$$\begin{aligned}U(\psi) &= \mathbb{P}_n\Big\{[Y-\gamma(O,A;\psi)]\,(S(A)-E[S(A)|O])\Big\}\\ &= \mathbb{P}_n\left\{\left[Y-\frac{1}{2}(A+1)\times(\psi_0+\psi_1 O)\right]\times\begin{pmatrix}(A+1)/2-P[A=1|O]\\ O((A+1)/2-P[A=1|O])\end{pmatrix}\right\}.\end{aligned}$$

The G-estimates (95 % CI), which can be found in closed-form, are $\hat{\psi}_0 = 0.847$ (0.337, 1.358) and $\hat{\psi}_1 = -0.014$ (-0.023, -0.005), so that the optimal rule is to treat all amblyopes who are no older than 61.7 months. Bootstrap re-sampling was used to estimate standard errors. The confidence interval of each parameter excludes 0, implying that there is a significant effect of treatment at the 5 % level. Using G-estimating Eq. (4.3) yields the same estimate of the optimal rule.

4.4.4.2 Analysis Using IMOR

Following Murphy (2003), we assume a quadratic regret, $\mu^f(O,A) = \beta_1(A + sign(O-\beta_2))^2/4$, which we will approximate with

$$\breve{\mu}^f(O,A) = \frac{\beta_1}{4}\left[A+2\left(\frac{e^{-30(O-\beta_2)}}{1+e^{-30(O-\beta_2)}}-\frac{1}{2}\right)\right]^2. \tag{4.8}$$

The expit function is scaled by -30 to reflect that treatment is to be recommended *below* a given age threshold, rather than above. Minimizing the LHS of Eq. (4.4) estimates β_1 (95% CI) as 0.000 [0,0.007), while β_2 is undefined since the scale parameter is not significantly different from zero, suggesting no effect of treatment. The confidence interval for β_1 may not be precise since the estimate is on the boundary of the parameter space.

The regret model implies a (discontinuous) blip whose form implies that it is *equally* disadvantageous to receive occlusion when one should not as it is to have occlusion withheld when it is needed. It further implies that the negative impact of inappropriate treatment is the same *regardless of a child's age*.

4.4.4.3 IMOR Using the Model $\mu(O,A)$

The G-estimation result, which suggests that occlusion *is* beneficial but less so at older ages, is in keeping with medical knowledge of neuro-development. Both the models and the methods of estimation varied between the two analyses described above, and so we now investigate further to discern the source of the differing results.

The linear blip of Eq. (4.7) implies a symmetric regret:

$$\begin{aligned}\mu(O,A) &= |\psi_0+\psi_1 O| \times (A - sign(\psi_0+\psi_1 O))^2/4 \\ &= |\beta - O| \times (A + sign(O-\beta))^2/4 \end{aligned} \tag{4.9}$$

when treatment should occur for *low* values of O, which, using G-estimation, is estimated to be

$$\begin{aligned}\mu(O,A;\hat{\psi}) &= |0.847-0.014O| \times (A+sign(O-61.7))^2/4 \\ &= |61.7-O| \times (A+sign(O-61.7))^2/4.\end{aligned}$$

Suppose that the model of the regret from the G-estimation approach, described in (4.9), is correct and take the optimal treatment to be: treat only patients who are no older than 62 months. The threshold β_2 in the SNMM described by $\breve{\mu}^f(O,A)$ corresponds to $-\psi_0/\psi_1 = 62$ from $\mu(O,A)$ in Eq. (4.9). To help visualize this, let $\beta_2 = 62$ and arbitrarily choose $\beta_1 = 0.4$; then the model $\mu^f(O,A)$ is a step function (Fig. 4.2), which assigns equal regret to all treatment regimes other than that which is optimal. If the model of Eq. (4.9) is correct, then $\mu^f(O,A)$ is not capturing its "peakedness" and it is in exactly this case that simulations have shown the IMOR method to perform less well (Murphy 2003).

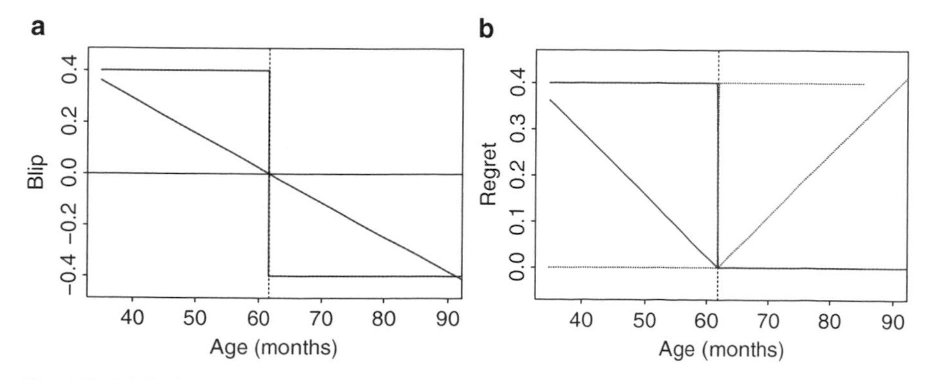

Fig. 4.2 (**a**) Optimal blip and (**b**) regret functions. The *blue lines* are under linear blip parameterization, the *red*, under $\mu^f(O,A)$, and the *dashed line* is the threshold for the optimal rule. In (**b**), the *solid lines* are regrets for $A = 1$, the *dotted lines*, for $A = -1$

Using IMOR to find β using model (4.9), i.e. $|\beta - O| \times (A + sign(O - \beta))^2/4$, gives estimates similar to those found via G-estimation: $\hat{\beta}$ (95 % CI) = 61.3 (58.6,64.1). Thus, when comparable blip and regret models are used, G-estimation and IMOR yielded similar estimates. Restricting the analysis to the children who were followed to 12 weeks resulted in the same decision rule (61 months), and varying the number of hours of occlusion required to define treatment also failed to substantially change the optimal decision rule.

4.4.5 *Simulation of a Two-Stage Occlusion Trial for Treatment of Amblyopia*

Suppose that children aged 36–96 months are treated for amblyopia by eye patching over 12 weeks, with a check-up at 8 weeks. The outcome is a utility function incorporating a child's visual acuity and a measure of psychological stress endured due to wearing an eye patch. Variables are distributed as follows:

Age: $O_1 \sim \text{Uniform}(36, 96)$
Week 8 visual acuity: $O_2 = O_1 + (1 - 0.8O_1)(A_1 + 1)/2 + \varepsilon$
Outcome under optimal treatment: $Y(A_1^{opt}, A_2^{opt}) = |\delta| + O_1/400 - O_2/30$

where $\varepsilon \sim \mathcal{N}(0, 0.05)$, $\delta \sim \mathcal{N}(0, 0.12)$ are independent of each other and of $\bar{A}_2, \bar{O}_2, Y$. Treatments A_j takes value 1 with probability p_j, where $p_1 = \text{expit}(2 - 0.03O_1)$ and $p_2 = \text{expit}(-0.1 + 0.5O_2)$. The optimal blips,

$$\gamma_1(H_1, A_1) = E[Y(A_1, A_2^{opt}) - Y(0, A_2^{opt})|H_1, A_1] = (18 - 0.3O_1)(A_1 + 1)/2,$$

$$\gamma_2(H_2, A_2) = E[Y(A_1, A_2) - Y(A_1, 0)|H_2, A_2] = (4 + 0.5O_2 + A_1)(A_2 + 1)/2$$

and corresponding regrets

$$\mu_1(H_1, A_1) = |18 - 0.3O_1|(A_1 - A_1^{opt})^2/4,$$

$$\mu_2(H_2, A_2) = |4 + 0.5O_2 + A_1|(A_2 - A_2^{opt})^2/4$$

give observed outcome $Y(A_1, A_2) = Y(A_1^{opt}, A_2^{opt}) - \mu_1(H_1, A_1) - \mu_2(H_2, A_2)$ under the assumption of additive local rank preservation.

In 1,000 simulations, both G-estimation and IMOR perform well in terms of bias (Table 4.2). The expected counterfactual model is mis-specified: when the optimal blip is linear, the expected counterfactual, $E[G_{\text{mod},j}(\psi)|H_j, A_{j-1}]$, is disjoint and piece-wise linear (Moodie et al. 2007). In these simulations, neither G-estimation with an incorrect model for $E[G_{\text{mod},j}(\psi)|H_j, A_{j-1}]$ nor IMOR dominates the other in terms of efficiency over all six decision rule parameters.

Table 4.2 Comparison of G-estimation and IMOR for two stages in 1,000 data sets of sample size 500: A hypothetical trial of occlusion therapy for treatment of amblyopia

	G-estimation				*IMOR*	
	Eq. (4.2)		Eq. (4.3)			
ψ	$\hat{\psi}$	SE	$\hat{\psi}$	SE	$\hat{\psi}$	SE
$n = 500$						
$\psi_{10} = 18.0$	17.845	2.554	17.984	0.717	17.996	0.561
$\psi_{11} = -0.3$	−0.298	0.038	−0.300	0.009	−0.300	0.008
$\psi_{20} = 3.0$	3.059	2.122	3.000	0.652	3.023	0.416
$\psi_{21} = 0.5$	0.456	3.001	0.507	0.857	0.475	0.635
$\psi_{22} = 2.0$	1.952	2.750	2.006	0.728	1.986	0.613
$\psi_{23} = 0.0$	0.016	4.630	−0.031	1.017	0.010	0.985
$n = 1{,}000$						
$\psi_{10} = 18.0$	17.914	1.734	17.998	0.470	18.019	0.381
$\psi_{11} = -0.3$	−0.299	0.026	−0.300	0.006	−0.300	0.006
$\psi_{20} = 3.0$	3.031	1.463	2.994	0.447	3.014	0.281
$\psi_{21} = 0.5$	0.469	2.068	0.506	0.582	0.483	0.432
$\psi_{22} = 2.0$	1.968	1.886	2.002	0.508	1.987	0.418
$\psi_{23} = 0.0$	0.028	3.171	−0.008	0.700	0.017	0.674
$n = 2{,}000$						
$\psi_{10} = 18.0$	17.916	1.197	17.997	0.327	18.006	0.269
$\psi_{11} = -0.3$	−0.299	0.018	−0.300	0.004	−0.300	0.004
$\psi_{20} = 3.0$	3.085	1.012	3.018	0.314	3.018	0.193
$\psi_{21} = 0.5$	0.386	1.432	0.473	0.412	0.473	0.297
$\psi_{22} = 2.0$	1.902	1.302	1.976	0.355	1.976	0.288
$\psi_{23} = 0.0$	0.144	2.196	0.030	0.487	0.038	0.463

4.5 Discussion

In this chapter, we have considered semi-parametric approaches to finding the optimal DTR via modeling contrasts of conditional mean outcomes: G-estimation and regret-based methods including an iterative minimization method and regression. We attempted to elucidate the connections between both the different types of models (blips, regrets, and Q-functions) as well as the estimation approaches themselves.

G-estimation can estimate the effects of treatments in longitudinal data and in particular, can estimate optimal DTRs even in the presence of measured confounding variables through the use of treatment models. G-estimation avoids the difficult task of specifying a complete likelihood for the longitudinal distribution of treatment, covariates, and response in each interval. G-estimation is similar, and in some cases identical, to Q-learning. It is very flexible, and allows the analyst to consider a larger set of potential treatment regimes than can typically be considered in marginal structural models considered in Sect. 5.2.

Regret-based methods of estimation are in many cases similar to G-estimation (and in some cases identical), and there is a simple transformation to allows conversion of a regret to a blip function and vice versa. Regret-regression is particularly appealing because, like Q-learning, it can be accomplished almost entirely using standard regression functions in any statistical software.

All of the methods that we have considered in this chapter are suitable for non-randomized data, and several of these can be made doubly-robust to lessen the dependence on model specification and often simultaneously improve precision. All methods rely on the validity of a number of assumptions, some of which are untestable but can be assessed at least informally using model diagnostics (see Sect. 9.2) and substantive knowledge of the health condition under consideration.

Chapter 5
Estimation of Optimal DTRs by Directly Modeling Regimes

In the previous chapters, we have considered methods of estimating the optimal DTRs that typically proceed in two steps: first, they model either the conditional mean outcomes (Q-learning) or *contrasts* between models for the mean outcomes under alternative treatments (G-estimation, A-learning, regret regression) at different stages, and then find the treatments that optimize the estimated mean or contrast models at each stage, ultimately leading to an optimal personalized treatment sequence. As an alternative estimation strategy, one can directly estimate the *value* or marginal mean outcome of each member in a pre-specified class of regimes $\mathscr{D}$, often indexed by some parameter $\psi \in \Psi$, and then pick the regimes that maximize the estimated value, i.e. the estimated optimal regime is given by

$$\hat{d}^{opt} = \arg\max_{d \in \mathscr{D}} \hat{V}^{d} \equiv \arg\max_{\psi \in \Psi} \hat{V}^{d(\psi)},$$

where $\hat{V}^{d}$ (or, $\hat{V}^{d(\psi)}$) is the estimated value function of the regime d (or, $d(\psi)$). Perhaps one of the simplest ways to conceptualize the indexing parameter ψ is to consider treatment rules of the form: "At stage j, change treatment when the *tailoring variable* (suitable summary of the available history H_j) falls below or above a threshold ψ". This class of methods is known as *policy search methods* in the RL literature (Ng and Jordan 2000). A variety of methods from the statistics literature, including *inverse probability weighting* (Robins et al. 2000) and *marginal structural models* (Robins et al. 2000; Hernán et al. 2000; Murphy et al. 2001), fall under this class of methods. The current chapter is devoted to a detailed description of these methods.

B. Chakraborty and E.E.M. Moodie, *Statistical Methods for Dynamic Treatment Regimes*, Statistics for Biology and Health 76, DOI 10.1007/978-1-4614-7428-9_5,

5.1 Estimating the Value of an Arbitrary Regime: Inverse Probability Weighting

The most crucial part of all the procedures mentioned above is the estimation of the value function for an arbitrary regime (or, treatment policy) d. The value of d can be estimated from a sample of n data trajectories of the form $\{O_1, A_1, \ldots, O_K, A_K, O_{K+1}\}$ in several ways. Note that the expectation in the expression of value in (3.6) is taken with respect to the distribution P_d, but the data trajectories are drawn from a distribution P_π, corresponding to the *exploration policy* π; see Chap. 3 for more details. When $d = \pi$, the estimation is relatively straightforward. For example, in a SMART, the investigator may be naturally interested in estimating the values of the regimes "embedded" in the study (these are the exploration policies). To make the discussion concrete, let us consider the hypothetical SMART design (with $K = 2$) in the addiction management context introduced in Chap. 2.

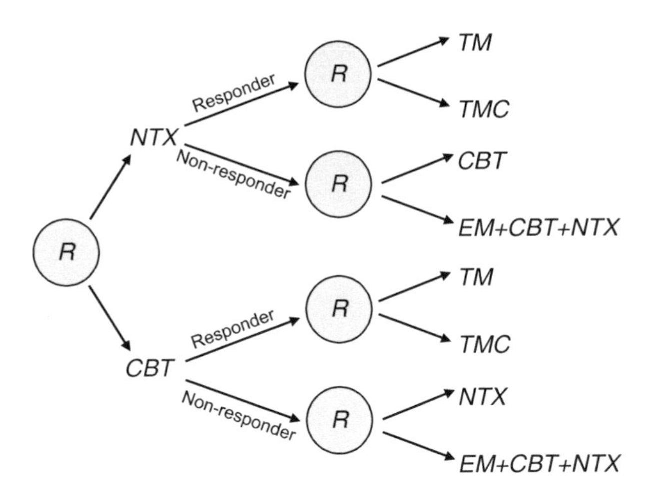

Fig. 5.1 Hypothetical SMART design schematic for the addiction management example (an "R" within a circle denotes randomization at a critical decision point)

There are eight embedded regimes in this study; see Fig. 5.1, which is a reproduction of Fig. 2.2. For example, one embedded regime is, "treat the patient with NTX at stage 1; give TM at stage 2 if the patient is a responder, and give CBT at stage 2 if the patient is a non-responder". Other embedded regimes can be described similarly. Estimating the value of any of these embedded regimes can be done by collecting all the subjects whose realized treatment experiences are consistent with the rules given by the embedded regime of interest, and computing the sample average of the primary outcome. When the regime to be evaluated, d, is not one of the embedded regimes in a study, the estimation is more complicated. Viewed from a causal inference perspective, this is a problem of estimating a *counterfactual expectation*, i.e. the expectation of the potential outcome under a particular regime, d. One can still estimate the desired expectation by using a change of probability measure, under the assumption that P_d is *absolutely continuous* with respect to P_π. The implication of *absolute continuity* is that any trajectory that can result in the implementation of the policy d, must also have a positive probability of occurring under the exploration policy π; this is equivalent to the *feasibility*[1] condition discussed in Chap. 2. Let Y be the primary outcome; in settings with stage-specific outcomes $Y_j(H_j, A_j, O_{j+1})$ as in Chap. 3, one can set $Y = \sum_{j=1}^{K} Y_j(H_j, A_j, O_{j+1})$. Then under the feasibility assumption, one can write the value function as

$$V^d = E_d Y = \int Y dP_d = \int Y \left(\frac{dP_d}{dP_\pi}\right) dP_\pi,$$

where $\frac{dP_d}{dP_\pi}$ is a version of the Radon-Nikodym derivative, and is given by the ratio of the two likelihoods (3.2) and (3.1). This ratio simplifies to

$$\prod_{j=1}^{K} \frac{\mathbb{I}[A_j = d_j(H_j)]}{\pi_j(A_j|H_j)}.$$

Note that the trick of changing the probability measure employs the same basic idea as *importance sampling* in Monte Carlo simulation. Thus, by changing the probability measure as above, the expression for value becomes

$$V^d = \int \Big(\prod_{j=1}^{K} \frac{\mathbb{I}[A_j = d_j(H_j)]}{\pi_j(A_j|H_j)}\Big) Y dP_\pi = \int w_{d,\pi} Y dP_\pi,$$

where

$$w_{d,\pi} = \prod_{j=1}^{K} \frac{\mathbb{I}[A_j = d_j(H_j)]}{\pi_j(A_j|H_j)}$$

is a weight function depending on the entire data trajectory (we deliberately suppressed the dependence on A_j and H_j for notational simplicity). A natural way to estimate V^d is by its empirical version $\hat{V}^d$,

$$\hat{V}^d = \mathbb{P}_n\left[w_{d,\pi} Y\right], \qquad (5.1)$$

where $\mathbb{P}_n$ denotes the empirical average over a sample of size n. Even though the expectation of the weight function is 1, it is preferable to normalize the weights by their sample mean to obtain a more stable estimate. The resulting estimator is known as the *inverse probability of treatment weighted* (IPTW) estimator (Robins

[1] While the term *feasibility* is commonly used in the causal inference literature, *absolute continuity* is an older concept in measure-theoretic probability.

et al. 2000), or more simply the inverse probability weighted or weighting (IPW) estimator, and is given by

$$\hat{V}^d_{IPTW} = \frac{\mathbb{P}_n\left[w_{d,\pi}Y\right]}{\mathbb{P}_n\left[w_{d,\pi}\right]}. \tag{5.2}$$

In the case where the data arise from a SMART, the exploration policy consisting of the randomization probabilities $\pi_j(A_j|H_j)$ is known by design. Hence, by the law of large numbers, the IPTW estimator is consistent. However, the IPTW estimator is highly variable due to the presence of the non-smooth indicator functions inside the weights.

Recently Zhang et al. (2012b) proposed a similar, doubly-robust estimator of the value function for a single-stage treatment regime, using *augmented* inverse probability of treatment weighting. Let a data trajectory be given by (H, A, Y) with the treatment $A \in \{-1, 1\}$, and $H \equiv O$ (since this is a one-stage setting). Let $d(H;\psi)$ denote a regime indexed by ψ, $\mu(A, H; \hat{\beta})$ an estimated model for the mean outcome as a function of baseline covariates H and treatment A, and $\pi(H;\hat{\gamma})$ an estimated propensity score. Then

$$\hat{V}^d_{AIPTW} = \mathbb{P}_n\left\{\frac{\mathscr{C}_\psi Y}{\pi_c(H;\psi,\hat{\gamma})} - \frac{\mathscr{C}_\psi - \pi_c(H;\psi,\hat{\gamma})}{\pi_c(H;\psi,\hat{\gamma})} m(H;\psi,\hat{\beta})\right\}$$

is the doubly-robust, augmented IPTW estimator of the mean outcome (value) under treatment rule $d(H;\psi)$ where

$$\begin{aligned}
\mathscr{C}_\psi &= \mathbb{I}[A = d(H;\psi)], \\
\pi_c(H;\psi,\hat{\gamma}) &= \pi(H;\hat{\gamma})\mathbb{I}[d(H;\psi) = 1] + (1 - \pi(H;\hat{\gamma}))\mathbb{I}[d(H;\psi) = -1], \\
m(H;\psi,\hat{\beta}) &= \mu(1, H;\hat{\beta})\mathbb{I}[d(H;\psi) = 1] + \mu(-1, H;\hat{\beta})\mathbb{I}[d(H;\psi) = -1].
\end{aligned}$$

Thus, for a specific value of ψ (denoting a specific regime), the contribution to the value function estimator for someone treated with $A = 1$ and for whom $d(H;\psi) = 1$ is

$$\left\{\frac{Y}{\pi(H;\hat{\gamma})} - \frac{1 - \pi(H;\hat{\gamma})}{\pi(H;\hat{\gamma})}\mu(1, X;\hat{\beta})\right\}$$

while for someone treated with $A = 1$ and for whom $d(H;\psi) = -1$ it is simply $\mu(-1, X;\hat{\beta})$. Similarly, the contribution to the value function estimator for someone who received $A = -1$ and for whom $d(H;\psi) = -1$ is

$$\left\{\frac{Y}{1 - \pi(H;\hat{\gamma})} - \frac{\pi(H;\hat{\gamma})}{1 - \pi(H;\hat{\gamma})}\mu(-1, X;\hat{\beta})\right\}$$

while for someone with $A = -1$ and $d(H;\psi) = 1$ it is $\mu(1, X;\hat{\beta})$. Thus, each individual contributes a convex combination of their observed outcome, Y, and their modeled outcome, $\mu(d(H;\psi), H;\hat{\beta})$ to the value estimator. In addition to being more robust to model mis-specification, doubly-robust estimators tend to be more efficient than their non-augmented counterparts (Robins 2004).

When the ultimate interest lies in picking a regime that is optimal, one can consider the estimated value as function of ψ, and then select the value of ψ, say ψ^{opt}, that maximizes $V^{\psi}_{AIPTW} \equiv V^{d}_{AIPTW}$. One can view this approach as a single-stage marginal structural modeling where the target of estimation becomes the marginal mean conditional on baseline covariates, i.e. $V^{\psi}_{AIPTW}(O_1)$, instead of the overall marginal mean V^{ψ}_{AIPTW}; see Sect. 3.3 to understand the distinction between the two. See Sect. 5.2 for details on the marginal structural modeling approach. Zhang et al. (2012b) also considered a similar estimator based on a standard IPTW formulation (i.e. without the augmentation term), but found its performance inferior to the optimal regime estimated via the augmented IPTW estimating function.

5.2 Marginal Structural Models and Weighting Methods

Marginal structural models (MSMs) were originally proposed to estimate the effect of static treatment regimes (Robins 1999a; Robins et al. 2000; Hernán et al. 2000), i.e., treatment regimens that are not tailored to evolving patient characteristics; however they are increasingly being applied to the problem of estimating optimal DTRs. These models are said to be *marginal* because they pertain to population-average effects (marginalizing over all time-varying covariates and/or intermediate outcomes, and possibly also over some or all baseline covariates), and *structural* because they describe causal (not associational) effects. The approach requires an initial investment in data manipulation, but is appealing because of the ease with which the models may be estimated using standard software. Furthermore, the approach provides a mechanism for evaluating the effect of small changes in the parameter indexing the regime (e.g. a decision rule threshold) on the average potential outcome in the population.

Although in discussing the estimation of marginal structural models, the focus in this text is on inverse probability weighting, estimation can also be performed by other means such as targeted maximum likelihood (Van der Laan and Rubin 2006; Neugebauer et al. 2010). In brief, targeted maximum likelihood estimation can estimate treatment effects for longitudinal data in the presence of time-dependent confounders; the method is doubly-robust and can be made to optimize asymptotic estimating efficiency, but may not be implemented as easily as IPTW in complex scenarios.

5.2.1 MSMs for Static Treatment Regimes

A marginal structural model is a model for the marginal expectation of a counterfactual outcome under a specified static treatment regime and, in great generality, we can express an *estimating function* for a MSM by

$$U^{IPW}(Y(\overline{a}), H_K|w, \beta) = w(\overline{A}|H_K)\frac{\partial}{\partial\beta}V^{\overline{a}}(O_1;\beta)[Y - V^{\overline{a}}(O_1;\beta)]$$

where O_1 denotes baseline covariates; any subset of O_1 may be used in modeling, including the empty set. Most often, $V^{\overline{a}}(O_1;\beta)$ is a specified as a linear combination of components of $\overline{a}$ and O_1, but recently more flexible, spline-based models have been considered (Xiao et al. 2012).

When the randomization probabilities in a study are unknown (e.g. a typical observational study), a nuisance model for the probability of receiving treatment must be fit first, to be able to estimate the parameters of an MSM. The treatment model is then used to weight individuals by the inverse probability of receiving the observed treatment (given history) in an unadjusted model for the outcome as a function of treatment. Stabilization of the inverse probability of treatment weights, as in equation (5.2), is commonly used to reduce the variability of MSM estimators that can arise when some combinations of covariates are rare (Sturmer et al. 2005). If the treatment model is correctly specified with respect to confounding variables, the estimator of the marginal effect of treatment has a causal interpretation.

As with all models for observational data, MSMs require strong assumptions to allow a casual interpretation of model parameters (Robins et al. 2000). As noted in Chap. 2, we require the assumptions of *no unmeasured confounding* (sequential randomization), *time ordering* (treatment precedes outcome) and *consistency*. In addition, we require *positivity*: that all combinations of covariates are possible (Robins et al. 2000; Mortimer et al. 2005).

The earliest use of MSMs for DTR estimation was undertaken to compare a DTR which assigned one of three levels of an intervention with a static regime corresponding to no intervention (Murphy et al. 2001). This approach used standard (static regime) MSM methodology to estimate the mean outcome under a small number of candidate treatment regimes. *History-adjusted* MSMs were next proposed as a means of estimating "statically optimal" DTRs; this approach requires assuming a different MSM at each stage to permit investigation of interactions between treatments and time-varying tailoring variables. Using notation from Sect. 3.3, this is equivalent to modeling $V^{\overline{a}}(H_j)$ for $1 \leq j \leq K$. A potential limitation of this approach is that it is possible to propose models at different stages which are not compatible. MSMs were further developed to allow estimation of the treatment tailoring threshold, allowing assessment of a much wider range of candidate treatment rules (Hernán et al. 2006; Petersen et al. 2007; Van der Laan and Petersen 2007a; Robins et al. 2008; Orellana et al. 2010a,b; Cotton and Heagerty 2011).

5.2.2 MSMs for Dynamic Treatment Regimes

Comparing multiple dynamic treatment regimes in a marginal structural modeling framework requires first the realization that an *individual study participant*'s observed treatment history may be compatible with several treatment regimes, at least for some part of the observation period. From a practical perspective, this implies an augmentation of the original data set to create multiple copies of the same individual for each regime with which their observed history is consistent; we follow Shortreed and Moodie (2012) in calling these copies *replicates*. For example, if an individual's data are consistent with regime $\bar{d}_K$ through stage j, we say that the replicate follows that regime through stage j; at the point where the individual's observed history is no longer compatible with regime $\bar{d}_K$, the replicate corresponding to that individual and threshold ψ is artificially censored. A weighted analysis of this augmented data set with artificial censoring mimics an analysis of a trial in which individuals are randomized to follow one of the treatment regimes of interest, under the assumptions of Sect. 2.1.3 as well as the assumptions of correct specification of the marginal response model.

MSMs for a Single-stage Treatment Rule

Zhao et al. (2012) and Zhang et al. (2012b) proposed closely related approaches that straddle the static and dynamic regime settings, in that they seek to estimate a personalized treatment rule, but do so in a single-stage setting only so that the regime is not truly dynamic, or changing, over time. The approach of Zhang et al. (2012b) has already been discussed in Sect. 5.1; we will discuss the approach of Zhao et al. (2012) in Sect. 5.3 while considering classification-based approach to estimating the value function.

MSMs for Multi-stage DTRs

As in the case of estimating the optimal treatment rule for a single stage of treatment, estimation of the optimal DTR for multi-stage treatments requires finding the regime d that maximizes the population average outcome $V^d(O_1) = E_d[Y|O_1] = E[Y(d)|O_1]$, or alternatively $V^d = E[Y(d)]$. Then

$$\begin{aligned} U^{IPW}(Y(\bar{d}), H_K|w, \beta) &= w(\bar{A}|H_K)\frac{\partial}{\partial \beta}V^{\bar{d}}(O_1;\beta)[Y - V^{\bar{d}}(O_1;\beta)] \\ &= w(\bar{A}|H_K)\frac{\partial}{\partial \beta}V^{\bar{a}}(O_1,\psi;\beta)[Y - V^{\bar{a}}(O_1,\psi;\beta)] \end{aligned}$$

is the estimating function for the marginal structural model, where $w = w(A|H_K)$ is a weight for a replicate in the augmented data set, and the threshold ψ is treated as a covariate in the outcome model, which is parameterized by β. The weight w is constructed by taking the product of the probability of receiving the assigned treatment regime and the probability of continued observation, i.e. of not being lost to follow-up (not censored) or artificially censored, of a replicate in the augmented data set under the assigned treatment regime. It is typically the case in MSM estimation of DTRs that, given a replicate's current covariates and a regime threshold ψ, the probability of continued observation at any stage j is equivalent to the time-dependent probability of being observed and treated, much as in the analysis of HIV treatment initiation by Cain et al. (2010). That is, censoring is a deterministic function of the history of treatment and the history of covariates in addition to the threshold ψ. Thus, for DTR analyses, it is usually the case that only censorship weights are required, unlike in the static-regime MSMs where both treatment and censoring models are needed to construct the weights.

The weights are often unknown; even when such probabilities are known, the probabilities may be estimated to improve efficiency of the estimators of ψ of the marginal model (Van der Laan and Robins 2003). This counter-intuitive phenomenon, examined in detail by Henmi and Eguchi (2004), can occur if the two components (that for the parameters of interest and that for the nuisance parameters) of the estimating functions are orthogonal; see Sect. 8.1.1 for details. The variance reduction can occur in fully parametric settings, but is more often observed in semi-parametric settings; in the context of semi-parametric estimation, we can gain some insight into the efficiency gain by realizing that estimating more components of the full likelihood, when done using correctly specified models, is in some senses "closer" to a fully parametric likelihood based approach and is therefore more efficient than a semi-parametric modeling approach. Provided the weights are estimated using consistent estimators of the treatment and censoring models which adequately eliminate confounding the optimal threshold ψ can be identified. This is accomplished by solving

$$\sum_{i=1}^{n^*} U^{IPW}(Y(\bar{d}), H_K | w, \beta) = 0 \tag{5.3}$$

where the subscript i is used to refer to an individual-regime pair in the augmented data set, that is a person and a value of the parameter ψ, and n^* is the total number of individual-regime pairs.

As in MSMs for static treatment regimes, stabilization of weights is preferable to the use of unstabilized weights (Robins et al. 2000), especially when weight variability is high: by reducing the variability of the weights, the variability of the entire estimation procedure is often controlled. Although better efficiency is typically observed with stabilized weights, it is not guaranteed. Furthermore, unlike in the context of static treatment regimes, the numerator weight used for stabilization in the dynamic treatment regimes context must condition only on baseline covariates but not on treatment received in previous stages (Cain et al. 2010). Additionally, truncation of the weights can decrease the chance that a small number of replicates will have undue influence on the results of the analysis. The weights for censoring are estimated using

$$\frac{P(C_{ij} = 0 | O_{1,i}, C_{i,j-1} = 0, \psi)}{P(C_{ij} = 0 | O_{1,i}, O_{ij}, C_{i,j-1} = 0, \psi)},$$

where $C_{ij} = 1$ denotes that a replicate was censored at stage j. Note that $C_j = 0$ implies $C_1 = C_2 = \ldots = C_{j-1} = 0$. These models are typically fit via logistic regression. Note that it is the models for the *denominators* of the weights that must contain all time-varying confounders for consistent estimation of the parameters of the MSM

(Robins 1999b). Furthermore, unlike in the stabilization of weights for marginal structural model estimation of static treatment regimes, the probabilities in the numerators cannot condition on treatment history (Cain et al. 2010).

We provide below an outline of the steps required to perform MSM estimation of a dynamic treatment regime of the form "change treatment when the tailoring variable O falls below ψ" for $\psi \in \Psi$. We use the term *original data* to refer to the data available in the study in question, which is in contrast to the *augmented data* which is obtained by replicating individuals from the original data for each regime (indexed by the threshold ψ) with which their data are compatible. The estimation procedure is as follows:

1. Create an augmented data set by replicating individuals enrolled in the original study data; recall that the term *replicate* is used to refer to a row in this augmented data set, i.e. a person-threshold pair.
2. Censor replicates in the augmented data (setting $C_{ij} = 1$) at the first stage j in which their data are no longer consistent with the ψ-regime in question. This is sometimes referred to as *artificial censoring*.
3. Estimate censoring models to account for the fact that artificial censoring may be (and typically is) informative. This ensures parameter estimates are not biased by any covariates that may be predictive of both censoring and the outcome. Using these models, construct stabilized censorship weights, taking the stage-specific probability of being observed for each replicate at stage j to be:

$$w_i(j) = \frac{P(C_{ij} = 0|O_{1,i}, C_{i,j-1} = 0, \psi)}{P(C_{ij} = 0|O_{1,i}, O_{ij}, C_{i,j-1} = 0, \psi)}.$$

   Then construct the final weight for each replicate i by taking the product over all observed stages, $w_i = \prod_j w_i(j)$.
4. Perform a weighted linear regression with weights w_i to obtain the coefficient estimates of the model $E[Y(d)|O_1] = V^{\bar{a}}(O_1, \psi; \beta)$. Typically, the model posited for $V^{\bar{a}}(O_1, \psi; \beta)$ will not be monotonic, but rather will allow for a flexion point, thus allowing the value to be maximized at some value ψ other than the boundaries of Ψ.

Cotton and Heagerty (2011) have proposed an approach that is closely related to the above algorithm, but rather than creating a replicate for each person-threshold pair, they propose generating m data sets in which patients are randomly assigned to one of the treatment regimes with which their data are compatible. Each of the m data sets is then analyzed as a single, complete data set in which regime membership is treated as known and unique. To date, no studies have been conducted to determine the relative performance of the two data-augmentation approaches to DTR MSM estimation.

5.2.3 *Simulation of a DTR MSM Analysis to Determine the Optimal Treatment Threshold*

To demonstrate the principle of estimating DTRs using MSMs, we provide a simulated example based on the work by Moodie (2009b). The general data-generating model of Bembom and Van der Laan (2007) is used, though somewhat simplified by restricting consideration to a two-treatment setting. The simulation considered data O_1, A_1, O_2, A_2, O_3 where O_j $(j = 1,2,3)$ is a health indicator (e.g. CD4 cell counts) and A_j $(j = 1,2)$ is an indicator of which of two treatments (coded -1 and 1) was received at stage j. The outcome was $Y = O_3 - O_1$, and the variable used for treatment switching was $S = O_2 - O_1$. Patients are assumed to have (unmeasured) susceptibility, U_0, to one treatment option with probability 0.7. Susceptibility, U_1, to the second treatment option occurs with probability 0.4 in those individuals susceptible to the first option and with probability 0.6 in those individuals not susceptible to the first option. See Fig. 5.2.

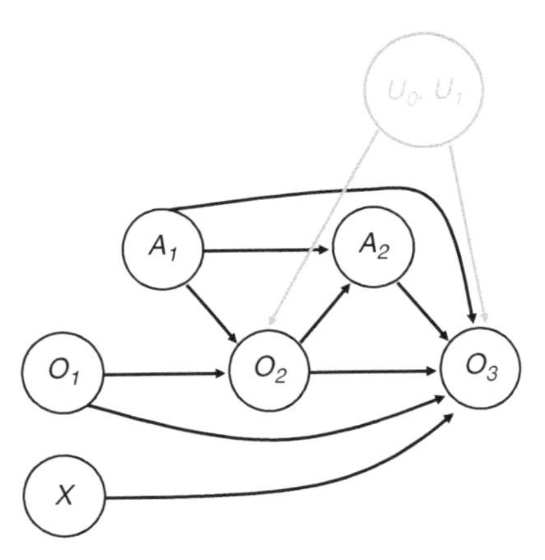

Fig. 5.2 Data-generating structure for the DTR MSM simulation

Following Bembom and Van der Laan (2007), O_1 was generated from a uniform (200, 800) distribution and O_j, $j = 2,3$, were generated from a normal distribution with mean π_j, variance 10^2 where

$$\pi_j = O_{j-1} - 40 + 50U_0\mathbb{I}[A_{j-1} = -1] + 60U_1\mathbb{I}[A_{j-1} = 1] + 1.2j\mathbb{I}[j = 3]X,$$

where X is a measured risk factor that is uniformly distributed on the range $(-6, 3)$. Treatment in the first stage, A_1, was randomly allocated with equal probability given to each option. In the second stage, treatment was again randomly allocated to all individuals for whom $S \geq -50$; all individuals with $S < -50$ switched treatments.

Denote the mean response under treatment rule "treat with $A_1 = a_1$ then switch to $A_2 = -a_1$ if $S < \psi$" by $V^{(a_1,\psi)}$. The true values of $V^{(a_1,\psi)}$ and of the optimal threshold were determined by Monte Carlo simulation. Bembom and Van der Laan (2007) were followed in assuming a simplifying, quadratic form for the relationship between the switching threshold, ψ, and the expected response. Figure 5.3 depicts

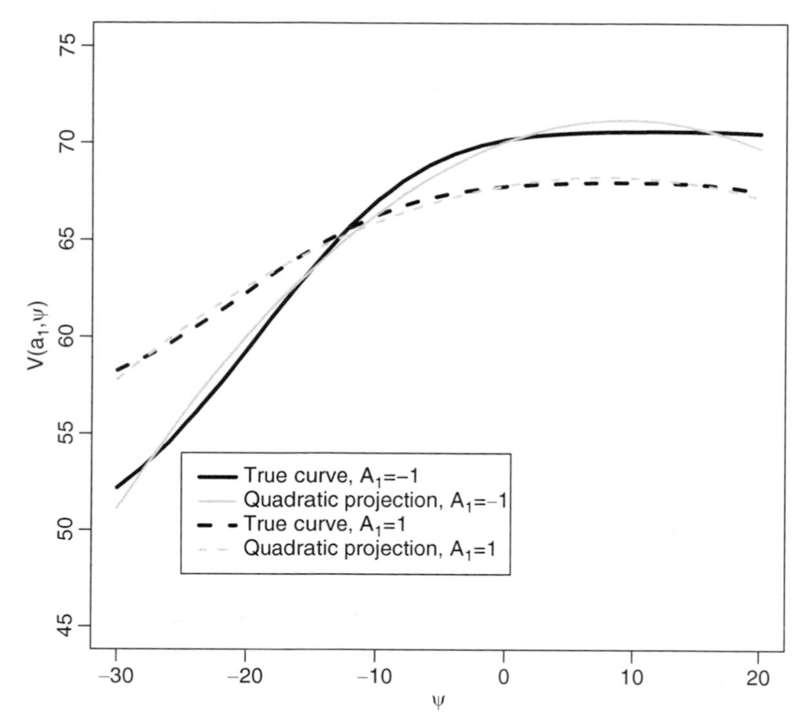

Fig. 5.3 The dependence of $V^{(a_1,\psi)}$ on the threshold ψ: truth (*thick black lines*) and projections onto a quadratic function (*thinner grey lines*)

the true dependence of the mean responses $V^{(-1,\psi)}$ and $V^{(1,\psi)}$ on the treatment-switching threshold ψ, and the projection of these functions onto quadratic models over the range of potential thresholds $(-30,\ldots,20)$. The true optimal rule is given by initial treatment $A_1 = -1$ followed by a switch to $A_2 = 1$ if the health indicator is not increased by at least 12; if the initial treatment is $A_1 = 1$, the optimal decision is to switch to treatment $A_2 = 1$ if the health indicator is not increased by at least 10. The projection of $V^{(a_1,\psi)}$ onto quadratic models, however, yields slightly less aggressive treatment rules: if initial treating is $A_1 = -1$, switch to $A_2 = 1$ if the health indicator is not increased by at least 8 while for initial treatment $A_1 = 1$, switch to $A_2 = -1$ if the indicator is not increased by at least 10.

Fifty-two candidate dynamic treatment regimes are evaluated, indexed by initial treatment and the switching threshold $\psi \in \{-30,-28,\ldots,18,20\}$, considering the following mean models:

$$\begin{aligned} E[Y|A_1,A_2,\psi;\gamma] &= \mathbb{I}[A_1=-1,A_2=1](\gamma_{01,0}+\gamma_{01,1}\psi+\gamma_{01,2}\psi^2)+\\ &\quad \mathbb{I}[A_1=1,A_2=-1](\gamma_{10,0}+\gamma_{10,1}\psi+\gamma_{10,2}\psi^2)\\ E[Y|A_1,A_2,\psi,X;\beta] &= \mathbb{I}[A_1=-1,A_2=1](\beta_{01,0}+\beta_{01,1}\psi+\beta_{01,2}\psi^2)+\\ &\quad \mathbb{I}[A_1=1,A_2=-1](\beta_{10,0}+\beta_{10,1}\psi+\beta_{10,2}\psi^2)+\beta_3 X, \end{aligned}$$

which we refer to as Model 1 and Model 2, respectively.

Results are presented in Table 5.1. Including the predictive variable in the response model leads to reduced mean squared error for the estimators of the parameters of the quadratic projection of the response onto the decision rule threshold. In terms of the decision rule itself, the median estimated optimal threshold over the 5,000 simulated data sets coincides for Models 1 and 2 and indeed the median values equal the values of the threshold that maximize the quadratic projection of the true dependence of the mean response onto ψ. However, the interval formed by taking the 2.5-th and 97.5-th percentiles in the distribution of thresholds is narrower for Model 2 than Model 1. For example, the interval formed over the simulated data sets for the optimal threshold for the regime $A_1 = -1, A_2 = 1, \psi$ is (6, 10) if X is included in the response model, and (4, 14) otherwise.

Table 5.1 Threshold rules for a continuous response estimated via MSMs. Bias, Monte Carlo standard error (SE), and root mean squared error (rMSE) of parameters estimating the dependence of the response, $V^{(a_1,\psi)}$, on the decision threshold ψ in a quadratic model. Model 1 omits the risk factor X from the response model; Model 2 does not. Summaries are based on 5,000 simulated data sets, for sample sizes $n = 100, 250, 500, 1{,}000$

		Model 1			*Model 2*		
		Bias (%)	SE[†]	rMSE[†]	Bias (%)	SE[†]	rMSE[†]
$A_1 = 0, A_2 = 1$							
$n = 100$	ψ	13.29	8.64	8.78	13.23	5.91	6.11
	ψ^2	9.16	0.42	0.43	9.42	0.31	0.32
$n = 250$	ψ	12.91	5.43	5.64	12.72	3.71	4.00
	ψ^2	8.85	0.26	0.27	8.56	0.20	0.21
$n = 500$	ψ	13.29	3.75	4.05	13.50	2.57	3.01
	ψ^2	8.67	0.18	0.19	8.64	0.14	0.15
$n = 1{,}000$	ψ	12.59	2.67	3.04	12.48	1.81	2.32
	ψ^2	8.38	0.13	0.14	8.24	0.10	0.11
$A_1 = 1, A_2 = 0$							
$n = 100$	ψ	6.64	12.44	12.54	7.11	9.26	9.42
	ψ^2	0.38	0.56	0.56	0.59	0.41	0.41
$n = 250$	ψ	6.69	7.72	7.89	6.54	5.77	5.98
	ψ^2	0.94	0.35	0.35	1.01	0.25	0.25
$n = 500$	ψ	7.02	5.41	5.67	6.75	4.06	4.38
	ψ^2	0.51	0.24	0.24	0.77	0.18	0.18
$n = 1{,}000$	ψ	7.09	3.86	4.23	6.99	2.93	3.39
	ψ^2	0.33	0.17	0.17	0.47	0.13	0.13

[†]Multiplied by 10^2

5.2.4 Treatment for Schizophrenia: An Illustration

The Clinical Antipsychotic Trials of Intervention and Effectiveness (CATIE) study was an 18-month multi-stage randomized trial (SMART) of 1,460 patients (Swartz et al. 2003; Stroup et al. 2003; Lieberman et al. 2005; McEvoy et al. 2006; Stroup et al. 2006). One of the primary scientific questions considered by the CATIE study was a comparison of the effectiveness of atypical antipsychotic drugs to a mid-potency typical (first generation) antipsychotic (Stroup et al. 2003). At entry into CATIE, patients were randomized to either the typical antipsychotic or to one of four possible atypical medications, three of which will be considered as a group in this analysis.[2]

Here, an analysis undertaken by Shortreed and Moodie (2012) will be presented. The goal of the analysis was to identify the optimal treatment regime so as to minimize schizophrenic symptoms while reducing exposure to the typical antipsychotic, which bears the risk of a debilitating and irreversible side effect. Two regimes were compared: the first is *always atypical* (*AA*), and the second is *typical and atypical* ($TA(\psi)$). The *AA* regime is a static regime, which calls for treatment with any one of the atypical antipsychotic drugs under study for 12 months, with switches between the three medications permitted as part of the regime should the patient and physician find the current medication ineffective or its side effects intolerable. $TA(\psi)$ is a dynamic regime, indexed by threshold ψ, in which any patients whose Positive and Negative Syndrome Scale (PANSS) score is at or above ψ at study entry will receive the typical (first generation) antipsychotic, while those with PANSS scores below ψ will receive an atypical antipsychotic medication. As part of this regime, during the follow-up period, those patients who begin on the typical antipsychotic will be switched to an atypical antipsychotic when symptom severity, as measured by the PANSS score, decreases beyond the threshold ψ. Thus, this regime assigns the typical antipsychotic to patients with high symptom severity in order to reduce symptoms as measured by the PANSS score; once the symptoms are under control, i.e. under the specified threshold, the patient's treatment is then switched to an atypical medication in order to reduce the patient's long term risk of side effects. As in the *AA* regime, once a patient initiates treatment with an atypical antipsychotic, changes between different atypical antipsychotic drugs are permitted under the $TA(\psi)$ regime.

We now apply the algorithm outlined in Sect. 5.2.2 to the CATIE context. The set of thresholds considered for initiating an atypical antipsychotic at baseline or switching away from the typical antipsychotic and onto an atypical antipsychotic consists of $\Psi = \{30, 35, 40, 45, 50, 55, 60, 65, 70\}$, with $\psi = 30$ representing the regime always treat with the typical antipsychotic as no PANSS scores in the sample lie below 30. The estimation procedure for a complete data set proceeds as follows:

1. Create the augmented data set, replicating individuals in the CATIE study. Replicates can correspond to the regime *AA* as well as each of the dynamic regimes under consideration indexed by threshold ψ, $TA(\psi)$. Each CATIE participant is replicated according to the number of regimes, as listed below (i)–(iii), that they follow for any length of time over the 12 months under consideration in this analysis.

   (a) *AA*: treat with an atypical antipsychotic, regardless of PANSS score;
   (b) $TA(30)$: always treat with the typical antipsychotic;

[2] The fourth was not FDA-approved at the time CATIE began enrollment; consequently more than a third of the study participants were not eligible to receive it. We therefore excluded all participants assigned to this drug in our analysis.

(c) $TA(\psi)$, $\psi \in (\Psi \backslash 30)$: treat with the typical antipsychotic at baseline if PANSS score is ψ or higher, then switch to an atypical antipsychotic when PANSS scores falls below ψ; if the PANSS score is below ψ at baseline, treat with an atypical antipsychotic for 12 months.
Note that if a replicate's baseline PANSS score is less than the threshold ψ^* and the individual was assigned the typical antipsychotic at enrollment in the CATIE trial this replicate is not deemed consistent with the regime $TA(\psi^*)$. Any replicate with a baseline PANSS score below the threshold ψ^* is considered to follow the regime $TA(\psi^*)$ only if their initial assigned treatment in the CATIE study was an atypical medication.

2. Censor CATIE replicates in the augmented data set at the month that any of the three following events occur:

(a) An individual, and thus all corresponding replicates, is randomized to a drug not considered in the current analysis.
(b) An individual, and thus all corresponding replicates, progresses to the unrandomized, unblinded stage of the trial prior to month 12.
(c) A replicate, for which the corresponding individual is initially assigned the typical antipsychotic, is censored for no longer following their assigned dynamic treatment regime. That is, given a PANSS threshold ψ, replicates may stop following the regime for one of two reasons:
  (i) Before choosing to switch off the typical antipsychotic, a replicate's PANSS score falls below the threshold ψ of their assigned regime.
  (ii) At the visit that treatment is switched from the typical antipsychotic, the PANSS score is equal to or greater than ψ.

Note that censoring individuals for reasons (a) and (b) could occur in any analysis of the CATIE data depending, of course, on the scientific question of interest; we refer to this as off-study censoring. Censoring for reason (c) is specific to the data augmented dynamic treatment regimes analysis, and we refer to this type as simply artificial censoring.

3. Estimate censoring models to ensure parameter estimates are not biased by any covariates that may be predictive of both censoring and 12-month outcome. Estimate stabilized censorship weights using the baseline variables listed below and a spline on month of observation with knots at months $1, 2, \ldots, 11$ to ensure continuity at the knots. Specifically, the baseline variables were:

- years on prescription antipsychotic medication;
- a binary indicator of hospitalization in the 3 months prior to CATIE entry;
- factors of the categorical variables site type, sex, race, marital status, education, employment;
- PANSS score;
- body-mass index;
- alcohol and drug use;
- Calgary depression score;
- presence and severity of movement disorders;

- quality of life;
- physical and mental functioning;
- and the threshold, ψ.

All baseline covariates are included in the numerator of the stabilized weights. In addition to the baseline variables, the model for the denominator of the weights includes baseline treatment, current (time-varying) values of body mass index, alcohol and drug use, PANSS score, Calgary depression score, presence and severity of movement disorders, quality of life, physical and mental functioning, medication adherence, date of observation, and previous month's treatment assignment. The baseline covariates are also included as linear terms in the final response model which was estimated using the weighted, augmented data set. Censorship models are estimated at each month, as individuals may switch treatment at any month in the CATIE study. Since not all variables were collected at every month, we use the last scheduled value for those covariates that were not collected at a particular monthly visit. Following convention, all weights were truncated at 10 to avoid excess variability (Cain et al. 2010; Van der Laan and Petersen 2007a).

4. Perform a weighted linear regression with the weights constructed as in the previous step to obtain the coefficient estimates of the model

$$
\begin{aligned}
E[Y(d)|O_1] &= V^{\bar{a}}(O_1, \psi; \beta) \\
&= \beta_1 \mathbb{I}[a = AA] + \mathbb{I}[a = TA(\psi)](\beta_2 + \beta_3\psi + \beta_4\psi^2) + \sum_{k=1}^{40} \beta_{4+k} O_{1,k}
\end{aligned}
$$

where $\{O_{1,k}\}$ is the collection of baseline variables used in the numerator of the stabilized censorship weights.

Missing data are handled by multiple imputation (Shortreed et al. 2010), while confidence intervals are constructed using a bootstrap procedure (Shao and Sitter 1996). Results are summarized in Fig. 5.4, which shows the predicted mean 12-month PANSS scores for an individual who is Caucasian and unmarried, who graduated from college, had not been hospitalized in the 3 months prior to CATIE, was not employed at entry into the CATIE study, had spent 13 years on prescription anti-psychotic medications prior to CATIE, was recruited from a university clinic, had an average baseline PANSS score (75.58), was classified as moderately ill by the clinician global impression of illness severity index, had no drug or alcohol use as judged by the clinician, had no movement disorder symptoms at baseline as measured by any of the three movement disorder scales, and had average baseline values of body-mass index (29.8), Calgary Depression score (4.7), quality of life score (2.8), and mental and physical function as measured by the SF-12. The coefficient estimates (95 % CI) are $\hat{\beta}_1$: 62.9 (50.9, 74.7); $\hat{\beta}_2$: 60.8 (58.2, 73.0); $\hat{\beta}_3$: $7.7 \times 10^{-1}(3.3 \times 10^{-1}, 1.02)$; $\hat{\beta}_4 : -6.0 \times 10^{-3}(-8.6, -2.0) \times 10^{-3}$. These results suggest that the treatment regimes "always treat with a typical antipsychotic" and "always treat with an atypical antipsychotic" are equivalent treatment strategies in order to reduce 12-month symptoms, as there was no significant difference between the predicted mean of these two regimes. As the threshold used for switching from the typical to an atypical antipsychotic is increased, 12-month PANSS score increases. The statistically significant threshold, ψ, indicates that there is merit to tailoring within the $TA(\psi)$ regime, and suggests that for most smaller values of ψ, reduced PANSS scores are observed at 12 months if initial therapy with the typical antipsychotic is continued rather than changing therapy depending on ψ.

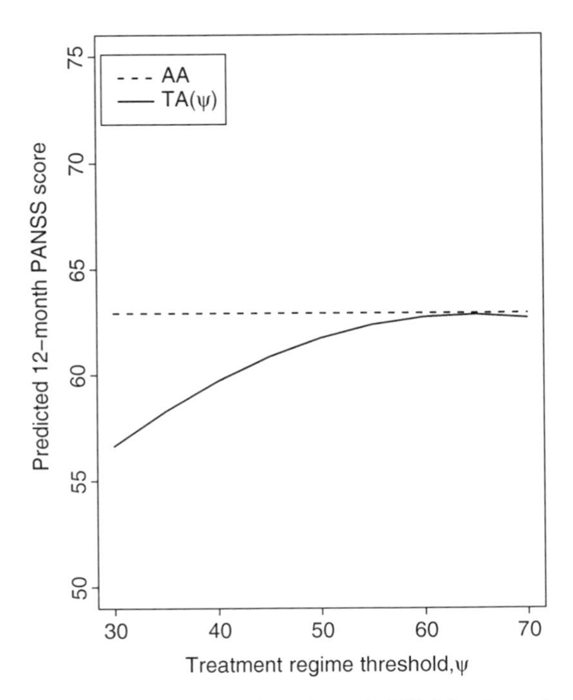

Fig. 5.4 Predicted 12-month PANSS scores from dynamic MSM for the regimes AA and $TA(\psi)$. The horizontal axis indicates the threshold values for the $TA(\psi)$ regime

5.3 A Classification Approach to Estimating DTRs

A change in perspective occurred with the use of marginal structural models to estimate dynamic treatment regimes, as focus shifted to parameterize and estimate the treatment rule directly, rather than to estimate a function of the mean or a contrast between means and then derive the implied treatment rules. This idea was taken a step further by Zhang et al. (2012a) and Zhao et al. (2012), who recast the estimation of the optimal decision rule as a classification problem for a single stage setting.

5.3.1 Contrast-Weighted Classification

It is first critical to note that the expected counterfactual outcome (i.e. value) under a treatment regime d can be expressed as a function of that regime and the contrast function $C(H) = \mu(H,1) - \mu(H,-1)$ where $\mu(H,A)$ is a model for the mean outcome as a function of the treatment A (coded as $-1/1$) and the covariate H:

$$V^d = E[Y(d)] = E\Big[\mathbb{I}[d(H) = 1]C(H)\Big] + E[\mu(H,-1)]$$

for $d(H) = 2 \cdot \mathbb{I}[\mu(H,1) > \mu(H,-1)] - 1$. Thus, if an estimate of the contrast function $C(H)$, say $\hat{C}(H)$, were available, the optimal regime could be found by taking:

$$d^{opt}(H) = \arg\max_d \mathbb{P}_n\left[d(H)\hat{C}(H)\right].$$

We briefly note that in a single stage case, an estimate of the contrast could be found by regression (Q-learning), where parameters in the mean outcome model $\mu(H,A;\beta)$ are estimated to give $\hat{C}_{reg}(H) = \mu(H,1;\hat{\beta}) - \mu(H,-1;\hat{\beta})$; or by G-estimation, where the contrast itself is modeled, yielding $\hat{C}_G(H)$; or indeed in any number of ways including the augmented IPW approach of Zhang et al. (2012b). Using either of the first two of these approaches, an optimal regime could be found by recommending treatment whenever the estimated contrast exceeds 0. The disadvantage to this approach is that there is strong reliance on correct specification of the model for the contrast (or the mean outcome); as we observed in Sect. 3.5, incorrect specification of the model can lead to considerable bias and very poor coverage.

The classification approach, then, aims to separate the estimation of the optimal regime from the modeling of the contrast to reduce the dependence of the optimal regime estimator on the specification of the contrast. Zhang et al. (2012a) and Rubin and van der Laan (2012) have independently shown that

$$\begin{aligned} d^{opt} &= \arg\max_d E\Big[\mathbb{I}[d(H) = 1]C(H)\Big] \\ &= \arg\min_d E\left[W(Z - d(H))^2\right] \end{aligned}$$

where $W = |C(H)|$ and $Z = sign(C(H))$. That is, they show that the optimal treatment decision is the one that minimizes the distance between the rule, $d(H)$, and the rule implied by the contrast, $Z = sign(C(H))$, where that distance is weighted by the relative importance of treating that individual, $W = |C(H)|$. That is, the goal is to minimize the error for the response Z using covariates H in the classification rule d. This can be accomplished using a host of different non-parametric classification methods (e.g. trees) and does not require a parametric form for the treatment regime. The authors further note that the augmented IPW estimator introduced in Sect. 5.1 is a special case of this type of classification-based estimator. In simulation, Zhang et al. (2012a) showed that the classification-based estimator of the optimal DTR using the augmented IPW estimate of the contrast performed very well, even when the true form of the decision rule was not characterized by a tree. However, the simulation results also demonstrated that the classification approach that took the estimated contrast from a regression or via non-augmented IPW often exhibited the worst performance. It is perhaps not surprising that the quality of the estimated contrast can seriously affect the classification-based estimator, as the estimated contrast is used to define the response, or target classification: $Z = sign(C(H))$.

5.3.2 *Outcome Weighted Learning*

Zhao et al. (2012) developed a method based on the IPTW approach to identifying the optimal regime and termed it *outcome weighted learning* (OWL), in recognition of the machine learning flavor present in the approach. Clearly the expected outcome (value) under a treatment rule d is given by

$$V^d_{IPTW} = E\left[\frac{\mathbb{I}[A = d(H)]}{A\pi(H) + (1-A)/2}Y\right]$$

where the treatment A is coded as $-1/1$ with $\pi(H) = P(A = 1|H)$. Note that the denominator reduces to the probability of being treated amongst those treated ($A = 1$), i.e. $\pi(H)$, and the probability of not being treated amongst those who were not ($A = -1$), i.e., $1 - \pi(H)$. Thus the optimal rule is given by

$$d^{opt}(H) = \underset{d}{\text{argmax}}\ V^d_{IPTW}.$$

Equivalently, this can be expressed as

$$\begin{aligned} d^{opt}(H) &= \underset{d}{\text{argmin}}\ E\left[\frac{\mathbb{I}[A \neq d(H)]}{A\pi(H) + (1-A)/2}Y\right] \\ &= \underset{d}{\text{argmin}}\ E\left[\frac{Y}{A\pi(H) + (1-A)/2}\mathbb{I}[A \neq d(H)]\right], \end{aligned}$$

which can be recognized as a weighted classification error. A natural estimator of the above is

$$\hat{d}^{opt}(H) = \underset{d}{\text{argmin}}\ \mathbb{P}_n\left[\frac{Y}{A\pi(H) + (1-A)/2}\mathbb{I}[A \neq d(H)]\right].$$

Since $d(H)$ can always be represented as $sign(f(H))$, for some suitable function f (exploiting the fact that A is coded $-1/1$), the above display is equivalent to finding

$$\hat{f}^{opt}(H) = \underset{f}{\text{argmin}}\ \mathbb{P}_n\left[\frac{Y}{A\pi(H) + (1-A)/2}\mathbb{I}[A \neq sign(f(H))]\right],$$

and then setting $\hat{d}^{opt}(H) = sign(\hat{f}^{opt}(H))$. In the machine learning literature, the objective function appearing on the right side of the above display is viewed as a weighted sum of 0–1 loss function, which is a non-smooth, non-convex function. It is well-known that such a function is difficult to minimize directly. One common approach to address this difficulty is to consider convex surrogate loss functions instead of the original non-convex 0–1 loss (Zhang 2004). Most of the modern classification methods, as well as the classical logistic regression method, in effect minimize such a convex surrogate loss function; see Hastie et al. (2009, Sect. 10.6) for a vivid discussion. In particular, Zhao et al. (2012) employed the popular *hinge loss* function that is used in the context of *support vector machines* (Cortes and Vapnik 1995). In addition, Zhao et al. (2012) penalized the hinge loss for complexity in the estimated f; this is a common technique to avoid overfitting the data. Thus, following the classification literature, Zhao et al. (2012) replaced the original minimization problem by the following convex surrogate minimization problem:

$$\hat{f}^{opt}(H) = \underset{f}{\operatorname{argmin}}\, \mathbb{P}_n \left[\frac{Y}{A\pi(H) + (1-A)/2}(1 - Af(H))^+ + \lambda_n ||f||^2 \right],$$

where $x^+ = \max(x, 0)$, $||f||$ is a suitable norm of f, and λ_n is a complexity parameter (tuning parameter) that can be chosen via cross-validation. The above can be solved by standard algorithms from the support vector machine literature; see either Hastie et al. (2009, Chap. 12) or the original paper by Zhao et al. (2012) for further details. In addition, Zhao et al. (2012) derived theoretical properties of the resulting estimator in terms of consistency, rate of convergence, and risk bounds. A thorough discussion of these theoretical properties are beyond the scope of this book.

5.4 Assessing the Merit of an Estimated Regime

An interesting question that has not yet been properly addressed in the existing literature is how best to define the merit of the estimated optimal regime $\hat{d}$, irrespective of the estimation procedure employed (e.g. Q-learning, G-estimation, MSM etc.). As in any estimation procedure, one would tend to think of bias and variance as natural metrics. However, since regimes are functions, rather than real numbers or vectors, bias and variance has to be defined, if possible, in terms of their associated values (mean potential outcomes) rather than directly. First let us consider the notion of variance since it is easy to conceptualize. Naturally, one can consider the variability in the value under the estimated regime or use cross-validation (Zhang et al. 2012a; Rubin and van der Laan 2012). More precisely, we can write,

$$\text{Var}(\hat{d}) = E\left(V^{\hat{d}} - E(V^{\hat{d}})\right)^2,$$

where the expectation is over the distribution of the entire sample. Thus, the above variance represents the variability of the value of $\hat{d}$ across different samples.

In the present context, bias is a more difficult concept. First, let $V^{opt} = \max_{d \in \mathscr{D}} V^d$ be the optimal value function (i.e. value of the optimal regime) within a pre-specified class of regimes $\mathscr{D}$. Then the bias of the estimated regime $\hat{d}$ can be defined as

$$\text{Bias}(\hat{d}) = E(V^{\hat{d}}) - V^{opt},$$

where the above expectation is over the distribution of the entire sample. The bias represents how much the expected value of the estimated regime, averaged over the distribution of the sample, differs from the best possible value. One can combine the bias and variance criteria into a mean squared error (MSE) type criterion of the estimated regime:

$$\text{MSE}(\hat{d}) = \text{Bias}^2(\hat{d}) + \text{Var}(\hat{d}) = E(V^{\hat{d}} - V^{opt})^2.$$

The MSE measures how "close" the estimated regime is to the truly optimal regime within the class under consideration, in a well-defined sense. It is not hard to imagine the existence of a bias-variance trade-off across different estimation procedures considered in this book; for example, the policy search or MSM-type methods considered in this chapter are likely to lead to less bias but more variance compared to Q-learning (which involves more parametric modeling).

A more traditional criterion for assessing the merit of an arbitrary (but fixed) regime from the reinforcement learning literature is the *generalization error*. The generalization error of a fixed regime d at a state (e.g. baseline covariate) o_1 is defined as the difference between the optimal value function and the value function under the regime of interest d. Thus,

$$\eta^d(o_1) = V^{opt}(o_1) - V^d(o_1).$$

However to assess the overall performance of a regime, one needs to combine the generalization errors over possible values of o_1. The traditional approach in reinforcement learning (Bertsekas and Tsitsiklis 1996) is to use the maximum generalization error, $\max_{o_1}(V^{opt}(o_1) - V^d(o_1))$, which represents the worst case scenario. Another option is to consider an average generalization error (Kearns et al. 2000; Kakade 2003; Murphy 2005b). An average generalization error is defined as

$$\eta^d = \int_{o_1} (V^{opt}(o_1) - V^d(o_1)) dP(o_1) = V^{opt} - V^d,$$

where P is a probability distribution over the possible values of o_1. In the context of medical decision making using DTRs, it is particularly appealing to use this average generalization error, since P represents the distribution of baseline covariates of subjects from a particular population of interest.

For an estimated regime $\hat{d}$, the MSE and the generalization error are related; it turns out that the MSE is the expected value of the squared average generalization error, i.e.,

$$\text{MSE}(\hat{d}) = E\eta^2(\hat{d}),$$

where the above expectation is taken with respect to the distribution of the sample.

While the concept of generalization error is simple and intuitive, its computation for a given estimation procedure is usually quite complex. Murphy (2005b) derived finite-sample upper bounds on the generalization error of Q-learning. The results are quite technical in nature, and hence beyond the scope of this book. We are not aware of the existence of any work that has considered generalization errors of other estimation procedures presented in this book. The next question is that of formal inference, e.g. testing for a significant difference between candidate regimes, arising from different procedures, in terms of their values; we will briefly re-visit this in Sect. 8.10. It is not clear whether such testing must be done through values, or whether a more direct approach can be devised.

5.5 Discussion

In this chapter, we have considered several approaches to estimating the optimal DTR by directly modeling the regimes as opposed to modeling the conditional mean models: IPTW, marginal structural models (MSMs), and classification-based methods. The fundamental difference between the approaches considered in the current chapter (e.g. MSM, weighting, and classification-based methods) and the approaches considered in previous chapters (e.g. Q-learning and G-estimation), lies in the primary target of estimation (and inference): the MSM, weighting, and classification-based approaches really target the parameters of the decision rule itself, rather than parameters of a model for the mean outcome (Q-learning) or for the contrast between models for the mean outcome under alternative treatments (G-estimation). While the approaches considered in the present chapter are typically non-parametric or semi-parametric, requiring only mild assumptions about the data distribution and hence are quite robust, the main drawback is the high variability of the value function estimates, and thereby the high variability in the resulting estimated regimes.

We attempted to elucidate the connections between the different estimation approaches introduced in this chapter: IPTW, MSM, and classification-based methods are deeply connected. Note that in a single-stage setting any mean model, $\mu(H,A;\beta)$ defines a class of treatment regimes. For example, the model

$$\mu(H,A;\beta) = \beta_0 + \beta_1 H + \beta_2 A + \beta_3 AH$$

defines regimes of the form $d(H;\beta) = \mathbb{I}\{\beta_2 + \beta_3 H > 0\} - \mathbb{I}\{\beta_2 + \beta_3 H \leq 0\}$. If β_3 is positive, this can be re-expressed as $d(H;\psi) = \mathbb{I}\{H > \psi\} - \mathbb{I}\{H \leq \psi\}$ for $\psi = -\beta_2/\beta_3$, where many values of the β vector can give rise to the same ψ (Zhang et al. 2012b). Thus, while developed independently, the single-stage regime estimator of Zhang et al. (2012b) is in fact based on the same principles of estimation as the multi-stage (longitudinal) DTR estimators of Hernán et al. (2006), Van der Laan and Petersen (2007a), Robins et al. (2008), Orellana et al. (2010a), and Orellana et al. (2010b): in both cases, the treatment threshold parameters are the direct targets of estimation, and are obtained through estimating the value (population average marginal outcome) as a function of the decision parameters, with the optimal rule being chosen by the indexing parameter which maximizes the mean marginal outcome.

Marginal structural models are appealing due to the simplicity of implementation as well as their familiarity among statisticians and epidemiologists who use these as a standard tool when estimating the impact of static treatment regimes in longitudinal data. Using MSMs, estimated via inverse probability weighting (augmented or not), allows the analyst to estimate the decision rule parameters directly.

All of the methods that we have considered in this chapter are suitable for non-randomized data; of course they rely on the validity of a number of assumptions, some of which are untestable but can be assessed at least informally using model diagnostics (see Sect. 9.2) and substantive knowledge of the health condition under consideration.

Chapter 6
G-computation: Parametric Estimation of Optimal DTRs

In this chapter, we will focus on fully parametric estimation of optimal DTRs by modeling the full, longitudinal distribution of the trajectories data. As noted in Chap. 3, optimal dynamic treatment regimes may be determined using dynamic programming. In a classic, likelihood-based framework, this requires modeling the complete longitudinal distribution of the data. If a joint distribution for the longitudinal data can be decomposed into its conditional components, it can be used to predict the expected outcome under a variety of treatment regimes using a Monte Carlo approach. The link between the models used in dynamic programming to those used in G-computation has been made previously (Lavori and Dawson 2004), and forms the basis of the likelihood-based methods of estimation.

6.1 Frequentist G-computation

The semi-parametric approaches to estimating DTRs of the previous two chapters relied on correct modeling of the propensity score, $\pi_j(A_j|H_j)$ (at least with respect to confounding variables). This is trivially satisfied in RCT settings, but could potentially be problematic in an observational study, where $\pi_j(A_j|H_j)$ is unknown and potentially difficult to model. In this case, one can proceed by expressing the value function V^d alternatively as

$$V^d = E\left\{ \sum_{\{(h_j,a_j):1\leq j\leq K\}} \mathbb{I}[d_1(h_1) = a_1, \ldots, d_K(h_K) = a_K] \right. \\ \left. \times \quad E\Big[\sum_{j=1}^{K} Y_j \Big| H_j = h_j, A_j = a_j\Big] \right\},$$

and then fitting a parametric model, say $\phi_j(h_j, a_j; \theta_j)$, for the inside conditional expectation. Note that in a single-stage setting, the above expression simply gives

B. Chakraborty and E.E.M. Moodie, *Statistical Methods for Dynamic Treatment Regimes*, Statistics for Biology and Health 76, DOI 10.1007/978-1-4614-7428-9_6,

$V^d = E\Big\{E[Y|H=h,A=d(h)]\Big\}$, which is estimated by $\mathbb{P}_n[Y|A=d(h),H=h] = \mathbb{P}_n\phi(h,d(h);\hat{\theta})$ where $\hat{\theta}$ is an estimator of θ. The resulting estimator is known as the *G-computation formula* (Robins 1986), and is given by

$$\hat{V}_G^d = \mathbb{P}_n\left[\sum_{\{(h_j,a_j):1\leq j\leq K\}} \mathbb{I}[d_1(h_1)=a_1,\ldots,d_K(h_K)=a_K]\,\phi_j(h_j,a_j;\hat{\theta}_j)\right]. \quad (6.1)$$

This estimator is consistent if the models $\phi_j(h_j,a_j;\hat{\theta}_j)$ are correctly specified. Like inverse probability weighting and G-estimation, G-computation can be highly variable due to the presence of non-smooth indicator functions; however in comparison to the (semi-parametric) IPTW estimator, the variability is reduced to some extent by employing the parametric model ϕ.

Note that unlike Q-learning or G-estimation, which are performed recursively in time (backwards induction methods), G-computation models and then simulates data forward in time. That is, in G-computation, a sequence of models for responses at stage j, $j=1,\ldots,K$ are posited and estimated from the observed data. Then, beginning at the first interval and using these models and their estimated parameters, given observed baseline data, data is simulated under a particular regime of interest, d, to generate a distribution of potential outcomes $O_2(d_1)$; next, the stage 2 model is used to simulate (or generate) potential outcomes in response to following the regime of interest, d, in the second stage, generating the distribution of potential outcomes $Y(d)$ in a two-stage setting; more generally, in the K-stage setting, the second stage of simulation would produce $O_3(d_1,d_2)$, and simulation would continue forward until the final stage outcome was simulated under regime $d = d_1(H_1), d_2(H_2), \ldots, d_K(H_K)$.

As noted earlier, when d is not one of the embedded DTRs in the study, estimating V^d is really a problem of counterfactual estimation. In his original work, Robins introduced the above method from a purely causal inference perspective as an approach to estimating counterfactual means, and more generally, entire counterfactual distributions. When the interest lies in estimating counterfactual distributions rather than means, instead of modeling the conditional expectation $E\Big(\sum_{j=1}^K Y_j\Big|H_j=h_j,A_j=a_j\Big)$, one must model the corresponding conditional likelihood, e.g. $\prod_{j=1}^{K+1} f_j(o_j|h_{j-1},a_{j-1})$ in Eq. (3.1). Thus the key idea underlying G-computation is to estimate the marginal mean (or distribution) of the outcome by first fitting models for conditional means (or conditional likelihoods) of stage-specific, time-varying outcomes given history and action, and then to substitute values corresponding to specific treatment patterns into Eq. (6.1) (or corresponding expression of the data likelihood). Note that in G-computation, a potentially greater part of the likelihood of the data is modeled (the states and responses), in contrast to some of the semi-parametric approaches of the previous two chapters, where efforts are focused on modeling the treatment allocation probabilities and the final outcome model. G-computation requires the assumption of *no unmeasured confounding* introduced in Chap. 2. See Robins and Hernán (2009) or Dawid and Didelez (2010) for a detailed exposition of G-computation.

6.1.1 Applications and Implementation of G-computation

G-computation has seen considerable use in the last decade. Thall et al. (2002) considered G-computation to evaluate a phase II clinical trial of prostate cancer treatment. Lavori and Dawson (2004) demonstrated (with R pseudocode) how to evaluate two-stage data, motivated by the treatment for major depressive disorder in the sequentially randomized STAR*D trial; see Chap. 2 for a brief description of this trial. Bembom and Van der Laan (2007) demonstrated the use of G-computation and compared results with marginal structural models (see Sect. 5.2) to examine the optimal chemotherapy for the treatment of prostate cancer, choosing from among four first-line treatments and the same four treatments offered as salvage therapy (Thall et al. 2007b).

One of the most complex and realistic implementations of G-computation using epidemiological data was performed by Taubman et al. (2009), who used more than 20 years of data from the Nurses' Health Study to examine the effect of composite lifestyle interventions on the risk of coronary heart disease. Similarly, Young et al. (2011) analyzed data from a large multi-country cohort study of HIV+ individuals to determine when to initiate antiretroviral therapy as a function of CD4 cell count, and Westreich et al. (2012) used G-computation to evaluate the impact of antiretroviral therapy on time to AIDS or death. The question was the same as that investigated by Cain et al. (2010) using a marginal structural modeling approach (albeit with different data). G-computation has also been adopted in the econometric literature (e.g. Abbring and Heckman 2007), where it has been used to explore the effects of television-watching on performance in math and reading (Huang and Lee 2010), and of spanking on behavior (Lee and Huang 2012).

Diggle et al. (2002) provided a simple expositional example on two stages where all variables are binary; in such a case, it is simple to implement G-computation non-parametrically (i.e. without using a parametric model for the conditional mean or distribution). More recently, Daniel et al. (2013) demonstrated the use of G-computation, as well as two semi-parametric approaches to estimating time-varying treatment effects, using simulated data. In the tutorial, a small by-hand example of a non-parametric implementation of G-computation is given as is a more complex scenario which requires parametric modeling. The supplementary material in the tutorial include a worked example in which there is loss to follow-up, so that the treatment of interest is redefined to be not simply treatment pattern $\bar{a}$, but rather receipt of treatment pattern $\bar{a}$ *and* continued observation. G-computation has been implemented as a SAS macro

`http://www.hsph.harvard.edu/causal/software/`

and as a Stata command (Daniel et al. 2011), facilitating dissemination and use of the method.

There are two potentially serious drawbacks to G-computation. The first is that in complex settings (many stages, or high dimensional intermediate observations), G-computation typically requires an estimate of the distribution of each intermediate outcome O_j, given each possible history up to that time point. Using a Monte Carlo approach to simulate the counterfactual distribution for complex longitudinal data with many stages can be computationally intensive, however algorithms have been proposed to reduce the computational burden (Neugebauer and Van der Laan 2006). The second, and more worrisome, limitation of G-estimation is that incorrect model specification can lead to biased results and incorrect conclusions in longitudinal settings with time-varying treatments, even when the "sharp" null hypothesis holds, i.e. when there is no treatment effect for any individual so that $Y(\bar{a}_K) - Y(\bar{a}'_K) = 0$ with probability 1 for all regimes $\bar{a}_K$ and $\bar{a}'_K$. This is known as the null paradox, and can occur even in sequentially randomized trials where randomization probabilities are known (Robins and Wasserman 1997).

6.1.2 Breastfeeding and Vocabulary: An Illustration

Background and Study Details

The PROmotion of Breastfeeding Intervention Trial (PROBIT) (Kramer et al. 2001), briefly introduced in Chap. 2, randomized hospitals and affiliated polyclinics in the Republic of Belarus to a breastfeeding encouragement intervention modeled on the WHO/UNICEF Baby-Friendly Hospital Initiative or to standard care. All study infants were born from June 17, 1996, to December 31, 1997, at term in one of 31 Belarusian maternity hospitals, weighing at least 2,500 g, initiated breastfeeding, and were recruited during their postpartum stay. This resulted in the enrollment of 17,046 mother-infants pairs who were followed regularly for the first year of life. In a later wave of PROBIT, follow-up interviews and examinations were performed on 13,889 (81.5 %) children at 6.5 years of age. One of the components of these visits was the administration of the Wechsler Abbreviated Scales of Intelligence (WASI), which consists of four subtests: vocabulary, similarities, block designs, and matrices. We focus our analysis on the vocabulary subtest.

Many studies from developed countries have observed higher cognitive scores on IQ and other tests among both children and adults who were breastfed compared with those who were formula-fed (Anderson et al. 1999). Based on an intention-to-treat analysis, PROBIT demonstrates that prolonged and exclusive breastfeeding improves children's cognitive development (Kramer et al. 2008). We consider 13,739 children (excluding 159 children from the follow-up due to missing data in the variables of interest from the first year of life). A simple random effects model controlling for within-hospital correlation reveals a statistically significant effect of the intervention on the vocabulary subset score of 7.5 points (95 % CI: 0.7 to 14.4 points) in these children and, as noted by Kramer et al. (2008), the intervention also served to significantly and meaningfully increase the duration and intensity of breastfeeding; for instance, 43.3 % of infants in the intervention group were exclusively breastfed at 3 months of age, as compared to 6.4 % of the infants in the control group. Here, we provide a demonstration of G-computation to examine the evidence that actual breastfeeding (rather than exposure to breastfeeding encouragement) increases verbal cognitive ability, and consider whether tailoring breastfeeding habits to infant growth can improve this outcome.

Analysis and Results

In this example, consider two key stages (intervals): birth to 3 months, and 3–6 months of age. The "treatment" or exposure of interest for our analysis is any breastfeeding measured in each of the stages. That is, A_1 takes the value 1 if the child was breastfed up to 3 months of age (and is set to -1 otherwise), and A_2 is the corresponding quantity for any breastfeeding from 3 to 6 months of age. Note that any breastfeeding allows for exclusive breastfeeding or breastfeeding with supplementation with formula or solid foods. The outcome, Y, is the vocabulary subtest score on the WASI measured at age 6.5 years. A single tailoring variable is considered at each stage: the birthweight of the infant at the first stage, and the infant's 3-month weight at the second stage.

Implementing G-computation to address the question of whether breastfeeding itself produces higher vocabulary subtest scores requires models for both the vocabulary subtest score, as well as for the 3-month weight. A linear model was used to fit the vocabulary subtest score on the log-scale (Y) as a function of baseline covariates (intervention group status, geographical location (eastern/rural, eatern/urban, western/rural, or western/urban), mother's education, mother's smoking status, family history of allergy, mother's age, mother's breastfeeding of any previous children, whether birth was by cesarean section, gender) as well as birthweight, 3 month weight, breastfeeding from 0 to 3 months (A_1), breastfeeding from 3 to 6 months (A_2), and the first-order interactions (i) $A_1 \times A_2$, (ii) A_1 by birthweight, and (iii) A_2 by 3-month weight. Note that O_1 includes all baseline covariates and the tailoring variable birthweight, while O_2 includes all variables in O_1 in additional to 3-month weight. Three-month weight was also fit on the log scale using a linear model that conditioned on the baseline covariates and birthweight, breastfeeding from 0 to 3 months (A_1), and the interaction between A_1 and birthweight.

The G-computation procedure used can be described by the following steps, for any regime of interest, $d = (d_1(h_1), d_2(h_2))$:

1. Fit an appropriate joint distribution model for the baseline variables O_1. For PROBIT, a non-parametric approach is adopted, and the empirical distribution was used.
2. Fit an appropriate model to the intermediate variable, O_2, as a function of O_1 and A_1. For PROBIT, a linear model on the log-transformed 3-month weight is used.
3. Fit an appropriate model to the response, Y, as a function of O_1, A_1, O_2, and A_2. For PROBIT, a linear model on the log-transformed subtest score is used.
4. Create a hypothetical population by drawing a random sample with replacement from the distribution of baseline covariates fit in Step (1).

5. Using coefficient estimates and randomly sampled residuals from the model fit in Step (2), determine the (counterfactual) intermediate variable $o_2(d_1)$ under treatment regime d_1 with history $h_1 = o_1$.
6. Using coefficient estimates and randomly sampled residuals from the model fit in Step (3), determine the response under treatment regime d with history $h_1 = o_1$, $h_2 = (o_1, d_1(h_1), o_2(d_1))$.

Using this approach, we can compare distributions under different treatment regimes, such as the static regimes "never breastfeed" or "breastfeed until at least 6 months of age", or the dynamic regime "breastfeed until three months of age, then continue only if 3-month weight exceeds 6.5 kg". Note that in steps 5 and 6, one could assume a likelihood for the potential outcomes, e.g. a normal distribution, rather than the less parametric approach of selecting a random residual.

Table 6.1 Parameter coefficients from a linear regression model for the log-transformed vocabulary subtest score of the WASI and log-transformed 3-month weight

	Vocab. score		Weight at 3 months	
	Est.	SD	Est.	SD
Intercept	4.315	0.047	1.312	0.020
Intervention	0.071	0.035	0.012	0.006
East Belarus (rural)	0.034	0.048	−0.015	0.008
West Belarus (urban)	0.008	0.053	−0.011	0.008
West Belarus (rural)	−0.002	0.044	−0.016	0.007
Attended some university	0.047	0.003	0.008	0.002
Completed university	0.099	0.004	0.009	0.003
Smoker	−0.008	0.008	0.002	0.005
Allergy	0.023	0.006	−0.003	0.004
Age	0.009	0.002	−0.001	0.001
Age^2	0.000	0.000	0.000	0.000
BF previously	−0.049	0.003	0.001	0.002
Did not BF	−0.042	0.003	−0.002	0.002
Cesarean	0.000	0.004	−0.005	0.002
Gender	−0.011	0.002	0.045	0.001
Birthweight	0.010	0.004	0.139	0.002
A_1: Breastfed 0–3 months	0.048	0.019	0.008	0.012
Weight at 3 months	0.017	0.002		
A_2: Breastfed 3–6 months	−0.121	0.057		
$A_1 \times$Birthweight	−0.012	0.005	0.001	0.004
$A_2 \times$Weight at 3 months	0.016	0.007		
$A_1 \times A_2$	0.019	0.037		

Results from regression models which account for within-hospital clustering are presented in Table 6.1; coefficient estimates from models which ignored clustering are very similar. Statistically significant effects of breastfeeding and its interaction with weight are found in the model for the log vocabulary score. However, when these models are subsequently used to produce samples from the counterfactual distribution of outcomes, it is evident that the impact of breastfeeding itself on the

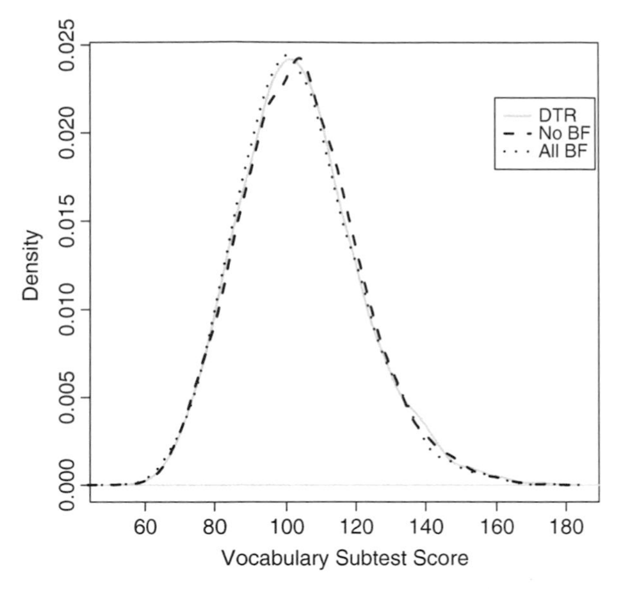

Fig. 6.1 Counterfactual vocabulary subtest score under three different breastfeeding regimes estimated by G-computation: a DTR (*gray, solid line*), no breastfeeding (*dashed line*) and breastfeeding until at least 6 months (*dotted line*)

vocabulary subtest score is minimal (see Fig. 6.1), with mean test scores varying by less than one point under the three regimes considered. These results are broadly in line with the findings of Moodie et al. (2012).

6.2 Bayesian Estimation of DTRs

A detailed presentation of the many modeling choices required for any particular application of a Bayesian estimation of a dynamic treatment regime is beyond the scope of this text, however a great number of resources are available to the interested reader (see, e.g. Chen et al. 2010).

6.2.1 Approach and Applications

Parametric frequentist methods of estimating optimal DTRs typically rely on the assumption that all models are correctly specified, while semi-parametric approaches are often able to relax some modeling assumptions. In the Bayesian setting, a number of different approaches have been proposed. Wathen and Thall (2008) considered at the outset a number of candidate models, and choose from among them using an approximate Bayes factor. Arjas and Saarela (2010) used model averaging over random draws from the space of possible models, so that inference is based on results from the averaged model. They argued that this is a distinct advantage of a Bayesian approach over frequentist methods (semi-parametric or otherwise), as it allows the analyst to incorporate uncertainty regarding model specification into the estimation procedure. As in the frequentist approaches, Bayesian estimation of optimal dynamic treatment regimes may be computationally burdensome in complex settings with many covariates and/or stages, although some advances have been made. For example, Wathen and Thall (2008) adapted the forward-sampling approach of Carlin et al. (1998) so as to be able to sample from the predictive distribution of the outcome under each of several regimes, where the distribution is estimated from the observed data, however in this case the "regimes" of interest were stopping rules for group sequential clinical trials.

Arjas and Saarela (2010) considered data on HIV treatment from the Multi-Center AIDS Cohort (Kaslow et al. 1987), focusing on a two-stage setting in which there is a single (continuous) tailoring variable at each stage, treatment is binary, and the outcome is a continuous variable. They postulated appropriate prior distributions for each component of the joint likelihood, and thus obtained the joint posterior distribution. Following this, the posterior predictive distribution was used to see how the outcomes of individuals drawn from the same population as those who formed the sample data were distributed under different treatment patterns. This approach uses the principles set forth by Arjas and Parner (2004), who suggested using summaries of the posterior predictive distributions as the main criterion for comparing different treatment regimes, leading to what they refer to as an "integrated causal analysis" in which the same probabilistic framework is used for inference about model parameters as well as for treatment comparisons and hence the choice of an optimal regime.

Lavori and Dawson (2000) used multiple imputations performed by an approximate Bayesian bootstrap (Rubin and Shenker 1991) to generate draws from the counterfactual distributions, and thereby allow a non-parametric means of comparing mean outcomes under different treatment strategies. Zajonc (2012) proposed a similar approach, though from a more overtly Bayesian perspective, and considers data from the North Carolina Education Research Data Center, examining the impact of honors programs on tenth grade mathematics test scores. Two stages with a binary exposure were considered; several baseline confounders, and two time-dependent variables were used in the analysis. Tailoring of the decision rule was performed in a variety of ways including using the single, continuous mathematics score at the start of each stage as well as by creating an index score that was a composite of five variables including sex, race, and test score. The approach was the same in spirit as that of Arjas and Saarela (2010), however the motivation was somewhat different. Like Lavori and Dawson (2000) and Zajonc (2012) framed the estimation problem as one of missing data, where the missing information is on the potential outcomes, and undertakes estimation through what is effectively a multiple imputation approach. Thus, Bayesian machinery was used to estimate the posterior predictive distribution of the potential outcomes, and the optimal regime was selected as that which maximized the expected posterior utility, where the utility was simply some analyst-defined function of the outcome and potentially other factors such as treatment cost.

The Bayesian posterior predictive approach to dynamic treatment regime estimation is in many ways similar to G-computation, but is more readily able to capture three primary sources of variability in estimators: (i) randomness in covariates and outcomes as specified by the predictive distribution for the outcome given data, (ii) potential randomness in the regime (if, for example, the DTR had a stochastic component such as "treat within three months of the occurrence of a particular health-related event"); and (iii) variability in the unknown model parameters (Arjas 2012). There have also been a number of applications of Bayesian predictive inference to examine questions of causation for non-continuous outcomes, many by Elja Arjas and colleagues. For example, Arjas and Andreev (2000) used a Bayesian nonparametric intensity model for recurrent events to study the impact of child-care setting on the number of ear infections.

6.2.2 Assumptions as Viewed in a Bayesian Framework

Although rarely discussed explicitly in Bayesian analyses, most implicitly require the assumption of no unmeasured confounding or exchangeability (Saarela et al. 2012b). Arjas and Saarela (2010) used this assumption so that in using the posterior predictive distribution to estimate mean response, the values of treatment at each stage could be set to specific values, i.e. they noted "we can switch from observed treatment values in the data to 'optional' or 'forced' in the predictions is again consequence of the no unmeasured confounders postulate" and that this "can be viewed as representing 'do'-conditioning (Pearl 2009)." Arjas and Saarela (2010) further related this condition to the assumption of missing at random (Little and Rubin 2002). Arjas (2012) elaborated on the mathematical conditions under which the forced 'do'-probabilities can be identified from observational data (what he terms a 'see'-study, following Lindley (2002)) and related these probabilistic statements to Rubin's causal model (1974) and to the sequential randomization design of Robins (1986), which rely on the potential outcomes framework. Zajonc (2012), too, linked the NUC assumption to the idea that the treatment mechanism may be considered ignorable, i.e. possibly dependent on observed data, but not on unobserved counterfactual quantities.

6.2.3 Breastfeeding and Vocabulary: An Illustration, Continued

We now return to the PROBIT trial, and re-analyze the data using a Bayesian predictive approach.

A Bayesian G-computation procedure is designed to complement and compare with the analysis performed in Sect. 6.1.2. A variety of summary measures of the counterfactual outcome under different regimes may be computed. For example, to estimate the counterfactual distribution of outcomes (see Fig. 6.1 for a frequentist version) for a regime of interest, $d = (d_1(h_1), d_2(h_2))$, we may:

1. Fit an appropriate joint distribution model for the baseline variables O_1. For PROBIT, a non-parametric approach is adopted, and the empirical distribution was used.
2. Fit an appropriate model to the intermediate variable, O_2, as a function of O_1 and A_1. For PROBIT, a linear model on the log-transformed 3-month weight is used with a normal, mean-zero, variance 10 (covariance 0) prior is used for all regression coefficients, β_2, and the (proper) Inverse Gamma prior with parameters 5, 0.2 is used for the variance parameters.
3. Fit an appropriate model to the response, Y, as a function of O_1, A_1, O_2, and A_2. As in the previous step, a normal (0,diag(10)) prior is used for regression coefficients, β_1, and an Inverse Gamma(5,0.2) prior is used for the variance parameters in the PROBIT analysis.
4. Draw a sample from the posterior predictive distribution of the counterfactual mean outcome using the following steps:

   (a) Draw a random sample of size 10,000 with replacement from the distribution of baseline covariates fit in Step (1) to create a hypothetical population.
   (b) For each member of the hypothetical population, draw a sample value from the posterior distribution of β_1 found in Step (2) and use this to determine the mean (counterfactual) intermediate variable $o_2(d_1)$, and call this $\mu_{o_2}(\beta_1)$. Next, draw a value of $o_2(d_1)$ from the posterior predictive distribution with mean $\mu_{o_2}(\beta_1)$.
   (c) Then, for each member of the hypothetical population, draw a sample value from the posterior distribution of β_2 found in Step (3) and use this to determine the mean (counterfactual) outcome, and call this $\mu_y(\beta_2)$. Draw a value of $y(d_1, d_2)$ from its posterior predictive distribution with mean $\mu_y(\beta_2)$.

Note that in this approach, the uncertainty in the estimation of the regression parameters β_1 and β_2 is incorporated into the sampling from the counterfactual means. Figure 6.2 compares the counterfactual distribution of vocabulary subtest scores under two static regimes "never breastfeed" and "breastfeed until at least 6 months of age". Note that these are nearly identical to their frequentist analogues, which is reassuring though not surprising given the large sample size.

The approach described above may be altered to produce the distributions of the *mean* counterfactual outcomes, averaging over the covariate space, rather than the distribution of the counterfactual outcomes themselves. To do this, follow Steps (1)–(3) as above. Perform Step (4), and then in (5) take the average counterfactual outcome. Repeat Steps (4) and (5) a large number of times; boxplots of 1,000 means of counterfactual distributions can be found in Fig. 6.3.

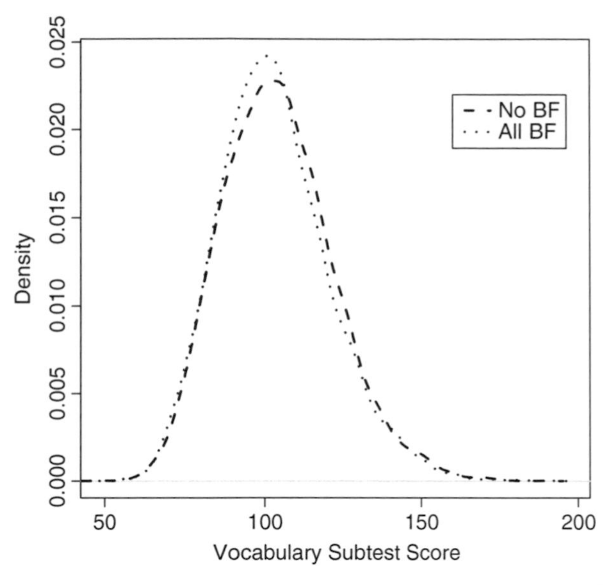

Fig. 6.2 Counterfactual vocabulary subtest score under two different breastfeeding regimes estimated by a Bayesian implementation of G-computation: no breastfeeding (*dashed line*) and breastfeeding until at least 6 months (*dotted line*)

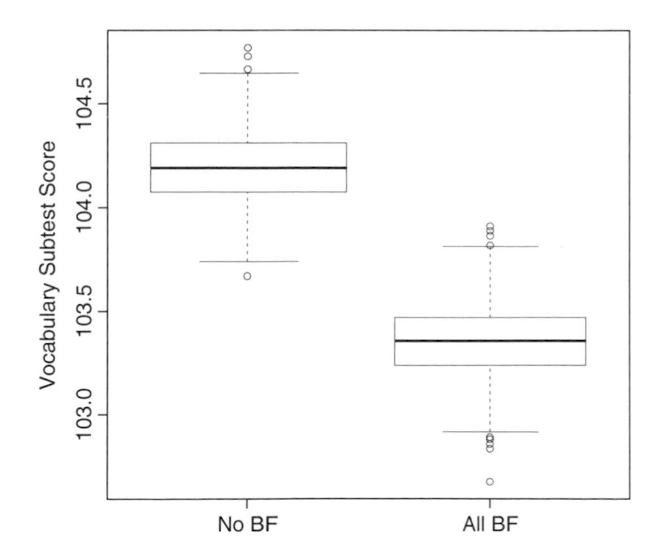

Fig. 6.3 Distribution of the mean counterfactual vocabulary subtest score under two breastfeeding regimes estimated by a Bayesian implementation of G-computation: no breastfeeding (*left*) and breastfeeding until at least 6 months (*right*)

6.3 Discussion

In this chapter, we have presented the fully parametric estimation approach of G-computation. We presented the approach in the frequentist setting, then turned our attention to the Bayesian DTR literature, describing the general approach which is effectively a G-computation based on posterior predictive distributions. We implemented G-computation in the PROBIT data, using both a frequentist and then a Bayesian approach; the conclusions of the two analyses were nearly identical, but the Bayesian calculations permitted the incorporation of the variability due to the estimation of the time-varying parameter distributions into the counterfactual response distributions. A Bayesian perspective on the variance of marginal structural models has recently been considered (Saarela et al. 2012a), but this has not yet been used in the context of DTRs.

Chapter 7
Estimation of DTRs for Alternative Outcome Types

Up to this point, our development has focused entirely on the continuous outcome setting. In this chapter, we will turn our attention to the developments that have been made for estimating DTRs for more difficult outcome types including multi-component rewards, time-to-event data, and discrete outcomes. As we shall see, the range of approaches considered in previous chapters have been employed, but additional care and thought must be devoted to appropriately handling additional complexities in these settings.

7.1 Trading Off Multiple Rewards: Multi-dimensional and Compound Outcomes

Most DTR applications involve simple, univariate outcomes or utilities such as symptom scores or even survival times. However, it may be the case that a single dimension of response is insufficient to capture the patient experience under treatment. Recently, for example, Wang et al. (2012) conducted an analysis of a SMART-design cancer treatment study in which the outcome was taken to be a compound score numerically combining information on treatment efficacy, toxicity, and the risk of disease progression. The optimal DTR using the composite endpoint was found to differ from that using simpler endpoints based on a binary or ternary variable indicating treatment success.

Lizotte et al. (2010) considered an approach based on *inverse preference elicitation*. They proposed to find optimal regimes that can vary depending on how a new patient is willing to trade off different outcomes, such as whether he is willing to tolerate some side-effects for a greater reduction in disease symptoms. Specifically, they considered a situation where there were two possible outcomes of interest, R_1 and R_2, whose respective desirability could be described via a weighted sum $Y = \delta R_1 + (1-\delta)R_2$ for $\delta \in [0,1]$. In this situation, Q-functions may be modeled as a function of the two possible outcomes and δ; for example, a linear model for the Q-function might be represented using

B. Chakraborty and E.E.M. Moodie, *Statistical Methods for Dynamic Treatment Regimes*, Statistics for Biology and Health 76, DOI 10.1007/978-1-4614-7428-9_7,

$$Q_j^{opt}(H_j,A_j) = \delta(\beta_{j1}^T H_{j0} + \psi_{j1}^T H_{j1} A_j) + (1-\delta)(\beta_{j2}^T H_{j0} + \psi_{j2}^T H_{j1} A_j).$$

Estimates of $\beta_j = (\beta_{j1}, \beta_{j2})$ and $\psi_j = (\psi_{j1}, \psi_{j2})$ may be obtained by OLS by setting δ to 0 or 1 (Lizotte et al. 2010). This conceptualization of the outcome addresses an important issue for researchers who may wish to propose not a single DTR, but one which may be adapted not only to patient covariates but also to the relative value patients place on different outcomes. For example, Thall et al. (2002) provided an analysis where the response is taken to be a linear combination of the probability of complete remission and the probability of death as judged by a physician with expertise. It would be possible to use the approach of Lizotte et al. (2010) to either leave δ unspecified so that future "users" or "recipients" of the DTR (i.e. patients) could select their preferred weighting on the risks of remission versus death.

As noted by Almirall et al. (2012b), using a linear combination of outcomes as the final response may not in all circumstances be clinically meaningful, but may provide an important form of sensitivity analysis when outcome measures are subjective.

7.2 Estimating DTRs for Time-to-Event Outcomes with Q-learning

While much of the DTR literature has focused on continuous outcomes, research and analyses have been conducted for time-to-event data as well. Here, we briefly review some key developments.

7.2.1 Simple Q-learning for Survival Data: IPW in Sequential AFT Models

Huang and Ning (2012) used linear regression to fit *accelerated failure time* (AFT) models (Cox and Oaks 1984) in a Q-learning framework to estimate the optimal DTR in a time-to-event setting. Consider a two-stage setting, where patients may receive treatment in at least one and possibly two stages of a study. That is, all patients are exposed to some level of the treatment (where we include a control condition as a possible level of treatment) at the first stage. After the first stage of treatment, one of three possibilities may occur to a study participant: (1) the individual is cured by the treatment and does not require further treatment; (2) the individual experiences the outcome event, or (3) the individual requires a second stage of treatment, e.g. because of disease recurrence. Let Y denote the total follow-up time for an individual. If the individual is cured, he is followed until the end of the study and then censored so that Y is the time from the start of treatment to the censoring time; if he experiences the outcome event, Y is the time at which the event occurs. Further, let R denote the time from the initial treatment to the start of the second stage treatment (assuming this to be the same as the time of disease recurrence), and let S denote the time from the start of the second stage treatment until end of follow-up (due to experiencing the event or the end of the study); then $Y = R + S$. Set $S = 0$ for those individuals who did not experience a second stage of treatment.

First, let us assume that there is no censoring. Then an AFT Q-learning algorithm for time-to-event outcomes proceeds much like that for continuous outcomes:

1. Stage 2 parameter estimation: Using OLS, find estimates $(\hat{\beta}_2, \hat{\psi}_2)$ of the conditional mean model $Q_2^{opt}(H_{2i}, A_{2i}; \beta_2, \psi_2)$ of the log-transformed time of follow-up from the start of the second stage, $\log(S_i)$, for those who experienced a second stage treatment.
2. Stage 2 optimal rule: By substitution, $\hat{d}_2^{opt}(h_2) = \arg\max_{a_2} Q_2^{opt}(h_2, a_2; \hat{\beta}_2, \hat{\psi}_2)$.
3. Stage 1 pseudo-outcome: Set $S_i^* = \max_{a_2} \exp(Q_2^{opt}(H_{2i}, a_2; \hat{\beta}_2, \hat{\psi}_2))$, $i = 1, \ldots, n$, which can be viewed as the time to event that would be expected under optimal second-stage treatment. Then calculate the pseudo-outcome,

$$\hat{Y}_{1i} = \begin{cases} Y_i \text{ if } S_i = 0 \\ R_i + S_i^* \text{ if } S_i > 0 \end{cases} \qquad i = 1, \ldots, n.$$

4. Stage 1 parameter estimation: Using OLS, find estimates

$$(\hat{\beta}_1, \hat{\psi}_1) = \arg\min_{\beta_1, \psi_1} \frac{1}{n} \sum_{i=1}^{n} \left(\log(\hat{Y}_{1i}) - Q_1^{opt}(H_{1i}, A_{1i}; \beta_1, \psi_1) \right)^2.$$

5. Stage 1 optimal rule: By substitution, $\hat{d}_1^{opt}(h_1) = \arg\max_{a_1} Q_1^{opt}(h_1, a_1; \hat{\beta}_1, \hat{\psi}_1)$.

In the presence of censoring, the regressions in steps 1 and 4 above can be performed with *inverse probability weighting* (IPW), where each subject is weighted by the inverse of the probability of not being censored. Because censoring time is a continuous measure, the probability of not being censored can be calculated from the estimated survival curve for censoring, e.g. by fitting a Cox proportional hazards model to estimate the distribution of the censoring times. Huang and Ning (2012) proved consistency and asymptotic normality of the regression parameters under a set of regularity conditions, illustrated good finite-sample performance of the methodology under varying degrees of censoring using a simulation study, and applied the methodology to analyze data from a study on the treatment of soft tissue sarcoma.

7.2.2 Q-learning with Support Vector Regression for Censored Survival Data

In Q-learning, the Q-functions need not always be modeled by linear models. In the RL literature, Q-functions had been modeled via regression trees or more sophisticated variations like *random forests* and *extremely randomized trees* (Ernst et al.

2005; Geurts et al. 2006; Guez et al. 2008) or via kernel-based regression (Ormoneit and Sen 2002). More recently in the DTR literature, Zhao et al. (2011) employed *support vector regression* (SVR) to model the Q-functions in the context of modeling survival time in a cancer clinical trial. These modern methods from the machine learning literature are often appealing due to their robustness and flexibility in estimating the Q-functions. Following Zhao et al. (2011), here we briefly present the SVR method to fit Q-functions.

Stepping outside the RL framework for a moment, consider a regression problem with the vector of predictors $x \in \mathbb{R}^m$ and the outcome $y \in \mathbb{R}$. Given the data $\{x_i, y_i\}_{i=1}^n$, the goal in SVR is to find a (regression) function $f : \mathbb{R}^m \to \mathbb{R}$ that closely matches the target y_i for the corresponding x_i. One of the popular loss functions is the so-called ε-insensitive loss function (Vapnik 1995), defined as: $\mathscr{L}(f(x_i), y_i) = (|f(x_i) - y_i| - \varepsilon)_+$, where $\varepsilon > 0$ and u_+ denotes the positive part of u. The ε-insensitive loss function ignores errors of size less than ε and grows linearly beyond that. Conceptually, this property is similar to that of the robust regression methods (Huber 1964); see Hastie et al. (2009, p. 435) for more details on this similarity, including a graphical representation.

In SVR, typically the regression function $f(\cdot)$ is assumed to take the form $f(x) = \theta_0 + \boldsymbol{\theta}^T \boldsymbol{\Phi}(x)$, where $\boldsymbol{\Phi}(x)$ is a vector of non-linear basis functions (or, features) of the original predictor vector x. Thus, while the regression function employs a linear model involving the transformed features $\boldsymbol{\Phi}(x)$, it can potentially become highly non-linear in the original predictor space, thereby allowing great flexibility and predictive power. It turns out that the problem of solving for unknown f is a convex optimization problem, and can be solved by quadratic programming using Lagrange multipliers (see, for example, Hastie et al. 2009, Chap. 12).

In the context of dynamic treatment regimes, the outcome of interest y (e.g. survival time from cancer) is often censored. The presence of censoring makes matters more complicated and the SVR procedure as outlined above cannot be used without modification. Shivaswamy et al. (2007) considered a version of SVR, without the ε-insensitive property, to take into account censored outcomes. Building on their work, Zhao et al. (2011) developed a procedure called ε-SVR-C (where C denotes censoring) that can account for censored outcomes and has the ε-insensitive property. Below we briefly present their procedure.

In general, we denote interval-censored survival (more generally, time-to-event) data by $\{x_i, l_i, u_i\}_{i=1}^n$, where l and u stand for the lower and upper bound of the interval under consideration. If a patient experiences the death event, then the corresponding observation is denoted by $\{x_i, y_i\}_{i=1}^n$ with $l_i = u_i = y_i$. Also, letting $u_i = +\infty$, one can easily construct a right-censored observation $\{x_i, l_i, +\infty\}$. Given the interval-censored data, consider the following loss function:

$$\mathscr{L}(f(x_i), l_i, u_i) = \max(l_i - \varepsilon - f(x_i), f(x_i) - u_i - \varepsilon)_+.$$

The shape of the loss function for both interval-censored data and right-censored data are displayed in Fig. 7.1.

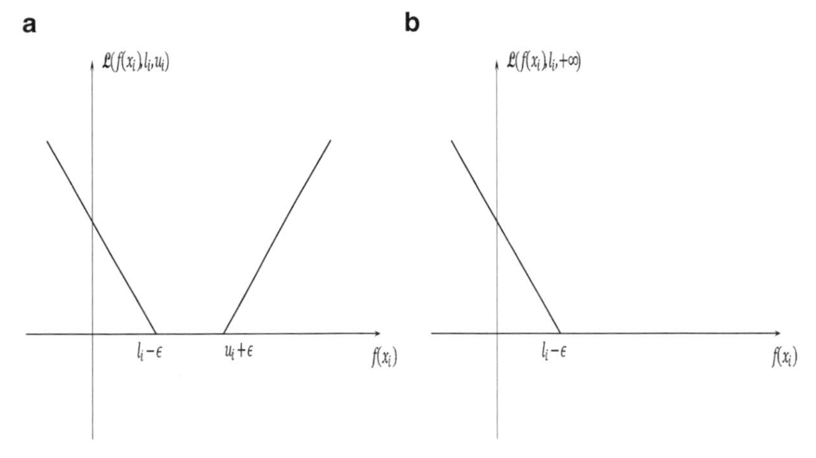

Fig. 7.1 ε-SVR-C loss functions for: (**a**) interval-censored data (*left panel*), and (**b**) right-censored data (*right panel*)

Defining the index sets $L = \{i : l_i > -\infty\}$ and $U = \{i : u_i < +\infty\}$, the ε-SVR-C optimization formulation is:

$$\min_{\theta,\theta_0,\xi,\xi'} \frac{1}{2}||\theta||^2 + C_E\Big(\sum_{i\in L}\xi_i + \sum_{i\in U}\xi_i'\Big), \quad \text{subject to}$$
$$(\theta_0 + \theta^T\Phi(x_i)) - u_i \le \varepsilon + \xi_i,\ i \in U;$$
$$l_i - (\theta_0 + \theta^T\Phi(x_i)) \le \varepsilon + \xi_i',\ i \in L;$$
$$\xi_i \ge 0,\ i \in L;$$
$$\xi_i' \ge 0,\ i \in U.$$

In the above display, ξ_i and ξ_i' are the so-called *slack variables* and C_E is the cost of error. By minimizing the regularization term $\frac{1}{2}||\theta||^2$ as well as the training error $C_E\Big(\sum_{i\in L}\xi_i + \sum_{i\in U}\xi_i'\Big)$, the ε-SVR-C algorithm can avoid both overfitting and underfitting of the training data.

Interestingly, the solution depends on the basis function Φ only through inner products $\Phi(x_i)^T\Phi(x_j)$, $\forall i,j$. In fact, one need not explicitly specify the basis function Φ; it is enough to specify the *kernel function* $K(x_i,x_j) = \Phi(x_i)^T\Phi(x_j)$. One popular choice of K used by Zhao et al. (2011) is the Gaussian (or radial basis) kernel, given by $K(x_i,x_j) = \exp(-\gamma||x_i - x_j||^2)$. Thus the above optimization problem is equivalent to the following dual problem:

$$\min_{\lambda,\lambda'} \frac{1}{2}(\lambda-\lambda')^T K(x_i,x_j)(\lambda-\lambda') - \sum_{i\in L}(l_i-\varepsilon)\lambda_i' + \sum_{i\in U}(u_i+\varepsilon)\lambda_i,$$
$$\text{subject to}$$
$$\sum_{i\in L}\lambda_i' - \sum_{i\in U}\lambda_i = 0,\ 0 \le \lambda_i,\lambda_i' \le C_E,\ i = 1,\ldots,n.$$

The tuning parameters γ (in the definition of K) and C_E are obtained by cross-validation to achieve good performance. Once the above formulation is solved to find the optimal values of λ_i and λ_i', say $\hat{\lambda}_i$ and $\hat{\lambda}_i'$, the regression function is given by $\hat{f}(x) = \sum_{i=1}^{n}(\hat{\lambda}_i' - \hat{\lambda}_i)K(x_i,x) + \hat{\theta}_0$. Due to the nature of the constraints in the above optimization problem, typically only a subset of values of $(\hat{\lambda}_i' - \hat{\lambda}_i)$ are non-zero, and the associated data points are called the *support vectors*.

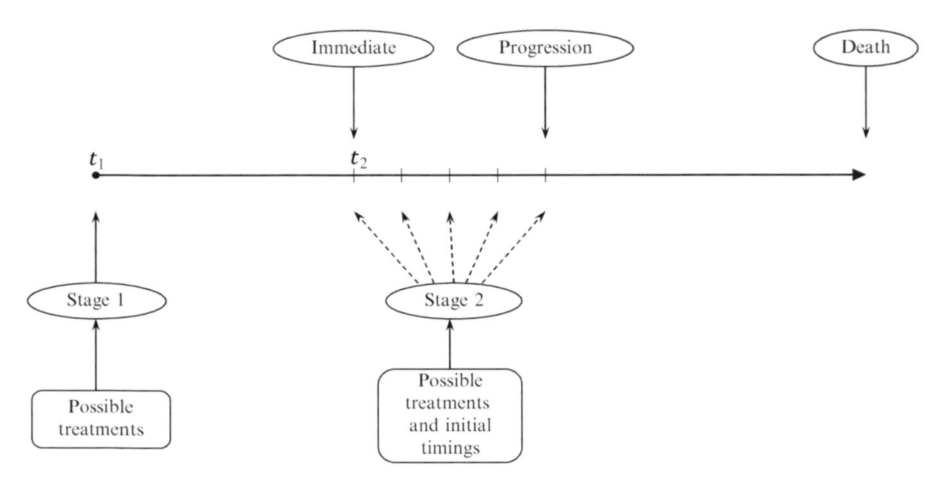

Fig. 7.2 Treatment plan and therapy options for advanced non-small cell lung cancer in a hypothetical SMART design

Zhao et al. (2011) implemented Q-learning in conjunction with the ε-SVR-C method described above in the context of a hypothetical two-stage SMART for treating advanced non-small cell lung cancer; see Fig. 7.2 for a schematic. In addition to the complexity of the problem of selecting optimal stage-1 and stage-2 treatments, another goal was to determine the optimal time to initiate the stage-2 treatment, either immediately or delayed, that would yield the longest overall survival time. Let t_1 and t_2 denote the time-points where the first and second stage treatment decisions are made, respectively. Let the time to disease progression, after initiation of the stage-1 treatment (chemotherapy), be denoted by T_P (for simplicity, it is assumed that $T_P \geq t_2$ with probability 1). Let T_M denote the targeted time after t_2 of initiating the stage-2 treatment. The actual time to initiate the stage-2 treatment is $(t_2 + T_M) \wedge T_P$. At the end of first-stage therapy, i.e. at time t_2, clinicians make a decision about the target start time T_M. Let T_D denote the time of death from the start of therapy (t_1), i.e. the overall survival time. Note that this scenario is more complex than that of the previous section; in the simpler setting of Huang and Ning (2012), $R = (t_2 + T_M) \wedge T_P$ and $S = T_D - R$ or, in the presence of censoring, S will be the time on study following initiation of second treatment (total time minus R).

Acknowledging the possibility of right censoring, denote the patient's censoring time by C and indicator of the event (i.e. of not being censored) by $\delta = \mathbb{I}[T_D \leq C]$. Assume that the censoring is independent of both the death time and the patient covariates. For convenience, define $T_1 = T_D \wedge t_2$ and $Y_D = \mathbb{I}[T_D \wedge C \geq t_2]$, and also $T_2 = (T_D - t_2)\mathbb{I}[T_D \geq t_2] = (T_D - t_2)\mathbb{I}[T_1 = t_2]$ and $C_2 = (C - t_2)\mathbb{I}[C \geq t_2]$. Note that $T_D = T_1 + T_2$, where T_1 is the time of life lived in $[t_1, t_2]$ and T_2 is the time of life lived after t_2.

As in previous chapters, let H_1 and H_2 denote the histories (e.g. current and past covariates, and also past treatments) available at first and second stage respectively. Also, let A_1 and A_2 denote the treatment choices at the two stages. In this study, the treatment decision at the second stage also involves an initiation time T_M, as discussed above. Thus the stage-2 treatment is two-dimensional, denoted compactly as (A_2, T_M). Define the optimal Q-functions for the two stages as follows:

$$Q_2^{opt}\big(H_2,(A_2,T_M)\big) = E\big[T_2\big|H_2,(A_2,T_M)\big],$$
$$Q_1^{opt}(H_1,A_1) = E\big[T_1 + \mathbb{I}[T_1 = t_2] \max_{(A_2,T_M)} Q_2^{opt}\big(H_2,(A_2,T_M)\big)\big|H_1,A_1\big].$$

In case of known Q-functions, the optimal DTR (d_1^{opt}, d_2^{opt}), using a backwards induction argument, would be

$$d_2^{opt}(h_2) = \arg\max_{(a_2,T_M)} Q_2^{opt}(h_2,(a_2,T_M)),$$
$$d_1^{opt}(h_1) = \arg\max_{a_1} Q_1^{opt}(h_1,a_1).$$

When the Q-functions are unknown, they are estimated using suitable models. In the present development, censored outcomes $(T_1 \wedge C, \delta_1 = \mathbb{I}[T_1 \leq C])$ and $(T_2 \wedge C_2, \delta_2 = \mathbb{I}[T_2 \leq C_2])$ are used at both stages. The exact algorithm to perform Q-learning with ε-SVR-C for censored survival data is as follows:

1. For those individuals with $Y_D = 1$ (i.e. those who actually go on to the second stage of treatment), perform right-censored regression using ε-SVR-C of the censored outcome $(T_2 \wedge C_2, \delta_2)$ on the stage-2 variables $(H_2, (A_2, T_M))$ to obtain $\hat{Q}_2^{opt}$.
2. Construct the pseudo-outcome

$$\hat{T}_D = T_1 + \mathbb{I}[T_1 = t_2] \max_{(A_2,T_M)} \hat{Q}_2^{opt}(H_2,A_2,T_M) = T_1 + \mathbb{I}[T_1 = t_2]\hat{T}_2 = T_1 + Y_D\hat{T}_2.$$

3. In fitting Q_1^{opt}, the pseudo-outcome $\hat{T}_D$ is assessed through the censored observation $(\tilde{X}, \tilde{\delta})$, with $\tilde{X} = T_1 \wedge C + Y_D\hat{T}_2 = \hat{T}_D \wedge \tilde{C}$ and $\tilde{\delta} = \mathbb{I}[\hat{T}_D \leq \tilde{C}]$, where $\tilde{C} = C\mathbb{I}[C < t_2] + \infty\mathbb{I}[C_2 \geq t_2]$. Perform ε-SVR-C of $(\tilde{X}, \tilde{\delta})$ on (H_1, A_1) to obtain $\hat{Q}_1^{opt}$.

Once the Q-functions are fitted, the estimated optimal DTR is given by $(\hat{d}_1^{opt}, \hat{d}_2^{opt})$, where the stage-specific optimal rules are given by

$$\hat{d}_2^{opt}(h_2) = \operatorname{argmax}_{(a_2,T_M)} \hat{Q}_2^{opt}(h_2,(a_2,T_M)),$$
$$\hat{d}_1^{opt}(h_1) = \operatorname{argmax}_{a_1} \hat{Q}_1^{opt}(h_1,a_1).$$

In the ε-SVR-C steps of the Q-learning algorithm, the tuning parameters C_E and γ are chosen via cross validation over a grid of values. Zhao et al. (2011) reported robustness of the procedure to relatively small values of ε; they set its value at 0.1 in their simulation study.

Zhao et al. (2011) evaluated the above method of estimating the optimal DTR with survival-type outcome in an extensive simulation study. In short, they considered a generative model, the parameters of which could be easily tweaked to reflect four different clinical scenarios resulting in four different optimal regimes. They generated data on 100 virtual patients from each of the 4 clinical scenarios, thus a total of 400 virtual patients. Then the optimal regime was estimated via Q-learning with ε-SVR-C. For evaluation purposes, an independent test sample of size 100 per clinical scenario (hence totaling 400) was also generated. Outcomes (overall survival) for these virtual test patients were evaluated for the estimated optimal regime as well as all possible (12) fixed regimes, using the generative model. Furthermore, they repeated the simulations ten times for the training sample (each of size 400). Then ten different estimated optimal regimes from these ten training samples were applied to the same test sample (of size 400) mentioned earlier. All the results for each of the 13 treatment regimes (12 fixed, plus the estimated optimal) were averaged over the 400 test patients. It was found that the true overall survival was substantially higher for the estimated optimal regime than any of the 12 fixed regimes. They also conducted additional simulations to check the sensitivity of the procedure to the sample size. It was found that for sample sizes ≥ 100, the procedure is very reliable in selecting the optimal regime.

7.3 Q-learning of DTRs for Discrete Outcomes

Moodie et al. (2013) recently tackled the challenging problem of Q-learning for discrete-valued outcomes, and took a less parametric approach to modeling the Q-functions by using generalized additive models (GAMs). Generalized additive models provide a user-friendly means to introducing greater flexibility in modeling the relationship between an outcome and covariates. GAMs are treated as penalized regression splines with different smoothing parameters allowed for each covariate, where the degree of smoothing is selected by generalized cross-validation (Wood 2006, 2011). The automatic parsimony that the approach ensures helps to control the dimensionality of the estimation problem, an important feature in the DTR setting where the covariate space is potentially very large.

Suppose we are in a setting where the outcome at the final stage is discrete, and there are no intermediate rewards. The outcome could represent, for instance, a simple indicator of success such as maintenance of viral load below a given threshold over the course of a study (a binary outcome), or the number of emergency room visits in a given period (a count, possibly Poisson-distributed). When the outcome Y is discrete, the Q-learning procedure must be adapted to respect the constraints on the outcome, for example, Y is bounded in $[0,1]$, or Y is non-negative. By definition, in a two-stage setting, we have $Q_2^{opt}(H_2, A_2) = E\left[Y \middle| H_2, A_2\right]$ at the final interval. A reasonable modeling choice would be to consider a generalized linear model (GLM). For instance, for a Bernoulli utility, we might choose a logistic model of the form $E\left[Y \middle| H_2, A_2\right] = \text{expit}\left(\beta_j^T H_{j0} + (\psi_j^T H_{j1})A_j\right)$, where $\text{expit}(x) = \exp(x)/(1+\exp(x))$ is the inverse-logit function. Similarly, for a non-negative outcome, we might choose a Poisson family GLM with the canonical link. The key is to choose a link function that is strictly increasing (or decreasing), since this allows maximization of the second-stage Q-function by a maximization of the linear specification in the mean. For example, in the binary outcome setting, since the inverse-logit function is strictly increasing, $\text{expit}\left(\beta_j^T H_{j0} + (\psi_j^T H_{j1})A_j\right)$ can be maximized by maximizing its argument, $\beta_j^T H_{j0} + (\psi_j^T H_{j1})A_j$. Therefore

$$Q_1^{opt}(H_1, A_1; \beta_1, \psi_1) = \max_{a_2} Q_2^{opt}(H_{2i}, a_2; \hat{\beta}_2, \hat{\psi}_2) = \text{expit}\left(\hat{\beta}_2^T H_{20,i} + |\hat{\psi}_2^T H_{21,i}|\right),$$

which is bounded by [0,1]. As in the continuous utility setting, the optimal regime at the first interval is defined by

$$\hat{d}_1^{opt}(h_1) = \arg\max_{a_1} Q_1^{opt}(h_1, a_1; \hat{\beta}_1, \hat{\psi}_1).$$

Continuing with the binary outcome example, we have

$$\arg\max_{a_1} Q_1^{opt}(h_1, a_1; \hat{\beta}_1, \hat{\psi}_1) = \arg\max_{a_1} \text{logit}\left(Q_1^{opt}(h_1, a_1; \hat{\beta}_1, \hat{\psi}_1)\right)$$

since the logit function is strictly increasing. We may therefore model the logit of $Q_1^{opt}(H_1, A_1; \beta_1, \psi_1)$ rather than the Q-function itself to determine the optimal DTR.

The Q-learning algorithm for a discrete outcome consists of the following steps:

1. Interval 2 parameter estimation: Using GLM regression with a strictly increasing link function, $f(\cdot)$, find estimates $(\hat{\beta}_2, \hat{\psi}_2)$ of the conditional mean model for the outcome Y, $Q_2^{opt}(H_{2i}, A_{2i}; \beta_2, \psi_2)$.
2. Interval 2 optimal rule: Set $\hat{d}_2^{opt}(h_2) = \arg\max_{a_2} Q_2^{opt}(h_2, a_2; \hat{\beta}_2, \hat{\psi}_2)$.
3. Interval 1 pseudo-outcome: Set

$$\tilde{Y}_{1i} = \max_{a_2} f(Q_2^{opt}(H_{2i}, a_2; \hat{\beta}_2, \hat{\psi}_2)), \; i = 1, \ldots, n.$$

4. Interval 1 parameter estimation: Using ordinary least squares regression, find estimates

$$(\hat{\beta}_1, \hat{\psi}_1) = \arg\min_{\beta_1, \psi_1} \frac{1}{n} \sum_{i=1}^{n} \left(\tilde{Y}_{1i} - Q_1^{opt}(H_{1i}, A_{1i}; \beta_1, \psi_1)\right)^2.$$

5. Interval 1 optimal rule: Set $\hat{d}_1^{opt}(h_1) = \arg\max_{a_1} Q_1^{opt}(h_1, a_1; \hat{\beta}_1, \hat{\psi}_1)$.

The estimated optimal DTR using Q-learning is given by $(\hat{d}_1, \hat{d}_2)$. In a binary outcome scenario, note that unlike in the continuous utility setting, the pseudo-outcome, $\tilde{Y}_{1i}$, does not represent the (expected) value of the second-interval Q-function under the optimal treatment but rather a transformation of that expected outcome.

We briefly consider a simulation study. The data for treatments (A_1, A_2), and covariates (C_1, O_1, C_2, O_2) were generated as in Sect. 3.5. We considered three outcome distributions: normal, Bernoulli, and Poisson, and two forms of the relationship between the outcome and the variables C_1 and C_2. The first setting corresponds to Scenario C of Sect. 3.5 (normal outcome, Q-functions linear in covariates); the second varies only in that a quadratic terms for C_1 and C_2 are included in the mean model. Similarly, settings three and four correspond to a Bernoulli outcome with Q-functions that are, respectively, linear and quadratic in C_1 and C_2, and the final pair of settings correspond to a Poisson outcome with Q-functions that are, respectively, linear and quadratic in the covariates. Results are presented in Table 7.1.

Overall, we observe very good performance of both the linear (correct) specification and the GAM specification of the Q-function when the true confounder-outcome relationship is linear: estimators are unbiased, and the use of the GAM for the Q-function exhibits reasonably variability even for the smaller sample size of 250. In fact the variability of the estimator resulting from a GAM for the Q-function is as low as the linear model-based estimator for the normal and Poisson outcomes, implying there is little cost for the additional flexibility in the cases. When the dependence of the utility on the confounding variables is quadratic, only the decision rule parameters resulting from a GAM for the Q-function exhibits little or no bias and good coverage rates.

Thus, it appears that Moodie et al. (2013) have taken a modest but promising step on the path to a more fully generalized Q-learning algorithm, with the consideration of a flexible, spline-based modeling approach for discrete outcomes. The next step of adapting Q-learning to allow discrete interval-specific outcomes is challenging, and remains an open problem.

7.4 Inverse Probability Weighted Estimation for Censored or Discrete Outcomes and Stochastic Treatment Regimes

Some of the seminal work in developing MSMs for DTR estimation was performed in a survival context, using inverse probability weighting combined with pooled logistic regression to approximate a Cox model for the estimation of the hazard ratio parameters (Hernán et al. 2006; Robins et al. 2008). The methods are gaining popularity in straightforward applications examining, for example, when to initiate dialysis (Sjölander et al. 2011) or antiretroviral therapy (Shepherd et al. 2010). These methods require little adaptation to the algorithm described in Sect. 5.2.2: as with continuous outcomes, data-augmentation is undertaken to create replicates of individuals that are compatible with each regime of interest. The only step that dif-

Table 7.1 Comparison of the performance Q-learning for normal, Bernoulli, and Poisson outcomes when the true Q-function is either linear or quadratic in the covariates: bias, Monte Carlo variance (MC var), Mean Squared Error (MSE) and coverage of 95 % bootstrap confidence intervals (Cover) of the first interval decision rule parameter ψ_{10}. Bias, variance, and MSE are each multiplied by 10.

Adjustment	$n = 250$				$n = 1{,}000$			
method	Bias	MC var	MSE	Cover	Bias	MC var	MSE	Cover
Normal outcome, Q-functions linear in covariates								
None	10.03	0.35	10.41	0.0	10.12	0.09	10.32	0.0
Linear	0.02	0.08	0.08	94.1	0.00	0.02	0.02	93.0
GAM	0.02	0.08	0.08	94.4	0.00	0.02	0.02	93.6
Normal outcome, Q-functions quadratic in covariates								
None	18.18	16.30	4.935	68.1	18.92	4.31	40.11	10.8
Linear	29.64	20.53	108.38	37.9	31.42	4.72	103.46	0.1
GAM	0.21	1.49	1.50	95.2	−0.11	0.40	0.40	92.7
Bernoulli outcome, Q-functions linear in covariates								
None	8.65	1.57	8.97	13.7	8.45	0.19	7.32	0.0
Linear	0.20	1.98	1.98	94.9	0.00	0.28	0.28	95.1
GAM	0.81	4.25	4.25	97.2	0.00	0.28	0.28	95.8
Bernoulli outcome, Q-functions quadratic in covariates								
None	3.77	0.65	2.07	64.8	3.71	0.15	1.53	10.8
Linear	1.54	0.87	1.11	92.5	1.56	0.20	0.44	79.7
GAM	0.06	2.63	2.63	97.2	−0.11	0.32	0.32	97.0
Poisson outcome, Q-functions linear in covariates								
None	8.97	0.70	8.74	5.6	9.49	0.23	9.23	0.0
Linear	0.14	0.11	0.11	93.9	0.14	0.02	0.03	93.8
GAM	0.13	0.11	0.11	95.7	0.14	0.02	0.03	94.5
Poisson outcome, Q-functions quadratic in covariates								
None	4.39	0.19	2.12	15.4	4.32	0.04	1.91	0.0
Linear	−1.01	0.27	0.38	90.1	−1.06	0.07	0.19	72.6
GAM	0.00	0.28	0.28	96.7	0.14	0.64	0.65	94.6

fers is the outcome regression model, which is adapted to the outcome type, using, for example a weighted Cox model or a weighted pooled logistic regression rather than weighted linear regression.

A separate but closely related body of work has focused on survival data primarily in two-phase cancer trials. In the trials which motivated the statistical developments, cancer patients were randomly assigned to one of several initial therapies and, if the initial treatments successfully induced remission, the patient was randomized to one of several maintenance therapies. A wide collection of methods have been developed in this framework, including weighted Kaplan-Meier censoring survivor curves and mean-restricted survival times (Lunceford et al. 2002), an improved estimator for the survival distribution which was shown to be the most efficient among regular, asymptotically linear estimators (Wahed and Tsiatis 2004, 2006). Log-rank tests and sample size calculations have since been developed (Feng and Wahed 2009). While these methods do address estimation of a dynamic regime of the form "what is the best initial treatment? what is the best subsequent treatment if the initial treatment fails?", these methods are typically used to select from among a small class of initial and maintenance treatment pairs, and have not been developed to select an optimal threshold from among a potentially large list of values.

The general MSM framework for DTR estimation has been further adapted to handle stochastic treatment assignment rules. For example, Cain et al. (2010) considered treatment rules which allowed for a grace period of m months in the timing of treatment initiation, i.e. a rule of the form "initiate treatment within m months of covariate O crossing threshold ψ" rather than "initiate treatment when covariate O crosses threshold ψ".

7.5 Estimating a DTR for a Binary Outcome Using a Likelihood Approach

Thall and colleagues have considered DTRs in several cancer treatment settings, where the typical treatment paradigm is "play the winner, drop the loser" (Thall et al. 2000): a patient given an initial course of a treatment will continue to receive that treatment if it is deemed to be sufficiently successful (e.g. due to partial tumor shrinkage or partial remission), will be switched to a maintenance therapy or follow-up if completely successful, and will be switched to an alternative treatment (sometimes referred to as a salvage therapy) if the initial treatment is unsuccessful. The definition of success on a particular course of treatment may depend on which course it is. For example, in prostate cancer, a success on the first course of treatment requires a decrease of at least 40 % in the cancer biomarker prostate-specific antigen (PSA) from baseline, while success in the second course requires a decrease of at least 80 % in PSA from the baseline value (and, in both cases, no evidence of disease progression).

In a prostate cancer treatment trial, Thall et al. (2000) took a parametric approach to estimating the best sequence of treatments with the goal of maximizing the probability of successful treatment, where success is a binary variable. Four treatment courses were considered. Patients were randomized to one of the four treatments, and if treatment failed, randomized to one of the remaining three options. That is, $\mathscr{A}_1 = \{1,2,3,4\}$ and $\mathscr{A}_2 = \mathscr{A}_1 \setminus a_1$ (where a_1 is the treatment actually given at the first stage). A patient was switched from a treatment after the first failure, or deemed to have had a successful therapy following two successful courses of the same treatment. Thus, the trial can be viewed as a two-stage trial in which patients can have at least one and at most two courses of treatment in the first stage, and at most two courses of treatment in the second stage for a total two to four courses of treatment.

The optimizing criterion for determining the best DTR was the probability of successful therapy. That is, the goal was to maximize $\xi(a,a') = \xi_a + (1-\xi_a)\xi_{a'|a}$, where ξ_a is the probability of a patient success in the first two courses with initial treatment a and $\xi_{a'|a}$ is the probability that the patient has two successful courses with treatment a' following initial (unsuccessful) treatment with a, i.e. under treatment strategy (a,a'). Parametric conditional probability models were posited to obtain estimates of $\xi(a,a')$ that were allowed to depend on the patient's state and treatment history. For example, letting Y_j take the value 1 if a patient experiences successful treatment on the jth course and 0 otherwise, patient outcomes through the first two courses of therapy can be characterized by the following probabilities:

$$\theta_1(a) = P(Y_1 = 1|A_1 = a)$$
$$\theta_2(1;(a,a)) = P(Y_2 = 1|Y_1 = 1, A_1 = A_2 = a)$$
$$\theta_2(0;(a',a)) = P(Y_2 = 1|Y_1 = 0, A_1 = a', A_2 = a)$$

which gives $\xi_a = \theta_1(a)\theta_2(1;(a,a))$. Logistic regression models were proposed for the above probabilities, i.e. logit(θ_j) were modeled as linear functions of treatment and covariate histories for each of the j courses of treatment. These probability models can be extended to depend on state variables such as initial disease severity as well. Once all these models are fitted, one can pick the best DTR, i.e. the best treatment pair (a,a') that maximizes the overall success probability $\xi(a,a')$.

7.6 Discussion

In this chapter, we have considered the estimation of DTRs for a variety of outcome types, including multi-dimensional continuous outcomes, time-to-event outcomes in the presence of censoring, as well as discrete outcomes. Methods used in the literature for such data include Q-learning, marginal structural models, and a fully parametric, likelihood-based approach. In the context of Q-learning, modeling of time-to-event data has been accomplished using accelerated failure time models (with censoring handled by inverse probability weighting) and using the less parametric approach of support vector regression. For discrete outcomes, Q-learning has also been combined with generalized additive models selected by generalized cross-validation, with promising results. The MSM approach has been implemented for discrete failure times only, but can easily be used in a continuous-time setting using a marginal structural Cox model. G-estimation can also be employed assuming an AFT (see Mark and Robins 1993; Hernán et al. 2005) to estimate DTRs, however the approach remains under-utilized, perhaps because of the relative lack of standard software with which it can be implemented.

Chapter 8
Inference and Non-regularity

Inference plays a key role in almost all statistical problems. In the context of DTRs, one can think of inference for mainly two types of quantities: (i) inference for the parameters indexing the optimal regime; and (ii) inference for the value function (mean outcome) of a regime – either a regime that was pre-specified, or one that was estimated. The literature contains several instances of estimation and inference for the value functions of one or more pre-specified regimes (Lunceford et al. 2002; Wahed and Tsiatis 2004, 2006; Thall et al. 2000, 2002, 2007a). However there has been relatively little work on inference for the value function of an estimated policy, mainly due to the difficulty of the problem.

Constructing confidence intervals (CIs) for the parameters indexing the optimal regime is important for the following reasons. First, if the CIs for some of these parameters contain zero, then perhaps the corresponding components of the patient history need not be collected to make optimal decisions using the estimated DTR. This has the potential to reduce the cost of data collection in a future implementation of the estimated optimal DTR. Thus in the present context, CIs can be viewed as a tool – albeit one that is not very sophisticated – for doing variable selection. Such CIs can be useful in exploratory data analysis when trying to interactively find a suitable model for, say, the Q-functions. Second, note that when linear models are used for the Q-functions, the difference in predicted mean outcomes corresponding to two treatments, e.g. a contrast of Q-functions or a blip function, becomes a linear combination of the parameters indexing the optimal regime. Point-wise CIs for these linear combinations can be constructed over a range of values of the history variables based on the CIs for individual parameters. These CIs can dictate when there is insufficient support in the data to recommend one treatment over another; in such cases treatment decisions can be made based on other considerations, e.g. cost, familiarity, burden, preference etc.

An additional complication in inference for the parameters indexing the optimal regime arises because of a phenomenon called *non-regularity*. It was Robins (2004) who first considered the problem of inference for the parameters of the optimal DTR in the context of G-estimation. As originally discussed by Robins, the treatment effect parameters at any stage prior to the last can be *non-regular* under

B. Chakraborty and E.E.M. Moodie, *Statistical Methods for Dynamic Treatment Regimes*, Statistics for Biology and Health 76, DOI 10.1007/978-1-4614-7428-9_8,

certain longitudinal distributions of the data. By non-regularity, we mean that the asymptotic distribution of the estimator of the treatment effect parameter does not converge uniformly over the parameter space; see below for further details. This technical phenomenon of non-regularity has considerable practical consequences; it often causes bias in estimation, and leads to poor frequentist properties of Wald-type or other standard confidence intervals. Any inference technique that aims to provide good frequentist properties such as appropriate Type I error and nominal coverage of confidence intervals has to address the problem of non-regularity. In this chapter, we consider various approaches to inference in the context of Q-learning and G-estimation.

8.1 Inference for the Parameters Indexing the Optimal Regime Under Regularity

All of the recursive methods of estimation considered in previous chapters, including Q-learning and G-estimation, can be viewed as two-step (substitution) estimators at each stage. At stage j, the first step of estimation requires finding the effect of treatment at all future stages, and then substituting these into the stage j estimating equation in order to find the estimator of ψ_j. For example, in the Q-learning context, for a two-stage example, the pseudo-outcome at the first stage equals $\hat{Y}_{1i} = Y_{1i} + \max_{a_2} Q_2^{opt}(H_{2i}, a_2; \hat{\beta}_2, \hat{\psi}_2)$ which relies on estimators of β_2 and ψ_2. Similarly, in the recursive implementation of G-estimation, the stage-1 estimating function includes $G_{\text{mod},1}(\psi_1) = Y + \left[\gamma_1(h_1, d_1^{opt}; \psi_1) - \gamma_1(h_1, a_1; \psi_1)\right] + \left[\gamma_2(h_2, d_2^{opt}; \hat{\psi}_2) - \gamma_2(h_2, a_2; \hat{\psi}_2)\right]$, which requires estimators of ψ_2 (as well as estimators of propensity score model parameters). At each stage, the decision rule parameters for that particular stage are treated as parameters of interest, and any other parameters including those for treatment models or subsequent treatment stages are considered nuisance parameters.

Newey and McFadden (1994) provide a discussion of the impact of the first-step estimation on the standard errors of the second-step estimates. Van der Laan and Robins (2003) also discuss the issue of second-step estimates' standard errors, arriving at the same standard error as Newey and McFadden found by a different, more measure-theoretic approach. We briefly review the theory of variance derivations for estimating equations, and apply these methods to Q-learning and G-estimation. Throughout this section, we consider only regular estimators, which in the DTR context implies that there is a unique optimal treatment for each possible treatment and covariate history at each stage. We will then consider the more challenging problem of non-regular estimators in Sect. 8.2 and subsequent sections.

8.1.1 A Brief Review of Variances for Estimating Equations

In this section, we provide a concise overview of the theory of estimating equations, since most methods of estimation discussed in this book are *M-estimators*, i.e. estimators which can be obtained as the minima of sums of functions of the data or are roots of an estimating function. In particular, as implemented in previous chapters, Q-learning and G-estimation are both M-estimators. This development will enable us to derive and discuss measures of variability and confidence of the estimators of decision rule parameters more precisely.

A function of the parameter and data, $U_n(\theta) = U_n(\theta, Y) = \mathbb{P}_n U(\theta, Y_i)$, which is of the same dimensionality as the parameter θ for which $E[U_n(\theta)] = 0$ is considered. $U_n(\theta)$ is said to be an *estimating function* (EF), and $\hat{\theta}$ is an *EF estimator* if it is a solution to the *estimating equation* $U_n(\theta) = 0$. That is, $\hat{\theta}$ is an EF estimator if $U_n(\hat{\theta}) = 0$. Note that the EF $U_n(\theta, Y)$ is itself a random variable, since it is a function of the random variable Y. To perform inference, we derive the frequency properties of the EF and can then transfer these properties to the resultant estimator with the help of a Taylor approximation and the delta method. Excellent resources on asymptotic theory of statistics are given by Van der Vaart (1998) and Ferguson (1996); or for a particular focus on semi-parametric methods, see Bickel et al. (1993) and Tsiatis (2006).

The corresponding estimating equation that defines the estimator $\hat{\theta}$ has the form

$$U_n(\hat{\theta}) = U_n(\hat{\theta}, Y) = \mathbb{P}_n U(\hat{\theta}, Y_i) = 0. \tag{8.1}$$

The estimating Eq. (8.1) is said to be unbiased if $E[U_n(\theta)] = 0$, and so

$$\begin{aligned} Var[U_n(\theta)] &= E\left[(U_n(\theta) - E[U_n(\theta)])(U_n(\theta) - E[U_n(\theta)])^T\right] \\ &= E[U_n(\theta)U_n(\theta)^T], \end{aligned}$$

which converges to some matrix Σ_U. Further, $U_n(\theta)$ is a sum of conditionally independent terms, so under standard regularity conditions

$$U_n(\theta) \rightarrow_d \mathcal{N}(0, \Sigma_U). \tag{8.2}$$

Using a first order Taylor expansion, we find

$$0 = U_n(\hat{\theta}_n) = U_n(\theta) + \left(\frac{\partial U_n(\theta)}{\partial \theta}\right)(\hat{\theta} - \theta) + o_p(1).$$

This gives that $(\hat{\theta} - \theta) = -\left(\frac{\partial U_n(\theta)}{\partial \theta}\right)^{-1} U_n(\theta) + o_p(1)$. From this, we can deduce that $\hat{\theta} \rightarrow_p \theta$ and

$$\sqrt{n}\,(\hat{\theta} - \theta) \rightarrow_d \mathrm{N}_p(0, A^{-1}\Sigma_U (A^T)^{-1}) \tag{8.3}$$

where $A = -E\left[\frac{\partial}{\partial\theta}U_n(\boldsymbol{\theta})\right]$. That is, $\hat{\boldsymbol{\theta}}$ is a consistent and asymptotically normally distributed estimator. The form of the variance in expression (8.3) has led to it being called the *sandwich estimator*, where A forms the "bread" and $\boldsymbol{\Sigma}_U$ is the "filling" of the sandwich.

It follows from Eq. (8.3) that $\sqrt{n}\boldsymbol{\Sigma}_{\hat{\theta}}^{-1/2}(\hat{\boldsymbol{\theta}} - \boldsymbol{\theta}) \rightarrow_d \mathrm{N}_p(0, \mathbf{I}_p)$ where $\boldsymbol{\Sigma}_{\hat{\theta}} = A^{-1}\boldsymbol{\Sigma}_U(A^T)^{-1}$ and $\mathbf{I}_p$ is the $p \times p$ identity matrix, implying that confidence intervals can be constructed, and significance tests performed, using a Wald statistic of the form $\sqrt{n}\boldsymbol{\Sigma}_{\hat{\theta}}^{-1/2}\hat{\boldsymbol{\theta}}$. In a more familiar form, this would give, for example, a 95 % confidence interval of $\hat{\boldsymbol{\theta}} \pm 1.96SE(\hat{\boldsymbol{\theta}})$ for a scalar-valued parameter $\boldsymbol{\theta}$ (for p-dimensional parameter $\boldsymbol{\theta}$, one can similarly construct component-wise CIs) and a test statistic $W = \sqrt{n}\boldsymbol{\Sigma}_{\hat{\theta}}^{-1/2}\hat{\boldsymbol{\theta}}$.

Confidence intervals for $\boldsymbol{\theta}$ can also be constructed directly using the EF and its standard error. From Eq. (8.2), we have $\boldsymbol{\Sigma}_U^{-1/2}U_n(\boldsymbol{\theta}) \rightarrow_d \mathcal{N}(0, \mathbf{I}_p)$. It is therefore the case that we can construct a *score* or *Rao* interval by searching for values $\boldsymbol{\theta}$ that satisfy $|\boldsymbol{\Sigma}_U^{-1/2}U_n(\boldsymbol{\theta})| \leq 1.96$. Unlike the Wald intervals, which rely only on the value of the estimated parameter and its standard error, score-based intervals may be more computationally burdensome as they may require a search over the space of $\boldsymbol{\theta}$. However, score-based intervals may exhibit better finite sample properties even when standard regularity conditions do not hold, since these intervals do not require derivatives of the EF (Robins 2004; Moodie and Richardson 2010).

Now suppose that $\boldsymbol{\theta}$ is vector-valued and can be partitioned such that $\boldsymbol{\theta} = (\boldsymbol{\psi}^T, \boldsymbol{\beta}^T)^T$ where $\boldsymbol{\psi}$ is of interest, and $\boldsymbol{\beta}$ contains nuisance parameters (such as, for example, parameters associated with predictive variables in Q-learning, or parameters from a propensity score model in G-estimation). If interest lies in performing significance tests about $\boldsymbol{\psi}$ leaving $\boldsymbol{\beta}$ unspecified, i.e. in testing null hypotheses of the form

$$\mathcal{H}_0 : \boldsymbol{\psi} = \boldsymbol{\psi}_0, \boldsymbol{\beta} = \text{`anything'}$$

versus the alternative hypothesis

$$\mathcal{H}_A : (\boldsymbol{\psi}, \boldsymbol{\beta}) \neq (\boldsymbol{\psi}_0, \boldsymbol{\beta})$$

then we have what is called a *composite* null hypothesis. Suppose further that the EF $U_n(\boldsymbol{\theta})$ can be decomposed into $U_n(\boldsymbol{\theta}) = \begin{pmatrix} U_n(\boldsymbol{\psi}) \\ U_n(\boldsymbol{\beta}) \end{pmatrix}$.

To derive the correct variance for the composite null hypothesis, consider a Taylor expansion of $U_n(\boldsymbol{\psi})$ about the limiting value, $\boldsymbol{\beta}$, of a consistent estimator, $\hat{\boldsymbol{\beta}}$, of the nuisance parameter $\boldsymbol{\beta}$:

$$U_{\text{adj}}(\boldsymbol{\psi}) = U_n(\boldsymbol{\psi}) + \left[\frac{\partial}{\partial\boldsymbol{\beta}}U_n(\boldsymbol{\psi})\right](\hat{\boldsymbol{\beta}} - \boldsymbol{\beta}) + o_p(1) \tag{8.4}$$

$$= U_n(\boldsymbol{\psi}) - \left[\frac{\partial}{\partial\boldsymbol{\beta}}U_n(\boldsymbol{\psi})\right]\left[\frac{\partial}{\partial\boldsymbol{\beta}}U_n(\boldsymbol{\beta})\right]^{-1}U_n(\boldsymbol{\beta}) + o_p(1). \tag{8.5}$$

From Eq. (8.4), it can be seen that $E[U_n(\psi)] = E[U_{\text{adj}}(\psi)]$ so $U_{\text{adj}}(\psi)$ is an unbiased EF; Eq. (8.5) follows from Eq. (8.4) via a substitution from a Taylor expansion of the EF for β about its limiting value. From Eq. (8.5), we can derive the asymptotic distribution of the parameter of interest ψ to be

$$\sqrt{n}\,(\hat{\psi} - \psi) \to_d \mathrm{N}_p(0, \Sigma_{\hat{\psi}})$$

where $\Sigma_{\hat{\psi}} = A_{\text{adj}}^{-1} \Sigma_{U_{\text{adj}}} (A_{\text{adj}}^T)^{-1}$ is the asymptotic variance of $\hat{\psi}$ with A_{adj} the probability limit of $-E\left[\frac{\partial}{\partial \psi} U_{\text{adj}}(\psi)\right]$ and $\Sigma_{U_{\text{adj}}}$ is the probability limit of $E\left[U_{\text{adj}}(\psi) U_{\text{adj}}(\psi)^T\right]$. Note that $\hat{\psi}$ is the substitution estimator defined by finding the solution to the EF where an estimate of the (vector) nuisance parameter $\hat{\beta}$ has been plugged into the equation in place of the true value, β.

It is interesting to consider the variance of the substitution estimator $\hat{\psi}$ with the estimator, say $\tilde{\psi}$, that would result from plugging in the true value of the nuisance parameter (a feasible estimator only when such true values are known). That is, we may wish to consider $\Sigma_{\hat{\psi}}$ and $\Sigma_{\tilde{\psi}}$. It turns out that no general statement regarding the two estimators' variances can be made, however there are special cases in which relationships can be derived (see Henmi and Eguchi (2004) for a geometric consideration of EF which serves to elucidate the variance relationships). For example, if the EF is the score function for θ in a parametric model, there is a cost (in terms of information loss or variance inflation) that is incurred for having to estimate the nuisance parameters. In contrast, in the semi-parametric setting where the score functions for ψ and β are orthogonal and that the score function is used as the EF for β, it can be shown that $\Sigma_{\tilde{\psi}} - \Sigma_{\hat{\psi}}$ is positive definite. That is, efficiency is *gained* by estimating rather than knowing the nuisance parameter β.

8.1.2 Asymptotic Variance for Q-learning Estimators

We now apply the theory of the previous section to Q-learning for the case where we use linear models parameterized by $\theta_j = (\psi_j, \beta_j)$ of the form $Q_j^{opt}(H_j, A_j; \beta_j, \psi_j) = \beta_j^T H_{j0} + (\psi_j^T H_{j1}) A_j$. For simplicity of exposition, we will focus on the two-stage setting, but extensions to the general, K-stage setting follow directly. Following the algorithm for Q-learning outlined in Sect. 3.4.1, we begin with a regression of Y_2 using the model $Q_2^{opt}(H_2, A_2; \beta_2, \psi_2) = \beta_2^T H_{20} + (\psi_2^T H_{21}) A_2$. Letting X_2 denote $(H_{20}, H_{21} A_2)$, this gives a linear regression of the familiar form $E[Y_2|X_2] = X_2 \theta_2$, with $Var[\hat{\theta}_2] = (X_2^T X_2)^{-1} \sigma^2$ where σ^2 denotes the variance of the residuals $Y_2 - X_2 \theta_2$. Confidence intervals can then be formed, and significance tests performed, for the vector parameter θ_2. If composite tests of the form $\mathscr{H}_0 : \psi_2 = 0$ are desired, hypothesizing that the variables contained in H_{21} are not significantly useful tailoring variables without specifying any hypothesized values for the value of β_2, then the Wald statistic should be scaled using $\mathscr{I}_{\psi_2 \psi_2 \cdot \beta_2}^{1/2} = (\mathscr{I}_{\psi_2 \psi_2} - \mathscr{I}_{\psi_2 \beta_2} \mathscr{I}_{\beta_2 \beta_2}^{-1} \mathscr{I}_{\beta_2 \psi_2})^{1/2}$, where

$$\begin{pmatrix} \mathscr{I}_{\psi_2\psi_2} & \mathscr{I}_{\psi_2\beta_2} \\ \mathscr{I}_{\beta_2\psi_2} & \mathscr{I}_{\beta_2\beta_2} \end{pmatrix}$$

is a block-diagonal matrix decomposition of the information of the regression parameters at the second stage, and similarly $\mathscr{I}^{1/2}_{\psi_2\psi_2\cdot\beta_2}$ should be used to determine the limits of a confidence interval.

Now, let us consider the first-stage estimator. First stage estimation proceeds by first forming the pseudo-outcome $Y_1 + \beta_2^T H_{20} + |\psi_2^T H_{21}|$, which we implement in practice using the estimate $\hat{Y}_1 = Y_1 + \hat{\beta}_2^T H_{20} + |\hat{\psi}_2^T H_{21}|$, and regressing this on $(H_{10}, H_{11}A_1)$ using the model $Q_1^{opt}(H_1, A_1; \beta_1, \psi_1) = \beta_1^T H_{10} + (\psi_1^T H_{11})A_1$. This two-stage regression-based estimation can be viewed as an estimating equation based procedure as follows. Define

$$\begin{aligned} U_{2,n}(\theta_2) &= \mathbb{P}_n\Big(Y_2 - Q_2^{opt}(H_2, A_2; \beta_2, \psi_2)\Big)\Big(\frac{\partial}{\partial\theta_2} Q_2^{opt}(H_2, A_2; \beta_2, \psi_2)\Big) \\ &= \mathbb{P}_n\Big(Y_2 - \beta_2^T H_{20} - (\psi_2^T H_{21})A_2\Big)(H_{20}^T, H_{21}^T A_2)^T, \\ U_{1,n}(\theta_1, \theta_2) &= \mathbb{P}_n\Big(Y_1 + \max_{A_2} Q_2^{opt}(H_2, A_2; \beta_2, \psi_2) - \\ &\qquad Q_1^{opt}(H_1, A_1; \beta_1, \psi_1)\Big)\Big(\frac{\partial}{\partial\theta_1} Q_1^{opt}(H_1, A_1; \beta_1, \psi_1)\Big) \\ &= \mathbb{P}_n\Big(Y_1 + \beta_2^T H_{20} + |\psi_2^T H_{21}| - \beta_1^T H_{10} - (\psi_1^T H_{11})A_1\Big)(H_{10}^T, H_{11}^T A_1)^T. \end{aligned}$$

Then the (joint) estimating equation for all the parameters from both stages of Q-learning is given by

$$\begin{pmatrix} U_{2,n}(\theta_2) \\ U_{1,n}(\theta_1, \theta_2) \end{pmatrix} = 0.$$

At the first stage, then, both the main effect parameters β_1 and all second stage parameters can be considered nuisance parameters. Collecting these into a single vector $\beta_1^\sharp = (\beta_1, \beta_2, \psi_2)$, we use a similar form to above, forming Wald test statistics or CIs for the tailoring variable parameters using $\mathscr{I}^{1/2}_{\psi_1\psi_1\cdot\beta_1^\sharp} = (\mathscr{I}_{\psi_1\psi_1} - \mathscr{I}_{\psi_1\beta_1^\sharp}\mathscr{I}^{-1}_{\beta_1^\sharp\beta_1^\sharp}\mathscr{I}_{\beta_1^\sharp\psi_1})^{1/2}$, where

$$\begin{pmatrix} \mathscr{I}_{\psi_1\psi_1} & \mathscr{I}_{\psi_1\beta_1^\sharp} \\ \mathscr{I}_{\beta_1^\sharp\psi_1} & \mathscr{I}_{\beta_1^\sharp\beta_1^\sharp} \end{pmatrix}$$

is a block-diagonal matrix decomposition of the inverse-variance of all parameters.

8.1.3 Asymptotic Variance for G-estimators

The variance of the optimal decision rule parameters $\hat{\psi}$ must adjust for the plug-in estimates of nuisance parameters in the estimating function of Eq. (4.3), $U(\psi) = \sum_{i=1}^{n}\sum_{j=1}^{K} U_j(\psi_j, \hat{\varsigma}_j(\psi_j), \hat{\alpha}_j)$. In the derivations that follow, we assume the parameters are not shared between stages, however the calculations are similar in the shared-parameter setting. Second derivatives of the estimating functions for all parameters are needed, and thus we require that each subject's optimal regime must be unique at every stage except possibly the first. If for any individual, the optimal treatment is not unique, then it is the case that $\gamma_j(h_j, a_j) = 0$, or equivalently that for a Q-function $\beta_j^T H_{j0} + (\psi_j^T H_{j1})(A_j + 1)/2$, $\psi_j^T H_{j1} = 0$. Provided the rule is unique, then the estimating functions used in each stage of estimation for G-estimation will be differentiable and so the asymptotic variance can be determined.

Robins (2004) derives the variance of $U(\psi, \varsigma(\psi), \alpha)$ by performing a first order Taylor expansion of the function about the limiting values of $\hat{\varsigma}(\psi)$ and $\hat{\alpha}$, ς and α:

$$
\begin{aligned}
U_{\text{adj}}(\psi) = U(\psi, \varsigma, \alpha) + E\left[\frac{\partial}{\partial \varsigma} U(\psi, \varsigma, \alpha)\right](\hat{\varsigma}(\psi) - \varsigma) + \\
E\left[\frac{\partial}{\partial \alpha} U(\psi, \varsigma, \alpha)\right](\hat{\alpha} - \alpha) + o_p(1)
\end{aligned}
$$

to obtain the adjusted G-estimating function, $U_{\text{adj}}(\psi)$, which estimates the parameters from all stages $j = 1, \ldots, K$ simultaneously. Of course, with the limiting values of the nuisance parameters unknown, this expression does not provide a practical EF. If $\dot{l}_\alpha$ and $\dot{l}_\varsigma$ denote the (score) EF for the treatment model and expected counterfactual model nuisance parameters, respectively, then we can again apply a Taylor expansion to find

$$
\begin{aligned}
\hat{\alpha} - \alpha &= -\left(E\left[\frac{\partial}{\partial \alpha}\dot{l}_\alpha(\alpha)\right]\right)^{-1} \dot{l}_\alpha(\alpha) + o_p(1), \\
\hat{\varsigma}(\psi) - \varsigma &= -\left(E\left[\frac{\partial}{\partial \varsigma}\dot{l}_\varsigma(\varsigma)\right]\right)^{-1} \dot{l}_\varsigma(\varsigma) + o_p(1).
\end{aligned}
$$

This gives

$$
\begin{aligned}
U_{\text{adj}}(\psi) = U(\psi, \varsigma, \alpha) - E\left[\frac{\partial}{\partial \varsigma} U(\psi, \varsigma, \alpha)\right]\left(E\left[\frac{\partial}{\partial \varsigma}\dot{l}_\varsigma(\varsigma)\right]\right)^{-1} \dot{l}_\varsigma(\varsigma) \\
- E\left[\frac{\partial}{\partial \alpha} U(\psi, \varsigma, \alpha)\right] E\left[\frac{\partial}{\partial \alpha}\dot{l}_\alpha(\alpha)\right]^{-1} \dot{l}_\alpha(\alpha).
\end{aligned}
$$

Thus the estimating function has variance $E[U_{\text{adj}}(\psi)^{\otimes 2}] = E[U_{\text{adj}}(\psi) U_{\text{adj}}(\psi)^T]$. It follows that the variance of the blip function parameters which index the decision rules, $\hat{\psi} = (\hat{\psi}_1^T, \hat{\psi}_2^T, \ldots, \hat{\psi}_K^T)^T$, is given by

$$\Sigma_{\hat{\psi}} = E\left[\left\{\left(E\left[\frac{\partial}{\partial\psi}U_{\text{adj}}(\psi,\varsigma,\alpha)\right]\right)^{-1}U_{\text{adj}}(\psi,\varsigma,\alpha)\right\}^{\otimes 2}\right].$$

Suppose at each of two stages, p different parameters are estimated. Then $\Sigma_{\hat{\psi}}$ is the $(2p)\times(2p)$ covariance matrix

$$\Sigma_{\hat{\psi}} = \begin{pmatrix} \Sigma_{\hat{\psi}}^{(11)} & \Sigma_{\hat{\psi}}^{(12)} \\ \Sigma_{\hat{\psi}}^{(21)} & \Sigma_{\hat{\psi}}^{(22)} \end{pmatrix}.$$

The $p\times p$ covariance matrix of $\hat{\psi}_2 = (\hat{\psi}_{20},\ldots,\hat{\psi}_{2(p-1)})$ that accounts for using the substitution estimates $\hat{\varsigma}_2$ and $\hat{\alpha}_2$ is $\Sigma_{\hat{\psi}}^{(22)}$, and accounting for substituting $\hat{\psi}_2$ as well as $\hat{\varsigma}_1$ and $\hat{\alpha}_1$ to estimate ψ_1 gives the $p\times p$ covariance matrix $\Sigma_{\hat{\psi}}^{(11)}$ for $\hat{\psi}_1 = (\hat{\psi}_{10},\ldots,\hat{\psi}_{1(p-1)})$.

However, as shown in Sect. 4.3.1, parameters can be estimated separately at each stage using G-estimation recursively at each stage. In such a case, it is possible to estimate the variances $\Sigma_{\hat{\psi}}^{(22)}$ and $\Sigma_{\hat{\psi}}^{(11)}$ of the stage-specific parameters recursively as well (Moodie 2009a). The development for the estimation of the diagonal components, $\Sigma_{\hat{\psi}}^{(jj)}$, of the covariance matrix $\Sigma_{\hat{\psi}}$ will be undertaken in a two-stage setting, but the extension to the K stage case follows directly.

Let $U_{\text{adj},1}(\psi_1,\psi_2)$ and $U_{\text{adj},2}(\psi_2)$ denote, respectively, the first and second components of $U_{\text{adj}}(\psi)$. At the second stage, use $U_{\text{adj},2}$ to calculate $\Sigma_{\hat{\psi}}^{(22)}$. To find the covariance matrix of $\hat{\psi}_1$, use a Taylor expansion of $U_1(\psi_1,\hat{\psi}_2,\hat{\varsigma}_1(\psi_1),\hat{\alpha}_1)$ about the limiting values of the nuisance parameters $(\psi_2,\varsigma_1,\alpha_1)$. After some simplification, this gives:

$$\begin{aligned} U_{\text{adj},1}^{\varepsilon}(\psi_1,\psi_2) = U_{\text{adj},1}(\psi_1,\psi_2) - E\left[\frac{\partial}{\partial\psi_2}U_1(\psi_1,\psi_2,\varsigma_1,\alpha_1)\right]\cdot \\ \left(E\left[\frac{\partial}{\partial\psi_2}U_{\text{adj},2}(\psi_2,\varsigma_2,\alpha_2)\right]\right)^{-1}U_{\text{adj},2}(\psi_2,\varsigma_2,\alpha_2) \\ +o_p(1). \end{aligned}$$

It then follows that $\sqrt{n}(\hat{\psi}_1-\psi_1)$ converges in distribution to

$$N\left(0,E\left[\left\{\left(E\left[\frac{\partial}{\partial\psi_1}U_{\text{adj},1}^{\varepsilon}\right]\right)^{-1}U_{\text{adj},1}^{\varepsilon}\right\}^{\otimes 2}\right]\right).$$

Thus, the diagonal components of $\Sigma_{\hat{\psi}}$ are obtained using a more tractable calculation.

Note that if there are $K>2$ stages, the similar derivations can be used, but require the use of $K-j$ adjustment terms to $U_{\text{adj},j}$ for the estimation and substitution of all future decision rule parameters, $\psi_{j+1},\ldots,\psi_K$. Note that $U_{\text{adj}}^{\varepsilon}$ and U_{adj}

produce numerically the same variance estimate at each stage: that is, the recursive variance calculation simply provides a more convenient and less computationally intensive approach by taking advantage of known independences (i.e. zeros in the matrix of derivatives of $U(\psi)$ with respect to ψ) which arise because decision rules do not share parameters at different stages. The asymptotic variances can lead to coverage below the nominal level in small samples, but perform well for samples of size 1,000 or greater in regular settings where differentiability of the EFs holds (Moodie 2009a).

8.1.4 Projection Confidence Intervals

Berger and Boos (1994) and Berger (1996) proposed a general method for constructing valid hypothesis tests in the presence of a nuisance parameter. One can develop an asymptotically exact confidence interval for the stage 1 parameter ψ_1 by inverting these hypothesis tests, based on the following nuisance parameter formulation. As we have noted above, many DTR parameter estimators are obtained via substitution because the true value of the stage 2 parameter ψ_2 is unknown and must be estimated (see Sect. 8.2 for details). Instead, if the true value of ψ_2 were known a priori, the asymptotic distribution of $\sqrt{n}(\hat{\psi}_1 - \psi_1)$ would be *regular* (in fact, normal), and standard procedures could be used to construct an asymptotically valid confidence interval although performance of such asymptotic variance estimators may be poor in small samples. Thus, while ψ_2 is not of primary interest for analyzing stage 1 decisions, it nevertheless plays an essential role in the asymptotic distribution of $\sqrt{n}(\hat{\psi}_1 - \psi_1)$. In this sense, ψ_2 is a nuisance parameter. This idea was used by Robins (2004) to construct a projection confidence interval for ψ_1.

The basic idea is as follows. Let $\mathscr{S}_{n,1-\alpha}(\psi_2)$ denote an asymptotically exact confidence interval for ψ_1 if ψ_2 were known, i.e., $P(\psi_1 \in \mathscr{S}_{n,1-\alpha}(\psi_2)) = 1-\alpha+o_P(1)$. Of course, the exact value of ψ_2 is not known, but since $\sqrt{n}(\hat{\psi}_2 - \psi_2)$ is regular and asymptotically normal, it is straightforward to construct a $(1-\varepsilon)$ asymptotic confidence interval for ψ_2, say $\mathscr{C}_{n,1-\varepsilon}$, for arbitrary $\varepsilon > 0$. Then, it follows that $\bigcup_{\gamma \in \mathscr{C}_{n,1-\varepsilon}} \mathscr{S}_{n,1-\alpha}(\gamma)$ is a $(1-\alpha-\varepsilon)$ confidence interval for ψ_1. To see this, note that

$$P\Big(\psi_1 \in \bigcup_{\gamma \in \mathscr{C}_{n,1-\varepsilon}} \mathscr{S}_{n,1-\alpha}(\gamma)\Big) \geq 1-\alpha+o_P(1)+P\big(\psi_2 \notin \mathscr{C}_{n,1-\varepsilon}\big) = 1-\alpha-\varepsilon+o_P(1). \tag{8.6}$$

Thus, the projection confidence interval is the union of the confidence intervals $\mathscr{S}_{n,1-\alpha}(\gamma)$ over all values $\gamma \in \mathscr{C}_{n,1-\varepsilon}$, and is an asymptotically valid $(1-\alpha-\varepsilon)$ confidence interval for ψ_1. The main downside of this approach is that it is potentially highly conservative. Also, its implementation can be computationally highly expensive.

8.2 Exceptional Laws and Non-regularity of the Parameters Indexing the Optimal Regime

The cumulative distribution function of the observed longitudinal data is said to be *exceptional* if, at some stage j, the optimal treatment decision depends on at least one component of covariate and treatment history *and* the probability that the optimal rule is not unique is positive (Robins 2004). The combination of three factors makes a law exceptional: (i) the form of the blip or Q-function model, (ii) the true value of the blip model parameters, and (iii) the distribution of treatments and state variables. For a law to be exceptional, then, condition (i) requires the blip or Q-function model to depend on at least one covariate such as prior treatment; conditions (ii) and (iii) require that the model takes the value zero with positive probability, that is, there is some subset of the population in which the optimal treatment is not unique. Exceptional laws may commonly arise in practice: under the hypothesis of no treatment effect, for a blip or Q-function that includes at least one component of treatment and state variable history, every distribution is an exceptional law. More generally, it may be the case that a treatment is ineffective in a sub-group of the population under study. Exceptional laws give rise to non-regular estimators.

The issue of non-regularity can be better understood with a simple but instructive example discussed by Robins (2004). Consider the problem of estimating $|\mu|$ based on n i.i.d. observations $X_1,\ldots,X_n$ from $\mathcal{N}(\mu,1)$. Note that $|\bar{X}_n|$ is the maximum likelihood estimator of $|\mu|$, where $\bar{X}_n$ is the sample average. It can be shown that the asymptotic distribution of $\sqrt{n}(|\bar{X}_n|-|\mu|)$ for $\mu=0$ is different from that for $\mu\neq 0$, and more importantly, the change in the distribution at $\mu=0$ happens abruptly. Thus $|\bar{X}_n|$ is a non-regular estimator of $|\mu|$. Also, for $\mu=0$,

$$\lim_{n\to\infty} E[\sqrt{n}(|\bar{X}_n|-|\mu|)] = \sqrt{\frac{2}{\pi}}.$$

Robins referred to this quantity as the *asymptotic bias* of the estimator $|\bar{X}_n|$. This asymptotic bias is one symptom of the underlying non-regularity, as discussed by Moodie and Richardson (2010).

We can graphically illustrate the asymptotic bias resulting from non-regularity using a class of generative models in which exceptional laws arise (see Sect. 8.8 for details). Thus there are many combinations of parameters that lead to (near-) non-regularity, and thereby bias in the parameter estimates. Hence it makes sense to study the prevalence and magnitude of bias over regions of the parameter space.

Moodie and Richardson (2010) employed a convenient way to study this bias in the context of G-estimation and the associated hard-threshold estimators using bias maps. We employ the same technique here in the Q-learning context; see Fig. 8.1. Bias maps show the absolute bias in $\hat{\psi}_{10}$ (parameter denoting main effect of treatment at stage 1) as a function of sample size n and one of the stage 2 parameters, ψ_{20}, ψ_{21}, or ψ_{22} (which are equal to the generative parameters γ_5, γ_6 and γ_7, respectively). The plots represent the average bias over 1,000 simulated data sets, computed over a range of 2 units (on a 0.1 unit grid) for each parameter at sample sizes $250, 300, \ldots, 1000$. From the bias maps, it is clear that there exist many regions

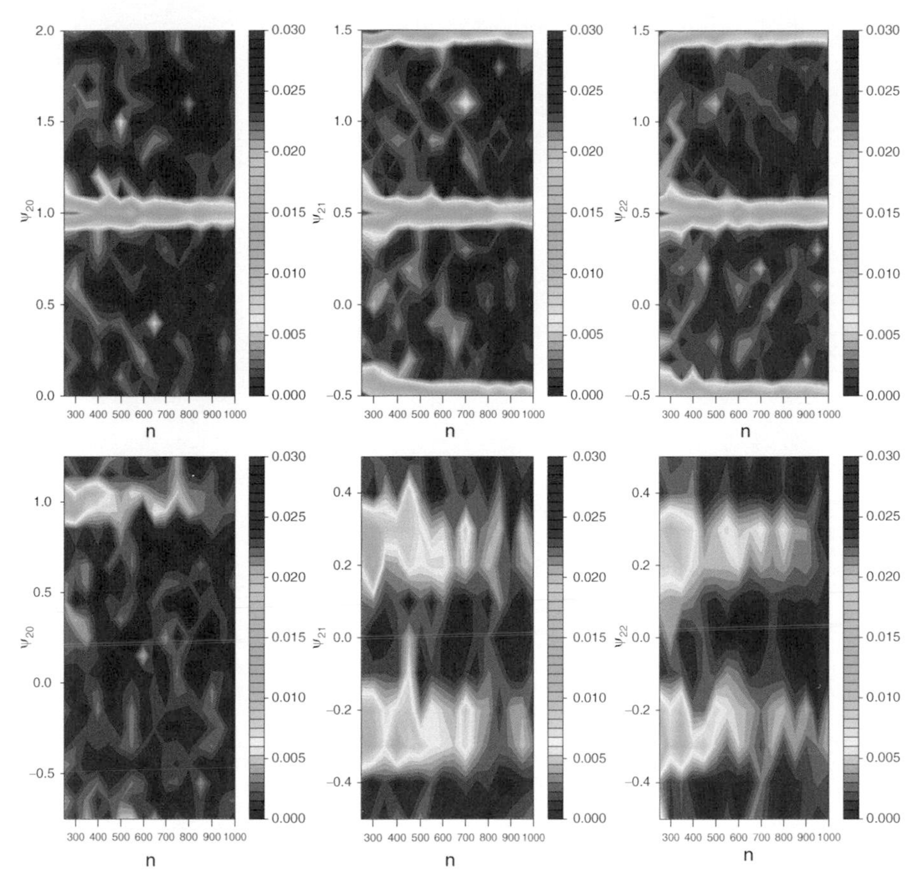

Fig. 8.1 Absolute bias of $\hat{\psi}_{10}$ in hard-max Q-learning in different regions (regular and non-regular) of the underlying parameter space. Different plots correspond to different parameter settings.

of the parameter space that lead to bias in $\hat{\psi}_{10}$, thereby reinforcing the necessity to address the problem through careful estimation and inference techniques.

As noted by Moodie and Richardson (2010), the bias maps can be used to visually represent the asymptotic results concerning DTR estimators. Consistency may be visualized by looking at a horizontal cross-section of a bias map: as sample size increases, the bias of the first-stage estimator will decrease to be smaller than any fixed, positive number at all non-regular parameter settings, even those that are nearly non-regular. However, as derived by Robins (2004), there exist sequences of data generating processes $\{\psi_{(n)}\}$ for which the second-stage parameters ψ_2 decrease with increasing n in such a way that the asymptotic bias of the first-stage estimator $\hat{\psi}_1$ is strictly positive. Contours of constant bias can be found along the lines on the bias map traced by plotting $g_2(\psi_2) = kn^{-1/2}$ against n, for some constant k. The asymptotic bias is bounded and, in finite samples, the value of the second-stage parameters (i.e. the "nearness" to non-regularity) and the sample size both determine the bias of the first-stage parameter estimator.

In many situations where the asymptotic distribution of an estimator is unavailable, bootstraping is used as an alternative approach to conduct inference. But the success of the bootstrap also hinges on the underlying smoothness of the estimator. When an estimator is non-smooth, the ordinary bootstrap procedure produces an inconsistent bootstrap estimator (Shao 1994). Inconsistency of bootstrap in the above toy example has been discussed by Andrews (2000). Poor performance of usual bootstrap CIs in the Q-learning context has been illustrated by Chakraborty et al. (2010). We first discuss non-regularity in the specific contexts of G-estimation and Q-learning, then, in the following sections, we consider several different approaches to inference that attempt to address the problem of non-regularity.

8.2.1 Non-regularity in Q-learning

With (3.8) as the model for Q-functions, the optimal DTR is given by

$$d_j^{opt}(H_j) = \arg\max_{a_j} (\psi_j^T H_{j1}) a_j = sign(\psi_j^T H_{j1}), \quad j = 1, 2, \tag{8.7}$$

where $sign(x) = 1$ if $x > 0$, and -1 otherwise. Note that the term $\beta_j^T H_{j0}$ on the right hand side of (3.8) does not feature in the optimal DTR. Thus for estimating optimal DTRs, the ψ_js are the parameters of interest, while β_js are nuisance parameters. These ψ_js are the policy parameters for which we want to construct confidence intervals.

Inference for ψ_2, the stage 2 parameters, is straightforward since this falls in the framework of standard linear regression. In contrast, inference for ψ_1, the stage 1 parameters, is complicated by the previously discussed problem of *non-regularity* resulting from the underlying non-smooth maximization operation in the estimation procedure. To further understand the problem, recall that the stage 1 pseudo-outcome in Q-learning for the i-th subject is

$$\hat{Y}_{1i} = Y_{1i} + \max_{a_2} Q_2^{opt}(H_{2i}, a_2; \hat{\beta}_2, \hat{\psi}_2) = Y_{1i} + \hat{\beta}_2^T H_{20,i} + |\hat{\psi}_2^T H_{21,i}|, \; i = 1, \ldots, n,$$

which is a non-smooth (the absolute value function is non-differentiable at zero) function of $\hat{\psi}_2$. Since $\hat{\psi}_1$ is a function of $\hat{Y}_{1i}$, $i = 1, \ldots, n$, it is in turn a non-smooth function of $\hat{\psi}_2$. As a consequence, the distribution of $\sqrt{n}(\hat{\psi}_1 - \psi_1)$ does not converge uniformly over the parameter space of (ψ_1, ψ_2) (Robins 2004). More specifically, the asymptotic distribution of $\sqrt{n}(\hat{\psi}_1 - \psi_1)$ is normal if ψ_2 is such that $P[H_2 : \psi_2^T H_{21} = 0] = 0$, but is non-normal if $P[H_2 : \psi_2^T H_{21} = 0] > 0$, and this change in the asymptotic distribution happens abruptly. A precise expression for the asymptotic distribution can be found in Laber et al. (2011). The parameter ψ_1 is called a *non-regular* parameter and the estimator $\hat{\psi}_1$ a *non-regular* estimator; see Bickel et al. (1993) for a precise definition of non-regularity. Because of this non-regularity, given the noise level present in small samples, the estimator $\hat{\psi}_1$ oscillates between the two asymptotic distributions across samples. Consequently, $\hat{\psi}_1$ becomes a biased estimator of ψ_1, and Wald type CIs for components of ψ_1 show poor coverage rates (Robins 2004; Moodie and Richardson 2010).

8.2.2 Non-regularity in G-estimation

Let us again consider a typical, two-stage scenario with linear optimal blip functions,

$$\gamma_1(h_1,a_1) = (\psi_{10}+\psi_{11}o_1)(a_1+1)/2, \text{ and}$$
$$\gamma_2(h_2,a_2) = (\psi_{20}+\psi_{21}o_2+\psi_{22}(a_1+1)/2+\psi_{23}o_2(a_1+1)/2)(a_2+1)/2.$$

Let $\eta_2 = \psi_{20}+\psi_{21}o_2+\psi_{22}(a_1+1)/2+\psi_{23}o_2(a_1+1)/2$ and similarly define $\hat{\eta}_2 = \hat{\psi}_{20}+\hat{\psi}_{21}o_2+\hat{\psi}_{22}(a_1+1)/2+\hat{\psi}_{23}o_2(a_1+1)/2$. The G-estimating function for ψ_2 is unbiased, so $E[\hat{\eta}_2] = \eta_2$. The sign of η_2 is used to decide optimal treatment at the second stage: $d_2^{opt} = sign(\eta_2) = sign(\psi_{20}+\psi_{21}o_2+\psi_{22}a_1+\psi_{23}o_2a_1)$ and $\hat{d}_2^{opt} = sign(\hat{\eta}_2)$ so that now the G-estimating equation solved for ψ_1 at the first interval contains:

$$\begin{aligned} G_{\text{mod},1}(\psi_1) &= Y-\gamma_1(o_1,a_1;\psi_1)+[\gamma_2(h_2,\hat{d}_2^{opt};\hat{\psi}_2)-\gamma_2(h_2,a_2;\hat{\psi}_2)] \\ &= Y-\gamma_1(o_1,a_1;\psi_1)+[(\hat{d}_2^{opt}-a_2)(\hat{\psi}_{20}+\hat{\psi}_{21}o_2+\hat{\psi}_{22}a_1+\hat{\psi}_{23}o_2a_1)/2] \\ &= Y-\gamma_1(o_1,a_1;\psi_1)+sign(\hat{\eta}_2)\hat{\eta}_2/2-a_2\hat{\eta}_2/2 \\ &\overset{E}{\geq} Y-\gamma_1(o_1,a_1;\psi_1)+sign(\eta_2)\eta_2/2-a_2\eta_2/2 = 0, \end{aligned}$$

where $\overset{E}{\geq}$ is used to denote "greater than or equal to in expectation". The quantity $\left[\gamma_2(h_2,d_2^{opt};\psi_2)-\gamma_2(h_2,a_2;\psi_2)\right]$ in $G_{\text{mod},1}(\psi_1)$ – or more generally, the sum $\sum_{k>j}\left[\gamma_k(h_k,d_k^{opt};\psi_k)-\gamma_k(h_k,a_k;\psi_k)\right]$ in $G_{\text{mod},j}(\psi_j)$ – corresponds conceptually to $|\mu|$ in the toy example with normally-distributed random variables X_i that was introduced at the start of the section. By using a biased estimate of $sign(\eta_2)\eta_2$ in $G_{\text{mod},1}(\psi_1)$, some strictly positive value is added into the G-estimating equation for ψ_1. The estimating function no longer has expectation zero and hence is asymptotically biased.

8.3 Threshold Estimators with the Usual Bootstrap

In this section, we will present two approaches to "regularize" the non-regular estimator (also called the *hard-max* estimator because of the maximum operation used in the definition) by thresholding and/or shrinking the effect of the term involving the maximum, i.e. $|\hat{\psi}_2^T H_{21}|$, towards zero. Usual bootstrap procedures in conjunction with these regularized estimators offer considerable improvement over the original hard-max procedure, as verified in extensive simulations. While these estimators are quite intuitive in nature, only limited theoretical results are available. We present these in the context of Q-learning, but these can equally be applied in a G-estimation setting.

8.3.1 The Hard-Threshold Estimator

The general form of the hard-threshold pseudo-outcome is

$$\hat{Y}_{1i}^{HT} = Y_{1i} + \hat{\beta}_2^T H_{20,i} + |\hat{\psi}_2^T H_{21,i}| \cdot \mathbb{I}[|\hat{\psi}_2^T H_{21,i}| > \lambda_i],\ i = 1,\ldots,n, \tag{8.8}$$

where λ_i (>0) is the threshold for the i-th subject in the sample (possibly depending on the variability of the linear combination $\hat{\psi}_2^T H_{21,i}$ for that subject). One way to operationalize this is to perform a preliminary test (for each subject in the sample) of the null hypothesis $\psi_2^T H_{21,i} = 0$ ($H_{21,i}$ is considered fixed in this test), set $\hat{Y}_{1i}^{HT} = \hat{Y}_{1i}$ if the null hypothesis is rejected, and replace $|\hat{\psi}_2^T H_{21,i}|$ with the "better guess" of 0 in the case that the test fails to reject the null hypothesis. Thus the hard-threshold pseudo-outcome can be written as

$$\hat{Y}_{1i}^{HT} = Y_{1i} + \hat{\beta}_2^T H_{20,i} + |\hat{\psi}_2^T H_{21,i}| \cdot \mathbb{I}\left[\frac{\sqrt{n}|\hat{\psi}_2^T H_{21,i}|}{\sqrt{H_{21,i}^T \hat{\Sigma}_{\hat{\psi}_2} H_{21,i}}} > z_{\alpha/2}\right] \tag{8.9}$$

for $i = 1,\ldots,n$, where $n^{-1}\hat{\Sigma}_{\hat{\psi}_2}$ is the estimated covariance matrix of $\hat{\psi}_2$. The corresponding estimator of ψ_1, denoted by $\hat{\psi}_1^{HT}$, will be referred to as the hard-threshold estimator. The hard-threshold estimator is common in many areas like variable selection in linear regression and wavelet shrinkage (Donoho and Johnstone 1994). Moodie and Richardson (2010) proposed this estimator for bias correction in the context of G-estimation, and called it the *Zeroing Instead of Plugging In* (ZIPI) estimator. In regular data-generating settings, ZIPI estimators converge to the usual recursive G-estimators and therefore are asymptotically consistent, unbiased and normally distributed. Furthermore, in any non-regular setting where there exist some individuals for whom there is a unique optimal regime, ZIPI estimators have smaller asymptotic bias than the recursive G-estimators provided parameters are not shared across stages (Moodie and Richardson 2010).

Note that $\hat{Y}_1^{HT}$ is still a non-smooth function of $\hat{\psi}_2$ and hence $\hat{\psi}_1^{HT}$ is a non-regular estimator of ψ_1. However, the problematic term $|\hat{\psi}_2^T H_{21}|$ is thresholded, and hence one might expect that the degree of non-regularity is somewhat reduced. An important issue regarding the use of this estimator is the choice of the significance level α of the preliminary test, which is an unknown tuning parameter. As discussed by Moodie and Richardson (2010), this is a difficult problem even in better-understood settings where preliminary test based estimators are used; no widely applicable data-driven method for choosing α in this setting is available. Chakraborty et al. (2010) studied the behavior of the usual bootstrap in conjunction with this estimator empirically.

8.3.2 The Soft-Threshold Estimator

The general form of the soft-threshold pseudo-outcome considered here is

$$\hat{Y}_{1i}^{ST} = Y_{1i} + \hat{\beta}_2^T H_{20,i} + |\hat{\psi}_2^T H_{21,i}| \cdot \left(1 - \frac{\lambda_i}{|\hat{\psi}_2^T H_{21,i}|^2}\right)^+, \; i = 1, \ldots, n, \quad (8.10)$$

where $x^+ = x\mathbb{I}[x > 0]$ stands for the positive part of a function, and λ_i (>0) is a tuning parameter associated with the i-th subject in the sample (again possibly depending on the variability of the linear combination $\hat{\psi}_2^T H_{21,i}$ for that subject). In the context of regression shrinkage (Breiman 1995) and wavelet shrinkage (Gao 1998), the third term on the right side of (8.10) is generally known as the *non-negative garrote* estimator. As discussed by Zou (2006), the non-negative garrote estimator is a special case of the *adaptive lasso* estimator. Chakraborty et al. (2010) proposed this soft-threshold estimator in the context of Q-learning.

Like the hard-threshold pseudo-outcome, $\hat{Y}_1^{ST}$ is also a non-smooth function of $\hat{\psi}_2$ and hence $\hat{\psi}_1^{ST}$ remains a non-regular estimator of ψ_1. However, the problematic term $|\hat{\psi}_2^T H_{21}|$ is thresholded and shrunk towards zero, which reduces the degree of non-regularity. As in the case of hard-threshold estimators, a crucial issue here is to choose a data-driven tuning parameter λ_i; see below for a choice of λ_i following a Bayesian approach. Figure 8.2 presents the hard-max, the hard-threshold, and the soft-threshold pseudo-outcomes.

Choice of Tuning Parameters

A hierarchical Bayesian formulation of the problem, inspired by the work of Figueiredo and Nowak (2001) in wavelets, was used by Chakraborty et al. (2010) to choose the λ_is in a data-driven way. It turns out that the estimator (8.10) with $\lambda_i = 3H_{21,i}^T \hat{\Sigma}_{\hat{\psi}_2} H_{21,i}/n$, $i = 1, \ldots, n$, where $n^{-1}\hat{\Sigma}_{\hat{\psi}_2}$ is the estimated covariance matrix of $\hat{\psi}_2$, is an approximate empirical Bayes estimator. The following theorem can be used to derive the choice of λ_i.

Theorem 8.1. *Let X be a random variable such that $X|\mu \sim N(\mu, \sigma^2)$ with known variance σ^2. Let the prior distribution on μ be given by $\mu|\phi^2 \sim N(0, \phi^2)$, with Jeffrey's noninformative hyper-prior on ϕ^2, i.e., $p(\phi^2) \propto 1/\phi^2$. Then an empirical Bayes estimator of $|\mu|$ is given by*

$$\begin{aligned} \widehat{|\mu|}^{EB} &= X\left(1 - \frac{3\sigma^2}{X^2}\right)^+ \left(2\Phi\left(\frac{X}{\sigma}\sqrt{\left(1 - \frac{3\sigma^2}{X^2}\right)^+}\right) - 1\right) \\ &+ \sqrt{\frac{2}{\pi}}\,\sigma\sqrt{\left(1 - \frac{3\sigma^2}{X^2}\right)^+} \exp\left\{-\frac{X^2}{2\sigma^2}\left(1 - \frac{3\sigma^2}{X^2}\right)^+\right\}, \quad (8.11) \end{aligned}$$

where $\Phi(\cdot)$ is the standard normal distribution function.

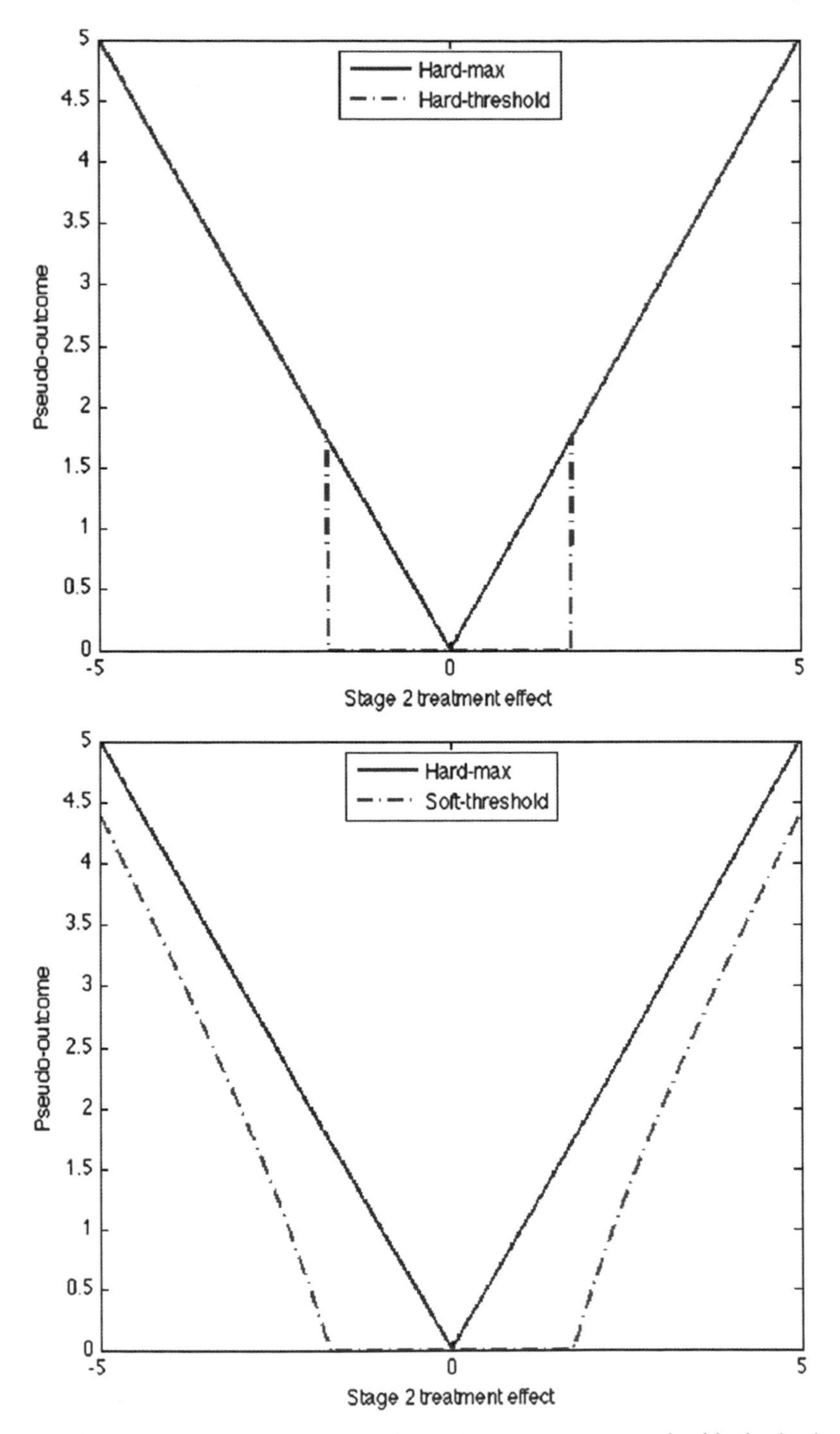

Fig. 8.2 Hard-threshold and soft-threshold pseudo-outcomes compared with the hard-max pseudo-outcome

The proof can be found in Chakraborty et al. (2010).

Clearly, $|\hat{\mu}|^{EB}$ is a thresholding rule, since $|\hat{\mu}|^{EB} = 0$ for $|X| < \sqrt{3}\sigma$. Moreover, when $|X/\sigma|$ is large, the second term of (8.11) goes to zero exponentially fast, and

$$\left(2\Phi\Big(\frac{X}{\sigma}\sqrt{\Big(1-\frac{3\sigma^2}{X^2}\Big)^+}\Big)-1\right) \approx (2\,\mathbb{I}[X>0]-1) = sign(X).$$

Consequently, the empirical Bayes estimator is approximated by

$$|\hat{\mu}|^{EB} \approx X\left(1-\frac{3\sigma^2}{X^2}\right)^+ sign(X) = |X|\left(1-\frac{3\sigma^2}{X^2}\right)^+. \tag{8.12}$$

Now for $i=1,\ldots,n$ separately, put $X = \hat{\psi}_2^T H_{21,i}$, and $\mu = \psi_2^T H_{21,i}$ (for fixed $H_{21,i}$); and plug in $\hat{\sigma}^2 = H_{21,i}^T \hat{\Sigma}_{\hat{\psi}_2} H_{21,i}/n$ for σ^2. This leads to a choice of λ_i in the soft-threshold pseudo-outcome (8.10):

$$\begin{aligned}\hat{Y}_{1i}^{ST} &= Y_{1i} + \hat{\beta}_2^T H_{20,i} + |\hat{\psi}_2^T H_{21,i}| \cdot \left(1 - \frac{3H_{21,i}^T\hat{\Sigma}_{\hat{\psi}_2}H_{21,i}}{n|\hat{\psi}_2^T H_{21,i}|^2}\right)^+, \\ &= Y_{1i} + \hat{\beta}_2^T H_{20,i} + |\hat{\psi}_2^T H_{21,i}| \cdot \left(1 - \frac{3H_{21,i}^T\hat{\Sigma}_{\hat{\psi}_2}H_{21,i}}{n|\hat{\psi}_2^T H_{21,i}|^2}\right) \cdot \mathbb{I}\left[\frac{\sqrt{n}|\hat{\psi}_2^T H_{21,i}|}{\sqrt{H_{21,i}^T\hat{\Sigma}_{\hat{\psi}_2}H_{21,i}}} > \sqrt{3}\right], \\ & \qquad i = 1,\ldots,n. \end{aligned} \tag{8.13}$$

The presence of the indicator function in (8.13) indicates that $\hat{Y}_{1i}^{ST}$ is a thresholding rule for small values of $|\hat{\psi}_2^T H_{21,i}|$, while the term just preceding the indicator function makes $\hat{Y}_{1i}^{ST}$ a shrinkage rule for moderate to large values of $|\hat{\psi}_2^T H_{21,i}|$ (for which the indicator function takes the value one).

Interestingly, the thresholding rule in (8.13) also provides some guidance for choosing the tuning parameter of the hard-threshold estimator. Note that the indicator function in (8.13) corresponds to a pretest that uses a critical value of $\sqrt{3} = 1.7321$; equating this value to $z_{\alpha/2}$ and solving for α, we get $\alpha = 0.0833$. Hence a hard-threshold estimator with tuning parameter $\alpha = 0.0833 \approx 0.08$ corresponds to the soft-threshold estimator without the shrinkage effect. Chakraborty et al. (2010) empirically showed that the hard-threshold estimator with $\alpha = 0.08$ outperformed other choices of this tuning parameter as reported in the original paper by Moodie and Richardson (2010).

8.3.3 Analysis of Smoking Cessation Data: An Illustration, Continued

To demonstrate the use of the soft-threshold method in a health application, here we present the analysis of the smoking cessation data described earlier in Sects. 2.4.1

and 3.4.3. The variables considered here are the same as those considered in Sect. 3.4.3. To find the optimal DTR, we applied both the hard-max and the soft-threshold estimators within the Q-learning framework. This involved:

1. Fit stage 2 regression ($n = 281$) of `FF6Quitstatus` using the model:

$$\begin{aligned}\texttt{FF6Quitstatus} = \beta_{20} &+ \beta_{21} \times \texttt{motivation} + \beta_{22} \times \texttt{source} \\ &+ \beta_{23} \times \texttt{selfefficacy} + \beta_{24} \times \texttt{story} \\ &+ \beta_{25} \times \texttt{education} + \beta_{26} \times \texttt{PQ6Quitstatus} \\ &+ \beta_{27} \times \texttt{source} \times \texttt{selfefficacy} \\ &+ \beta_{28} \times \texttt{story} \times \texttt{education} \\ &+ \left(\psi_{20} + \psi_{21} \times \texttt{PQ6Quitstatus}\right) \times \texttt{FFarm} + \texttt{error}.\end{aligned}$$

2. Construct the hard-max pseudo-outcome ($\hat{Y}_1$) and the soft-threshold pseudo-outcome ($\hat{Y}_1^{ST}$) for the stage 1 regression by plugging in the stage 2 estimates:

$$\begin{aligned}\hat{Y}_1 = \texttt{PQ6Quitstatus} &+ \hat{\beta}_{20} + \hat{\beta}_{21} \times \texttt{motivation} + \hat{\beta}_{22} \times \texttt{source} \\ &+ \hat{\beta}_{23} \times \texttt{selfefficacy} + \hat{\beta}_{24} \times \texttt{story} \\ &+ \hat{\beta}_{25} \times \texttt{education} + \hat{\beta}_{26} \times \texttt{PQ6Quitstatus} \\ &+ \hat{\beta}_{27} \times \texttt{source} \times \texttt{selfefficacy} + \hat{\beta}_{28} \times \texttt{story} \times \texttt{education} \\ &+ \left|\hat{\psi}_{20} + \hat{\psi}_{21} \times \texttt{PQ6Quitstatus}\right|;\end{aligned}$$

   and

$$\begin{aligned}\hat{Y}_1^{ST} = \texttt{PQ6Quitstatus} &+ \hat{\beta}_{20} + \hat{\beta}_{21} \times \texttt{motivation} + \hat{\beta}_{22} \times \texttt{source} \\ &+ \hat{\beta}_{23} \times \texttt{selfefficacy} + \hat{\beta}_{24} \times \texttt{story} \\ &+ \hat{\beta}_{25} \times \texttt{education} + \hat{\beta}_{26} \times \texttt{PQ6Quitstatus} \\ &+ \hat{\beta}_{27} \times \texttt{source} \times \texttt{selfefficacy} + \hat{\beta}_{28} \times \texttt{story} \times \texttt{education} \\ &+ \left|\hat{\psi}_{20} + \hat{\psi}_{21} \times \texttt{PQ6Quitstatus}\right| \\ &\times \left(1 - \frac{3\mathrm{Var}(\hat{\psi}_{20} + \hat{\psi}_{21} \times \texttt{PQ6Quitstatus})}{|\hat{\psi}_{20} + \hat{\psi}_{21} \times \texttt{PQ6Quitstatus}|^2}\right)^+.\end{aligned}$$

   Note that in this case one can construct both versions of the pseudo-outcomes for everyone who participated at stage 1, since there are no variables from post-stage 1 required to do so.

3. Fit stage 1 regression ($n = 1,401$) of the pseudo-outcome using a model of the form:

$$\begin{aligned}\hat{Y}_1 \text{ or } \hat{Y}_1^{ST} = \beta_{10} &+ \beta_{11} \times \texttt{motivation} \\ &+ \beta_{12} \times \texttt{selfefficacy} + \beta_{13} \times \texttt{education}\end{aligned}$$

$$+\left(\psi_{10}^{(1)}+\psi_{11}^{(1)}\times\texttt{selfefficacy}\right)\times\texttt{source}$$
$$+\left(\psi_{10}^{(2)}+\psi_{11}^{(2)}\times\texttt{education}\right)\times\texttt{story}+\texttt{error}.$$

No significant treatment effect was found at the second stage regression, indicating the likely existence of non-regularity. At stage 1, for either estimator, 95 % confidence intervals were constructed by *centered percentile bootstrap* (Efron and Tibshirani 1993) using 1,000 bootstrap replications. The stage 1 analysis summary is presented in Table 8.1. In this case, the hard-max and the soft-threshold estimators produced similar results.

Table 8.1 Regression coefficients and 95 % bootstrap confidence intervals at stage 1, using both the hard-max and the soft-threshold estimators (significant effects are in bold)

	Hard-max		Soft-threshold	
Variable	Coefficient	95 % CI	Coefficient	95 % CI
motivation	0.04	(−0.00, 0.08)	**0.04**	(0.00, 0.08)
selfefficacy	**0.03**	(0.00, 0.06)	**0.03**	(0.00, 0.06)
education	−0.01	(−0.07, 0.06)	−0.01	(−0.07, 0.06)
source	−0.15	(−0.35, 0.06)	−0.15	(−0.35, 0.06)
source × selfefficacy	**0.03**	(0.00, 0.06)	**0.03**	(0.00, 0.06)
story	0.05	(−0.01, 0.11)	0.05	(−0.01, 0.11)
story × education	**−0.07**	(−0.13, −0.01)	**−0.07**	(−0.13, −0.01)

From the above analysis, it is found that at stage 1 subjects with higher level of `motivation` or `selfefficacy` are more likely to quit. The highly personalized level of `source` is more effective for subjects with a higher `selfefficacy` ($\geq$7), and deeply tailored level of `story` is more effective for subjects with lower `education` ($\leq$ high school); these two conclusions can be drawn from the interaction plots (with confidence intervals) presented in Fig. 3.2 (see Sect. 3.4.3). Thus to maximize each individual's chance of quitting over the two stages, the web-based smoking cessation intervention should be designed in future such that: (1) smokers with high `self-efficacy` ($\geq$7) are assigned to highly personalized level of `source`, and (2) smokers with lower `education` are assigned to deeply tailored level of `story`.

8.4 Penalized Q-learning

In the threshold methods considered earlier, the stage 1 pseudo-outcomes can be viewed as *shrinkage functionals* of the least squares estimators of the stage 2 parameters. However, they are not optimizers of any explicit objective function (except in the special case of only one covariate or an orthonormal design). The *Penalized Q-learning* (hereafter referred to as *PQ-learning*) approach, recently proposed by Song et al. (2011), applies the shrinkage idea with Q-learning by considering an explicit penalized regression at stage 2. The main distinction between the penalization used here and that used in the context of variable selection is in the "target" of penalization: while penalties are applied to each variable (covariate) in a variable selection context, they are applied on each subject in the case of PQ-learning.

Let $\theta_j = (\beta_j^T, \psi_j^T)^T$ for $j = 1, 2$. PQ-learning starts by considering a penalized least squares optimization at stage 2; it minimizes the objective function

$$W_2(\theta_2) = \sum_{i=1}^{n} \left(Y_{2i} - Q_2^{opt}(H_{2i}, A_{2i}; \beta_2, \psi_2)\right)^2 + \sum_{i=1}^{n} J_{\lambda_n}\left(|\psi_2^T H_{21,i}|\right)$$

with respect to θ_2 to obtain the stage 2 estimates $\hat{\theta}_2$, where $J_{\lambda_n}(\cdot)$ is a pre-specified penalty function and λ_n is a tuning parameter. The penalty function can be taken directly from the variable selection literature; in particular Song et al. (2011) uses the *adaptive lasso* (Zou 2006) penalty, where $J_{\lambda_n}(\theta) = \lambda_n \theta / |\hat{\theta}|^\alpha$ with $\alpha > 0$ and $\hat{\theta}$ being a $\sqrt{n}$-consistent estimator of θ. Furthermore, as in the adaptive lasso procedure, the tuning parameter λ_n is taken to satisfy $\sqrt{n}\lambda_n \to 0$ and $n\lambda_n \to \infty$. The rest of the Q-learning algorithm (hard-max version) is unchanged in PQ-learning.

The above minimization is implemented via *local quadratic approximation* (LQA), following Fan and Li (2001). The procedure starts with an initial value $\hat{\psi}_{2(0)}$ of ψ_2, and then uses LQA for the penalty terms in the objective function:

$$J_{\lambda_n}\left(|\psi_2^T H_{21,i}|\right) \approx J_{\lambda_n}\left(|\hat{\psi}_{2(0)}^T H_{21,i}|\right) + \frac{1}{2} \frac{J'_{\lambda_n}\left(|\hat{\psi}_{2(0)}^T H_{21,i}|\right)}{|\hat{\psi}_{2(0)}^T H_{21,i}|} \left((\psi_2^T H_{21,i})^2 - (\hat{\psi}_{2(0)}^T H_{21,i})^2\right)$$

for ψ_2 close to $\hat{\psi}_{2(0)}$. Hence the objective function can be locally approximated, up to a constant, by

$$\sum_{i=1}^{n} \left(Y_{2i} - Q_2^{opt}(H_{2i}, A_{2i}; \beta_2, \psi_2)\right)^2 + \frac{1}{2} \sum_{i=1}^{n} \frac{J'_{\lambda_n}\left(|\hat{\psi}_{2(0)}^T H_{21,i}|\right)}{|\hat{\psi}_{2(0)}^T H_{21,i}|} (\psi_2^T H_{21,i})^2.$$

When Q-functions are approximated by linear models as in (3.8), the above minimization problem has a closed form solution:

$$\begin{aligned}
\hat{\psi}_2 &= [\mathbf{X}_{22}(\mathbf{I} - \mathbf{X}_{21}(\mathbf{X}_{21}^T \mathbf{X}_{21})^{-1} \mathbf{X}_{21}^T + \mathbf{D})\mathbf{X}_{22}]^{-1} \mathbf{X}_{22}^T (\mathbf{I} - \mathbf{X}_{21}(\mathbf{X}_{21}^T \mathbf{X}_{21})^{-1} \mathbf{X}_{21}^T) Y_2, \\
\hat{\beta}_2 &= (\mathbf{X}_{21}^T \mathbf{X}_{21})^{-1} \mathbf{X}_{21}^T (\mathbf{Y}_2 - \mathbf{X}_{22} \hat{\psi}_2),
\end{aligned}$$

where $\mathbf{X}_{22}$ is the matrix with i-th row equal to $H_{21,i}^T A_{2i}$, $\mathbf{X}_{21}$ is the matrix with i-th row equal to $H_{20,i}^T$, $\mathbf{I}$ is the $n \times n$ identity matrix, $\mathbf{D}$ is an $n \times n$ diagonal matrix with $D_{ii} = \frac{1}{2} J'_{\lambda_n}\left(|\hat{\psi}_{2(0)}^T H_{21,i}|\right) / |\hat{\psi}_{2(0)}^T H_{21,i}|$, and Y_2 is the vector of Y_{2i} values. The above minimization procedure can be continued for more than one step or until convergence. However, as discussed by Fan and Li (2001), either the one-step or multi-step procedure will be as efficient as the fully iterative procedure as long as the initial estimators are good enough.

Inference for θ_js in the context of PQ-learning is conducted via asymptotic theory. Under a set of regularity conditions, Song et al. (2011) proved that:

1. $\hat{\theta}_2$ is a $\sqrt{n}$-consistent estimator for the true value of θ_2.
2. *Oracle Property*: With probability tending to 1, PQ-learning can identify the individuals for whom the stage 2 treatment effect is zero.
3. Both $\hat{\theta}_2$ and $\hat{\theta}_1$ are asymptotically normal.

Variance Estimation

Song et al. (2011) provided a sandwich type plug-in estimator for the variance of $\hat{\theta}_2$:

$$\widehat{cov}(\hat{\theta}_2) = (\hat{I}_{20} + \hat{\Sigma})^{-1}\hat{I}_{20}(\hat{I}_{20} + \hat{\Sigma})^{-1},$$

where $\hat{I}_{20} \equiv \mathbb{P}_n[\nabla^2_{\theta_2\theta_2}(Y_2 - Q_2^{opt}(H_2, A_2; \theta_2))^2]$ is the empirical Hessian matrix and $\hat{\Sigma} = diag\{\mathbf{0}, \mathbb{P}_n J''_{\lambda_n}(|\hat{\psi}_2^T H_{21}|) H_{21} H_{21}^T\}$. The above variance formula can be further approximated by ignoring $\hat{\Sigma}$, in which case $\widehat{cov}(\hat{\theta}_2) = \hat{I}_{20}^{-1}$. Song et al. (2011) reported having used this reduced formula in their simulation studies and achieved good empirical performance. Likewise, the estimated variance for $\hat{\theta}_1$ is given by:

$$\widehat{cov}(\hat{\theta}_1) = \hat{I}_{10}^{-1}\Big[cov\Big\{\nabla_{\theta_1} Q_1^{opt}(H_1, A_1; \hat{\theta}_1)\Big(Y_1 + \max_{a_2} Q_2^{opt}(H_2, a_2; \hat{\theta}_2) - Q_1^{opt}(H_1, A_1; \hat{\theta}_1)\Big) + \mathbb{P}_n Z_1 \bar{S}_2^{\,T} \widehat{cov}(\hat{\theta}_2) \bar{S}_2 Z_1^T\Big\}\Big]\hat{I}_{10}^{-1},$$

where $\hat{I}_{10} \equiv \mathbb{P}_n[\nabla^2_{\theta_1\theta_1}(Y_1 + \max_{a_2} Q_2^{opt}(H_2, a_2; \hat{\theta}_2) - Q_1^{opt}(H_1, A_1; \theta_1))^2]$ is the empirical Hessian matrix.

There are a few characteristics of the PQ-learning approach that demand some discussion. First, this approach offers a data-analyst the ability to calculate standard errors using explicit formulae, which should be less time-consuming than a bootstrap procedure. However in the present era of fast computers, the difference in computing time between analytic and bootstrap approaches is gradually diminishing. Second, the asymptotic theory of PQ-learning assumes a finite support for the H_{21} values, which is achieved when only discrete covariates are used in the analysis. Thus, if there are important continuous covariates in a study, one must first discretize the continuous covariates before being able to use PQ-learning. Third, the success of PQ-learning in addressing non-regularity crucially depends on the "oracle property" described above; this property dictates that after the penalized regression in stage 2, all subsequent inference will be the same as if the analyst knew which subjects had no treatment effect. However this property does not say anything about very small effects that are not exactly zero but are indistinguishable from zero in finite samples due to noise in the data (e.g. in "near non-regular" cases; see Sect. 8.8). It has been widely argued (see e.g. Leeb and Pötscher 2005; Pötscher 2007; Pötscher and Schneider 2008; Laber and Murphy 2011) that characterizing non-regular settings by a condition like $P[H_2 : \psi_2^T H_{21} = 0] > 0$ is really a working assumption to reflect the uncertainty about the optimal treatment for patients with 'small' – rather than zero – treatment effects. Such situations may be better handled by a local asymptotic framework. From this perspective, the PQ-learning method is still non-regular as it is not consistent under local alternatives; see Laber et al. (2011) for further details on this issue.

8.5 Double Bootstrap Confidence Intervals

The *double bootstrap* (see, e.g. Davison and Hinkley 1997; Nankervis 2005) is a computationally intensive method for constructing CIs. Chakraborty et al. (2010) implemented this method for inference in the context of Q-learning. Empirically it was found to offer valid CIs for the policy parameters in the face of non-regularity. Below we present a brief description.

Let $\hat{\theta}$ be an estimator of a parameter θ and $\hat{\theta}^*$ be its bootstrap version. As is well-known, the $100(1-\alpha)\%$ percentile bootstrap CI is given by $\left(\hat{\theta}^*_{(\frac{\alpha}{2})}, \hat{\theta}^*_{(1-\frac{\alpha}{2})}\right)$, where $\hat{\theta}^*_\gamma$ is the 100γ-th percentile of the bootstrap distribution. Then the double (percentile) bootstrap CI is calculated as follows:

1. Draw B_1 first-step bootstrap samples from the original data. For each first-step bootstrap sample, calculate the bootstrap version of the estimator $\hat{\theta}^{*b}$, $b = 1, \ldots, B_1$.
2. Conditional on each first-step bootstrap sample, draw B_2 second-step (nested) bootstrap samples and calculate the double bootstrap versions of the estimator, e.g., $\hat{\theta}^{**bm}$, $b = 1, \ldots, B_1$, $m = 1, \ldots, B_2$.
3. For $b = 1, \ldots, B_1$, calculate $u^{*b} = \frac{1}{B_2}\sum_{m=1}^{B_2} \mathbb{I}[\hat{\theta}^{**bm} \leq \hat{\theta}]$, where $\hat{\theta}$ is the estimator based on the original data.
4. The double bootstrap CI is given by $\left(\hat{\theta}^*_{\hat{q}(\frac{\alpha}{2})}, \hat{\theta}^*_{\hat{q}(1-\frac{\alpha}{2})}\right)$, where $\hat{q}(\gamma) = u^*_{(\gamma)}$, the 100γ-th percentile of the distribution of u^{*b}, $b = 1, \ldots, B_1$.

Next we attempt to provide some intuition[1] about the double bootstrap using the *bagged* hard-max estimator. *Bagging* (Breiman 1996), a nickname for *bootstrap aggregating*, is a well-known ensemble method used to smooth "unstable" estimators, e.g. decision trees in classification. Bagging was originally motivated by Breiman as a variance-reduction technique; however Bühlmann and Yu (2002) showed that it is a smoothing operation that also reduces the mean squared error of the estimator in the case of decision trees, where a "hard decision" based on an indicator function is taken. Note that in the context of Q-learning, the hard-max pseudo-outcome can be re-written as

$$\hat{Y}_{1i} = Y_{1i} + \hat{\beta}_2^T H_{20,i} + |\hat{\psi}_2^T H_{21,i}|$$

[1] This is unpublished work, but the first author was pointed to this direction by Dr. Susan Murphy (personal communication).

$$= Y_{1i} + \hat{\beta}_2^T H_{20,i} + (\hat{\psi}_2^T H_{21,i}) \cdot \left(2 \cdot \mathbb{I}[\hat{\psi}_2^T H_{21,i} > 0] - 1\right). \quad (8.14)$$

The second term in (8.14) contains an indicator function (as in a decision tree). Hence one can expect that the bagged version of the hard-max estimator will effectively "smooth out" the effect of this indicator function (e.g. replace the hard decision by a soft decision) and hence should reduce the degree of non-regularity. More precisely, bagging would effectively replace the indicator $\mathbb{I}[\hat{\psi}_2^T H_{21,i} > 0]$ by $\Phi\left(\frac{\sqrt{n}\hat{\psi}_2^T H_{21,i}}{\sqrt{H_{21,i}^T \hat{\Sigma}_{\hat{\psi}_2} H_{21,i}}}\right)$; see Bühlmann and Yu (2002) for details. The bagged hard-max estimator of ψ_1 can be calculated as follows:

1. Construct a bootstrap sample of size n from the original data.
2. Compute the bootstrap version $\hat{\psi}_1^*$ of the usual hard-max estimator $\hat{\psi}_1$.
3. Repeat steps 1 and 2 above B_2 times yielding $\hat{\psi}_1^{*1}, \ldots, \hat{\psi}_1^{*B_2}$. Then the bagged hard-max estimator is given by $\hat{\psi}_1^{Bag} = \frac{1}{B_2}\sum_{b=1}^{B_2} \hat{\psi}_1^{*b}$.

When it comes to constructing CIs, the effect of considering a usual bootstrap CI using B_1 replications along with the bagged hard-max estimator (already using B_2 bootstrap replications) is, in a way, equivalent to considering a double bootstrap CI in conjunction with the original (un-bagged) hard-max estimator.

8.6 Adaptive Bootstrap Confidence Intervals

Laber et al. (2011) recently developed a novel *adaptive bootstrap* procedure to construct confidence intervals for linear combinations $c^T\theta_1$ of the stage 1 coefficients in Q-learning, where $\theta_1^T = (\beta_1^T, \psi_1^T)$ and $c \in \mathbb{R}^{\dim(\theta_1)}$ is a known vector. This method is asymptotically valid and gives good empirical performance in finite samples. In this procedure, Laber et al. (2011) considered the asymptotic expansion of $c^T\sqrt{n}(\hat{\theta}_1 - \theta_1)$ and decomposed it as:

$$c^T\sqrt{n}(\hat{\theta}_1 - \theta_1) = \mathbb{W}_n + \mathbb{U}_n,$$

where the first term is smooth and the second term is non-smooth. While $\mathbb{W}_n$ is asymptotically normally distributed, the distribution of $\mathbb{U}_n$ depends on the underlying data-generating process "non-smoothly". To illustrate the effect of this non-smoothness, fix $H_{21} = h_{21}$. If $h_{21}^T\psi_2 > 0$, then $\mathbb{U}_n$ is asymptotically normal with mean zero. On the other hand, $\mathbb{U}_n$ has a non-normal asymptotic distribution if $h_{21}^T\psi_2 = 0$. Thus, the asymptotic distribution of $c^T\sqrt{n}(\hat{\theta}_1 - \theta_1)$ depends abruptly on both the true parameter ψ_2 and the distribution of patient features H_{21}. In particular, the asymptotic distribution of $c^T\sqrt{n}(\hat{\theta}_1 - \theta_1)$ depends on the frequency of patient features $H_{21} = h_{21}$ for which there is no treatment effect (i.e. features for which $h_{21}^T\psi_2 = 0$). As discussed earlier in this chapter, this non-regularity complicates the construction of CIs for $c^T\theta_1$.

The *adaptive bootstrap* confidence intervals are formed by constructing smooth data-dependent upper and lower bounds on $\mathbb{U}_n$, and thereby on $c^T\sqrt{n}(\hat{\theta}_1 - \theta_1)$, by means of a preliminary hypothesis test that partitions the data into two sets: (i) patients for whom there appears to be a treatment effect, and (ii) patients in whom it appears there is no treatment effect, and then drawing bootstrap samples from these upper and lower bounds. The actual bounds are rather complex and difficult to present without going into the details, so the explicit forms will not be presented here. Instead, we focus on communicating the key ideas.

The bounds are formed by finding limits for the error of the overall approximation due to misclassification of patients in the partitioning step. The idea of conducting a preliminary hypothesis test prior to forming estimators or confidence intervals is known as *pretesting* (Olshen 1973). In fact, the hard-threshold estimator (Moodie and Richardson 2010) discussed earlier uses the same notion of pretest. As in the case of hard-thresholding, Laber et al. (2011) conducted a pretest for each *individual* in the data set as follows. Each pretest is based on

$$T_n(h_{21}) \triangleq \frac{n(h_{21}^T\hat{\psi}_2)^2}{h_{21}^T\hat{\Sigma}_{\hat{\psi}_2}h_{21}},$$

where $\hat{\Sigma}_{\hat{\psi}_2}/n$ is the estimated covariance matrix of $\hat{\psi}_2$. Note that $T_n(h_{21})$ corresponds to the usual test statistic when testing the null hypothesis: $h_{21}^T\psi_2 = 0$. The pretests are performed using a cutoff λ_n, which is a tuning parameter of the procedure and can be varied; to optimize performance, Laber et al. (2011) used $\lambda_n = \log\log n$ in their simulation study and data analysis.

Let the upper and lower bounds on $c^T\sqrt{n}(\hat{\theta}_1 - \theta_1)$ discussed above be given by $\mathscr{U}(c)$ and $\mathscr{L}(c)$ respectively; both of these quantities are functions of λ_n. Laber et al. (2011) showed that the limiting distributions of $c^T\sqrt{n}(\hat{\theta}_1 - \theta_1)$ and $\mathscr{U}(c)$ are equal in the case $H_{21}^T\psi_2 \neq 0$ with probability one. Similarly, the limiting distributions of $c^T\sqrt{n}(\hat{\theta}_1 - \theta_1)$ and $\mathscr{L}(c)$ are equal in the case $H_{21}^T\psi_2 \neq 0$ with probability one. That is, when there is a large treatment effect for almost all patients then the upper (or lower) bound is tight. However, when there is a non-null subset of patients for which there is no treatment effect, then the limiting distribution of the upper bound is stochastically larger than the limiting distribution of $c^T\sqrt{n}(\hat{\theta}_1 - \theta_1)$. This adaptivity between non-regular and regular settings is a key feature of this procedure.

Next we discuss how to actually construct the CIs by this procedure. By construction of $\mathscr{U}(c)$ and $\mathscr{L}(c)$, it follows that

$$c^T\hat{\theta}_1 - \frac{\mathscr{U}(c)}{\sqrt{n}} \leq c^T\theta_1 \leq c^T\hat{\theta}_1 - \frac{\mathscr{L}(c)}{\sqrt{n}}.$$

The distributions of $\mathscr{U}(c)$ and $\mathscr{L}(c)$ are approximated using the bootstrap. Let $\hat{u}$ be the $1-\alpha/2$ quantile of the bootstrap distribution of $\mathscr{U}(c)$, and let $\hat{l}$ be the $\alpha/2$ quantile of the bootstrap distribution of $\mathscr{L}(c)$. Then $[c^T\hat{\theta}_1 - \hat{u}/\sqrt{n}, c^T\hat{\theta}_1 - \hat{l}/\sqrt{n}]$ is the adaptive bootstrap CI for $c^T\theta_1$.

Through a series of theorems, Laber et al. (2011) proved the consistency of the bootstrap in this context, and in particular that

$$P\left(c^T\hat{\theta}_1 - \hat{u}/\sqrt{n} \leq c^T\theta_1 \leq c^T\hat{\theta}_1 - \hat{l}/\sqrt{n}\right) \geq 1 - \alpha + o_P(1).$$

The above probability statement is with respect to the bootstrap distribution. Furthermore, if $P(H_{21}^T\psi_2 = 0) = 0$, then the above inequality can be strengthened to equality. This result shows that the adaptive bootstrap method can be used to construct valid (though potentially conservative) confidence intervals regardless of the underlying parameters of the generative model. Moreover, in settings where there is a treatment effect for almost every patient (e.g. regular settings), the adaptive procedure delivers asymptotically exact coverage.

The theory behind adaptive bootstrap CIs uses a *local asymptotic* framework. This framework provides a medium through which a glimpse of finite-sample behavior can be assessed, while retaining the mathematical convenience of large samples. A thorough technical discussion of this framework is beyond the scope of this book; hence here we presented only the key results without making exact statements of the assumptions and theorems. The procedure discussed here can be extended to more than two stages and more than two treatments per stage; see Laber et al. (2011) for details. The main downside to this procedure lies in its complexity – not just in the theory but also in its implementation. Constructing the smooth upper and lower bounds involves solving very difficult nonconvex optimization problems, making it a computationally expensive procedure. This conceptual and computational complexity may be a potential barrier for its wide-spread dissemination.

8.7 *m*-out-of-*n* Bootstrap Confidence Intervals

The m-out-of-n bootstrap is a well-known tool for producing valid confidence sets for non-smooth functionals (Shao 1994; Bickel et al. 1997). This method is the same as the usual nonparametric bootstrap (Efron 1979) except that the resample size, historically denoted by m, is of a smaller order of magnitude than the original sample size n. More precisely, m depends on n, tends to infinity with n, and satisfies $m = o(n)$. Intuitively, the m-out-of-n bootstrap works asymptotically by letting the empirical distribution tend to the true generative distribution at a faster rate than the analogous convergence of the bootstrap empirical distribution to the empirical distribution. In essence, this allows the empirical distribution to reach its limit 'first' so that bootstrap resamples behave as if they were drawn from the true generative distribution. Unfortunately, the choice of the resample size m has long been a difficult obstacle since the condition $m = o(n)$ is purely asymptotic and thus provides no guidance for finite samples. Data-driven approaches for choosing m in various contexts were given by Hall et al. (1995), Lee (1999), Cheung et al. (2005), and Bickel and Sakov (2008). However, these choices were not directly connected with data-driven measures of non-regularity. Chakraborty et al. (2013) recently proposed a method for choosing the resample size m in the context of Q-learning that is directly connected to an estimated degree of non-regularity. This method of choosing m is adaptive in that it leads to the usual n-out-of-n bootstrap in a regular setting and the m-out-of-n bootstrap otherwise. This methodology, developed for producing asymptotically valid confidence intervals for parameters indexing estimated optimal DTRs, is conceptually and computationally simple, making it more appealing to data analysts. This should be contrasted with methods of Robins (2004) and Laber et al. (2011), both of which involve solving difficult non-convex optimization problems (see Laber et al. 2011, for a discussion).

Intuitively, the choice of the resample size m should reflect the degree of non-smoothness in the underlying generative model. The non-smoothness in Q-learning arises when there is an amassing of points on or near the boundary $\{h_{21} : h_{21}^T \psi_2 = 0\}$. Define $p \triangleq P(H_{21}^T \psi_2 = 0)$, and consider the situation where non-regularity does not exist, i.e. $p = 0$. Then $\sqrt{n}(\hat{\theta}_1 - \theta_1)$ is asymptotically normal and the n-out-of-n bootstrap is consistent. However, if $p > 0$, given that $\hat{\psi}_2$ is not exactly equal to the true value, the quantity $\hat{\theta}_1$, as a function of $\hat{\psi}_2$, oscillates with a rate $n^{-1/2}$ around a point where abrupt changes of the asymptotic distribution occur. This is also true for its bootstrap analogue $\hat{\theta}_{1,m}^{(b)}$ while the oscillating rate is $m^{-1/2}$. With a large p, indicating a high degree of non-regularity, it is hoped that this bootstrap analogue oscillates with a rate much slower than $n^{-1/2}$. Therefore, a reasonable class of resample sizes is given by

$$m \triangleq n^{f(p)},$$

where $f(p)$ is a function of p satisfying the following conditions:

(i) $f(p)$ is monotone decreasing in p, takes values in $(0,1]$ and satisfies $f(0) = 1$; and
(ii) $f(p)$ is continuous and has bounded first derivative.

One still needs to estimate $f(p)$ from data since p is unknown. Define the plug-in estimator for p, $\hat{p} = \mathbb{P}_n \mathbb{I}[n(H_{21}^T \hat{\psi}_2)^2 \leq \tau_n(H_{21})]$ for cutoff $\tau_n(H_{21})$ (see below), where $\mathbb{P}_n$ denotes the empirical average. Thus, naturally, one can use the resample size

$$\hat{m} \triangleq n^{f(\hat{p})}. \tag{8.15}$$

Chakraborty et al. (2013) showed that $\hat{m}/n^{f(p)} \to 1$ almost surely, and thus $\hat{m} \xrightarrow{P} \infty$ and $\hat{m}/n \xrightarrow{P} 0$. For implementation, they proposed a simple form of $f(p)$ satisfying conditions (i) and (ii),

$$\hat{m} \triangleq n^{\frac{1+\alpha(1-\hat{p})}{1+\alpha}}, \tag{8.16}$$

where $\alpha > 0$ is a tuning parameter that can be either fixed at a constant or chosen adaptively using the double bootstrap (see below for the algorithm). Note that for fixed n, $\hat{m}$ is a monotone decreasing function of $\hat{p}$, taking values in the interval $[n^{\frac{1}{1+\alpha}}, n]$. Thus, α governs the smallest acceptable resample size.

Another potentially important tuning parameter is $\tau_n(H_{21})$. For a given patient history h_{21}, the indicator $\mathbb{I}[n(h_{21}^T \hat{\psi}_2)^2 \leq \tau_n(h_{21})]$ can be viewed as the acceptance region of the null hypothesis $h_{21}^T \psi_2 = 0$. Thus, a natural choice for $\tau_n(h_{21})$ is $\left(h_{21}^T \hat{\Sigma}_{21} h_{21}\right) \cdot \chi^2_{1,1-\nu}$, where $n^{-1}\hat{\Sigma}_{21}$ is the plug-in estimator of the asymptotic covariance matrix of $\hat{\psi}_2$ and $\chi^2_{1,1-\nu}$ is the $(1-\nu) \times 100$ percentile of a χ^2 distribution with 1 degree of freedom. Chakraborty et al. (2013) used $\nu = 0.001$ in their simulations, and also showed robustness of results to this choice of ν via a thorough sensitivity analysis.

As before, let $c \in \mathbb{R}^{\dim(\theta_1)}$ be a known vector. To form a $(1-\eta) \times 100\,\%$ confidence interval for $c^T \theta_1$, first find $\hat{l}$ and $\hat{u}$, the $(\eta/2) \times 100$ and $(1-\eta/2) \times 100$ percentiles of $c^T \sqrt{m}(\hat{\theta}_1^{(b)} - \hat{\theta}_1)$ respectively, where $\hat{\theta}_1^{(b)}$ is the m-out-of-n bootstrap analog of $\hat{\theta}_1$ (the dependence of $\hat{\theta}_1^{(b)}$ on m is implicit in the notation). The confidence interval is then given by $(c^T \hat{\theta}_1 - \hat{u}/\sqrt{m}, c^T \hat{\theta}_1 - \hat{l}/\sqrt{m})$.

Next we describe the double bootstrap procedure for choosing the tuning parameter α employed to define m. Suppose $c^T \theta_1$ is the parameter of interest, and its estimate from the original data is $c^T \hat{\theta}_1$. Consider a grid of possible values of α; Chakraborty et al. (2013) used $\{0.025, 0.05, 0.075, \ldots, 1\}$ in their simulation study and data analysis. The exact algorithm follows.

1. Draw B_1 usual n-out-of-n first-stage bootstrap samples from the data and calculate the corresponding bootstrap estimates $c^T \hat{\theta}_1^{(b_1)}$, $b_1 = 1, \ldots, B_1$. Fix α at the smallest value in the grid.
2. Compute the corresponding values of $\hat{m}^{(b_1)}$ using Eq. (8.16), $b_1 = 1, \ldots, B_1$.
3. Conditional on each first-stage bootstrap sample, draw B_2 $\hat{m}^{(b_1)}$-out-of-n second-stage (nested) bootstrap samples and calculate the double bootstrap versions of the estimate $c^T \hat{\theta}_1^{(b_1 b_2)}$, $b_1 = 1, \ldots, B_1$, $b_2 = 1, \ldots, B_2$.
4. For $b_1 = 1, \ldots, B_1$, compute the $(\eta/2) \times 100$ and $(1-\eta/2) \times 100$ percentiles of $\left\{c^T \sqrt{\hat{m}^{(b_1)}}\left(\hat{\theta}_1^{(b_1 b_2)} - \hat{\theta}_1^{(b_1)}\right), b_2 = 1, \ldots, B_2\right\}$, say $\hat{l}_{\text{DB}}^{(b_1)}$ and $\hat{u}_{\text{DB}}^{(b_1)}$ respectively. Construct the *double centered percentile bootstrap* CI from the b_1-th first-stage bootstrap data as $\left(c^T \hat{\theta}_1^{(b_1)} - \hat{u}_{\text{DB}}^{(b_1)}/\sqrt{\hat{m}^{(b_1)}}, c^T \hat{\theta}_1^{(b_1)} - \hat{l}_{\text{DB}}^{(b_1)}/\sqrt{\hat{m}^{(b_1)}}\right)$, $b_1 = 1, \ldots, B_1$.
5. Estimate the coverage rate of the double bootstrap CI from all the first-stage bootstrap data sets as

$$\frac{1}{B_1} \sum_{b_1=1}^{B_1} \mathbb{I}\left[c^T \hat{\theta}_1^{(b_1)} - \hat{u}_{\text{DB}}^{(b_1)}/\sqrt{\hat{m}^{(b_1)}} \leq c^T \hat{\theta}_1 \leq c^T \hat{\theta}_1^{(b_1)} - \hat{l}_{\text{DB}}^{(b_1)}/\sqrt{\hat{m}^{(b_1)}}\right].$$

6. If the above coverage rate is at or above the nominal rate, up to Monte Carlo error, then pick the current value of α as the final value. Otherwise, update α to its next higher value in the grid.
7. Repeat steps 2–6, until the coverage rate of the double bootstrap CI, up to Monte Carlo error, attains the nominal coverage rate, or the grid is exhausted.[2]

[2] If this unlikely event does occur, one should examine the observed values of $\hat{p}$. If the values of $\hat{p}$ are concentrated close to zero, ν may be increased; if not, the maximal value in the grid should be increased.

Chakraborty et al. (2013) proved the consistency of the m-out-of-n bootstrap in this context, and in particular that

$$P\left(c^T\hat{\theta}_1 - \hat{u}/\sqrt{\hat{m}} \le c^T\theta_1 \le c^T\hat{\theta}_1 - \hat{l}/\sqrt{\hat{m}}\right) \ge 1 - \eta + o_P(1).$$

The above probability statement is with respect to the bootstrap distribution. Furthermore, if $P(H_{21}^T\psi_2 = 0) = 0$, then the above inequality can be strengthened to equality. This result shows that the m-out-of-n bootstrap method can be used to construct valid (though potentially conservative) confidence intervals regardless of the underlying parameters or generative model. Moreover, in settings where there is a treatment effect for every patient (regular setting), the adaptive procedure delivers asymptotically exact coverage. Unlike the theoretical setting of adaptive CIs of Laber et al. (2011), the theory of m-out-of-n bootstrap does not involve a local asymptotic framework (in fact it is not consistent under local alternatives).

The m-out-of-n bootstrap procedure for two stages in the context of Q-learning with linear models has been implemented in the R package `qLearn` that is freely available from the Comprehensive R Archive Network (CRAN):

`http://cran.r-project.org/web/packages/qLearn/index.html.`

8.8 Simulation Study

In this section, we consider a simulation study to provide an empirical evaluation of the available inference methods discussed in this chapter. Nine generative models are used in these evaluations, each of them having two stages of treatment and two treatments at each stage. Generically, these models can be described as follows:

- $O_i \in \{-1,1\}, A_i \in \{-1,1\}$ for $i = 1,2$;
- $P(A_1 = 1) = P(A_1 = -1) = 0.5$, $P(A_2 = 1) = P(A_2 = -1) = 0.5$;
- $O_1 \sim \text{Bernoulli}(0.5)$, $O_2|O_1,A_1 \sim \text{Bernoulli}(\text{expit}(\delta_1 O_1 + \delta_2 A_1))$;
- $Y_1 \equiv 0$,
  $Y_2 = \gamma_1 + \gamma_2 O_1 + \gamma_3 A_1 + \gamma_4 O_1 A_1 + \gamma_5 A_2 + \gamma_6 O_2 A_2 + \gamma_7 A_1 A_2 + \varepsilon$,

where $\varepsilon \sim \mathcal{N}(0,1)$ and $\text{expit}(x) = e^x/(1+e^x)$. This class is parameterized by nine quantities $\gamma_1, \gamma_2, \ldots, \gamma_7, \delta_1, \delta_2$.

The form of the above class of generative models, developed by Chakraborty et al. (2010), is useful as it allows one to influence the degree of non-regularity present in the example problems through the choice of γs and δs, and in turn evaluate performance in these different scenarios. Recall that in Q-learning, non-regularity occurs when more than one stage 2 treatment produces exactly or nearly the same optimal expected outcome for a set of patient histories that occur with positive probability. In the model class above, this occurs if the model generates histories for which $\gamma_5 A_2 + \gamma_6 O_2 A_2 + \gamma_7 A_1 A_2 \approx 0$, i.e., if it generates histories for which Q_2 depends weakly or not at all on A_2. By manipulating the values of γs and δs, we can control: (i) the probability of generating a patient history such that $\gamma_5 A_2 + \gamma_6 O_2 A_2 + \gamma_7 A_1 A_2 = 0$, and (ii) the standardized effect size $E(\gamma_5 + \gamma_6 O_2 + \gamma_7 A_1)/\sqrt{\text{Var}(\gamma_5 + \gamma_6 O_2 + \gamma_7 A_1)}$. These two quantities, denoted by p and ϕ, respectively, can be thought of as *measures of non-regularity*. Note that for fixed parameter values, the linear combination $(\gamma_5 + \gamma_6 O_2 + \gamma_7 A_1)$ that governs the non-regularity in an example generative model can take only four possible values corresponding to the four possible (O_2, A_1) cells. The cell probabilities can be easily calculated; the formulae are provided in Table 8.2. Using the quantities presented in Table 8.2, one can write

$$E[\gamma_5 + \gamma_6 O_2 + \gamma_7 A_1] = q_1 f_1 + q_2 f_2 + q_3 f_3 + q_4 f_4,$$
$$E[(\gamma_5 + \gamma_6 O_2 + \gamma_7 A_1)^2] = q_1 f_1^2 + q_2 f_2^2 + q_3 f_3^2 + q_4 f_4^2.$$

From these two, one can calculate $Var[\gamma_5 + \gamma_6 O_2 + \gamma_7 A_1]$, and subsequently the effect size ϕ.

Table 8.2 Distribution of the linear combination $(\gamma_5 + \gamma_6 O_2 + \gamma_7 A_1)$

(O_2, A_1) cell	Cell probability (averaged over O_1)	Value of the linear combination
$(1,1)$	$q_1 \equiv \frac{1}{4}\Big(expit(\delta_1 + \delta_2) + expit(-\delta_1 + \delta_2)\Big)$	$f_1 \equiv \gamma_5 + \gamma_6 + \gamma_7$
$(1,-1)$	$q_2 \equiv \frac{1}{4}\Big(expit(\delta_1 - \delta_2) + expit(-\delta_1 - \delta_2)\Big)$	$f_2 \equiv \gamma_5 + \gamma_6 - \gamma_7$
$(-1,1)$	$q_3 \equiv \frac{1}{4}\Big(expit(\delta_1 - \delta_2) + expit(-\delta_1 - \delta_2)\Big)$	$f_3 \equiv \gamma_5 - \gamma_6 + \gamma_7$
$(-1,-1)$	$q_4 \equiv \frac{1}{4}\Big(expit(\delta_1 + \delta_2) + expit(-\delta_1 + \delta_2)\Big)$	$f_4 \equiv \gamma_5 - \gamma_6 - \gamma_7$

Table 8.3 provides the parameter settings; the first six of these settings were constructed by Chakraborty et al. (2010), and were described therein as "non-regular," "near-non-regular," and "regular." Example 1 is a setting where there is no treatment effect for any subject (any possible history) in either stage. Example 2 is similar to example 1, where there is a very weak stage 2 treatment effect for every subject, but it is hard to detect the very weak effect given the noise level in the data. Example 3 is a setting where there is no stage 2 treatment effect for half the subjects in the population, but a reasonably large effect for the other half of subjects. In example 4, there is a very weak stage 2 treatment effect for half the subjects in the population, but a reasonably large effect for the other half of subjects (the parameters are close to those in example 3). Example 5 is a setting where there is no stage 2 treatment effect for one-fourth of the subjects in the population, but others have a reasonably large effect. Example 6 is a completely regular setting where there is a reasonably large stage 2 treatment effect for every subject in the population. Song et al. (2011) also used these six examples for empirical evaluation of their PQ-learning method.

To these six, Laber et al. (2011) added three further examples labeled A, B, and C. Example A is an example of a strongly regular setting. Example B is an example of a non-regular setting where the non-regularity is strongly dependent on the stage 1 treatment. In example B, for histories with $A_1 = 1$, there is a moderate effect of

A_2 at the second stage. However, for histories with $A_1 = -1$, there is no effect of A_2 at the second stage, i.e., both actions at the second stage are equally optimal. In example C, for histories with $A_1 = 1$, there is a moderate effect of A_2, and for histories with $A_1 = -1$, there is a small effect of A_2. Thus example C is a "near-non-regular" setting that behaves similarly to example B.

Table 8.3 Parameters indexing the example models

Example	γ^T	δ^T	Type	Regularity Measures	
1	$(0,0,0,0,0,0,0)$	$(0.5,0.5)$	Non-regular	$p=1$	$\phi=0/0$
2	$(0,0,0,0,0.01,0,0)$	$(0.5,0.5)$	Near-non-regular	$p=0$	$\phi=\infty$
3	$(0,0,-0.5,0,0.5,0,0.5)$	$(0.5,0.5)$	Non-regular	$p=1/2$	$\phi=1.0$
4	$(0,0,-0.5,0,0.5,0,0.49)$	$(0.5,0.5)$	Near-non-regular	$p=0$	$\phi=1.02$
5	$(0,0,-0.5,0,1.0,0.5,0.5)$	$(1.0,0.0)$	Non-regular	$p=1/4$	$\phi=1.41$
6	$(0,0,-0.5,0,0.25,0.5,0.5)$	$(0.1,0.1)$	Regular	$p=0$	$\phi=0.35$
A	$(0,0,-0.25,0,0.75,0.5,0.5)$	$(0.1,0.1)$	Regular	$p=0$	$\phi=1.035$
B	$(0,0,0,0,0.25,0,0.25)$	$(0,0)$	Non-regular	$p=1/2$	$\phi=1.00$
C	$(0,0,0,0,0.25,0,0.24)$	$(0,0)$	Near-non-regular	$p=0$	$\phi=1.03$

The Q-learning analysis models used in the simulation study are given by

$$\begin{aligned} Q_2^{opt}(H_2, A_2; \beta_2, \psi_2) &= H_{20}^T \beta_2 + H_{21}^T \psi_2 A_2, \\ Q_1^{opt}(H_1, A_1; \beta_1) &= H_{10}^T \beta_1 + H_{11}^T \psi_1 A_1, \end{aligned}$$

where the following patient history vectors are used:

$$\begin{aligned} H_{20} &= (1, O_1, A_1, O_1 A_1)^T, \\ H_{21} &= (1, O_2, A_1)^T, \\ H_{10} &= (1, O_1)^T, \\ H_{11} &= (1, O_1)^T. \end{aligned}$$

So the models for the Q-functions are correctly specified. For the purpose of inference, the focus is on ψ_{10} and ψ_{11}, the parameters associated with stage 1 treatment A_1 in the analysis model. They can be expressed in terms of γs and δs, the parameters of the generative model, as follows:

$$\begin{aligned} \psi_{10} &= \gamma_3 + q_1|f_1| - q_2|f_2| + q_3|f_3| - q_4|f_4|, \\ \text{and } \psi_{11} &= \gamma_4 + q_1'|f_1| - q_2'|f_2| - q_3'|f_3| + q_4'|f_4|, \end{aligned}$$

where $q_1' = q_3' = \frac{1}{4}(expit(\delta_1 + \delta_2) - expit(-\delta_1 + \delta_2))$, and $q_2' = q_4' = \frac{1}{4}(expit(\delta_1 - \delta_2) - expit(-\delta_1 - \delta_2))$.

Below we will present simulation results to compare the performances of ten competing methods of constructing CIs for the stage 1 parameters of Q-learning. We will be reporting the results for *centered percentile* bootstrap (CPB) (Efron and Tibshirani 1993) method. Let $\hat{\theta}$ be an estimator of θ and $\hat{\theta}^{(b)}$ be its bootstrap version. Then the $100(1-\alpha)\,\%$ CPB confidence interval is given by $\left(2\hat{\theta}-\hat{\theta}^{(b)}_{(1-\frac{\alpha}{2})}, 2\hat{\theta}-\hat{\theta}^{(b)}_{(\frac{\alpha}{2})}\right)$, where $\hat{\theta}^{(b)}_{\gamma}$ is the 100γ-th percentile of the bootstrap distribution. The competing methods are listed below:

(i) CPB interval in conjunction with the (original) hard-max estimator (CPB-HM);
(ii) CPB interval in conjunction with the hard-threshold estimator with $\alpha = 0.08$ (CPB-HT$_{0.08}$);
(iii) CPB interval in conjunction with the soft-threshold estimator (CPB-ST);
(iv) Double bootstrap interval in conjunction with the hard-max estimator (DB-HM);
(v) Asymptotic confidence interval in conjunction with the PQ-learning estimator (PQ);
(vi) Adaptive bootstrap confidence interval (ACI);
(vii) m-out-of-n CPB interval with fixed $\alpha = 0.1$, in conjunction with the hard-max estimator ($\hat{m}_{0.1}$-CPB-HM);
(viii) m-out-of-n CPB interval with data-driven α chosen by double bootstrap, in conjunction with the hard-max estimator ($\hat{m}_{\hat{\alpha}}$-CPB-HM);
(ix) m-out-of-n CPB interval with fixed $\alpha = 0.1$, in conjunction with the soft-threshold estimator ($\hat{m}_{0.1}$-CPB-ST);
(x) m-out-of-n CPB interval with data-driven α chosen by double bootstrap, in conjunction with the soft-threshold estimator ($\hat{m}_{\hat{\alpha}}$-CPB-ST)

The comparisons are conducted on a variety of settings represented by examples 1–6, A–C, using $N = 1{,}000$ simulated data sets, $B = 1{,}000$ bootstrap replications, and the sample size $n = 300$. However, the double bootstrap CIs are based on $B_1 = 500$ first-stage and $B_2 = 100$ second-stage bootstrap iterations, due to the increased computational burden. Note that here we simply compile the results from the original papers instead of implementing and running them afresh. As a consequence, the results for all the methods across all examples are not available.

We focus on the coverage rate and width of CIs for the parameter ψ_{10} that denotes the main effect of treatment; see Table 8.4 for coverage and Table 8.5 for width of CIs. Different authors also reported results for the stage 1 interaction parameter ψ_{11}; however the effect of non-regularity is less pronounced on this parameter, and hence less interesting for the purpose of illustration of non-regularity and comparison of competing methods.

First, let us focus on Table 8.4. As expected from the inconsistency of the usual n-out-of-n bootstrap in the present non-regular problem, the CPB-HM method shows the problem of under-coverage in most of the examples. While CPB-HT$_{0.08}$, by virtue of bias correction via thresholding (see Moodie and Richardson 2010), performs well in Ex. 1–4, it fares poorly in Ex. 5–6 (and was never implemented in Ex. A–C). Similarly CPB-ST performs well, again by virtue of bias correction via thresholding (see Chakraborty et al. 2010), except in Ex. 6, A, and B. The computationally expensive double bootstrap method (DB-HM) performs well across the first six examples (but was never tried on Ex. A–C). The PQ method (see Song et al. 2011) performs well across the first six examples (but was never tried on

Ex. A–C). PQ-learning is probably the cheapest method computationally, because CIs are constructed by asymptotic formulae rather than any kind of bootstrapping. The ACI, as known from the work of Laber et al. (2011), is a consistent bootstrap procedure that is conservative in some of the highly non-regular settings but delivers coverage rates closer to nominal as the settings become more and more regular (as the degree of non-regularity as measured by p decreases). The behavior of the m-out-of-n bootstrap method with fixed $\alpha = 0.1$ ($\hat{m}_{0.1}$-CPB-HM) is quite similar to that of ACI in that these CIs are conservative in highly non-regular settings, but become close-to-nominal as the settings become more regular. Both ACI and $\hat{m}_{0.1}$-CPB-HM deliver nominal coverage in the two strictly regular settings (Ex. 6, Ex. A) and the one mildly non-regular ($p = \frac{1}{4}$) setting (Ex. 5) considered. However, $\hat{m}_{0.1}$-CPB-HM is computationally much less expensive (about 180 times) than ACI which involves solving a very difficult optimization problem. Interestingly, the m-out-of-n bootstrap with data-driven α via double bootstrap ($\hat{m}_{\hat{\alpha}}$-CPB-HM) offers an extra layer of adaptiveness; fine-tuning α via double bootstrapping reduces the conservatism present in the case of ACI and $\hat{m}_{0.1}$-CPB-HM, and provides nominal coverage in all the examples. However, it is computationally expensive (comparable to ACI). The $\hat{m}_{0.1}$-CPB-ST method performs similarly to the other versions of m-out-of-n bootstrap methods, except perhaps a bit more conservately in non-regular examples. However, this conservatism is reduced in the $\hat{m}_{\hat{\alpha}}$-CPB-ST method. The performances of the last two methods of inference show that the use of m-out-of-n bootstrap is not limited to the original hard-max estimator, but can also be successfully used in conjunction with other non-smooth estimators like the soft-threshold estimator. See Chakraborty et al. (2013) for further discussion on the m-out-of-n bootstrap methods in this context.

Table 8.4 Monte Carlo estimates of coverage probabilities of confidence intervals for the main effect of treatment (ψ_{10}) at the 95 % nominal level. Estimates significantly below 0.95 at the 0.05 level are marked with ∗. Examples are designated *NR* non-regular, *NNR* near-non-regular, *R* regular

$n = 300$	Ex. 1	Ex. 2	Ex. 3	Ex. 4	Ex. 5	Ex. 6	Ex. A	Ex. B	Ex. C
	NR	NNR	NR	NNR	NR	R	R	NR	NNR
CPB-HM	0.936	0.932*	0.928*	0.921*	0.933*	0.931*	0.944	0.925*	0.922*
CPB-HT$_{0.08}$	0.950	0.953	0.943	0.941	0.932*	0.885*	–	–	–
CPB-ST	0.962	0.961	0.947	0.946	0.942	0.918*	0.918*	0.931*	0.938
DB-HM	0.936	0.936	0.948	0.944	0.942	0.950	–	–	–
PQ	0.951	0.940	0.952	0.955	0.953	0.953	–	–	–
ACI	0.994	0.994	0.975	0.976	0.962	0.957	0.950	0.977	0.976
$\hat{m}_{0.1}$-CPB-HM	0.984	0.982	0.956	0.955	0.943	0.949	0.953	0.971	0.970
$\hat{m}_{\hat{\alpha}}$-CPB-HM	0.964	0.964	0.953	0.950	0.939	0.947	0.944	0.955	0.960
$\hat{m}_{0.1}$-CPB-ST	0.993	0.993	0.979	0.976	0.954	0.943	0.939	0.972	0.977
$\hat{m}_{\hat{\alpha}}$-CPB-ST	0.971	0.976	0.961	0.956	0.949	0.935	0.926*	0.971	0.967

Table 8.5 presents the Monte Carlo estimates of the mean width of CIs. Mean widths corresponding to CPB-HT$_{0.08}$, DB-HM and PQ were not reported in the original papers in which they appeared. Among the rest of the methods, as expected,

Table 8.5 Monte Carlo estimates of the mean width of confidence intervals for the main effect of treatment (ψ_{10}) at the 95 % nominal level. Widths with corresponding coverage significantly below nominal are marked with $*$. Examples are designated *NR* non-regular, *NNR* near-non-regular, *R* regular

$n = 300$	Ex. 1 NR	Ex. 2 NNR	Ex. 3 NR	Ex. 4 NNR	Ex. 5 NR	Ex. 6 R	Ex. A R	Ex. B NR	Ex. C NNR
CPB-HM	0.269	0.269*	0.300*	0.300*	0.320*	0.309*	0.314	0.299*	0.299*
CPB-HT$_{0.08}$	–	–	–	–	–	–	–	–	–
CPB-ST	0.250	0.250	0.293	0.293	0.319	0.319*	0.323*	0.303*	0.304
DB-HM	–	–	–	–	–	–	–	–	–
PQ	–	–	–	–	–	–	–	–	–
ACI	0.354	0.354	0.342	0.342	0.341	0.327	0.327	0.342	0.342
$\hat{m}_{0.1}$-CPB-HM	0.346	0.347	0.341	0.341	0.340	0.341	0.332	0.342	0.343
$\hat{m}_{\hat{\alpha}}$-CPB-HM	0.331	0.331	0.321	0.323	0.330	0.336	0.322	0.328	0.328
$\hat{m}_{0.1}$-CPB-ST	0.324	0.324	0.336	0.336	0.343	0.352	0.343	0.353	0.353
$\hat{m}_{\hat{\alpha}}$-CPB-ST	0.273	0.275	0.306	0.306	0.328	0.349	0.331*	0.330	0.332

CIs constructed via the usual n-out-of-n method (CPB-HM and CPB-ST) have the least width; however these are often associated with under-coverage. The widths of the CIs from the last five methods are quite comparable, with $\hat{m}_{\hat{\alpha}}$-CPB-HM and $\hat{m}_{\hat{\alpha}}$-CPB-ST offering narrower CIs more often.

Given the above findings, it is very hard to declare an overall winner. From a purely theoretical standpoint, the ACI method (Laber et al. 2011) is arguably the strongest since it uses a local asymptotic framework. However it is conceptually complicated, computationally expensive, and often conservative in finite samples. In terms of finite sample performance, both versions of the m-out-of-n bootstrap method (Chakraborty et al. 2013) are at least as good as (and often better than) the ACI method; moreover, they are conceptually very simple and hence may be more attractive to practitioners. The version with fixed α ($\hat{m}_{0.1}$-CPB-HM), while similar to ACI in conservatism, is computationally much cheaper. On the other hand, the version with data-driven choice of α ($\hat{m}_{\hat{\alpha}}$-CPB), while computationally as demanding as the ACI, overcomes the conservatism and provides nominal coverage in all the examples. Nonetheless, m-out-of-n bootstrap methods are valid only under fixed alternatives, not under local alternatives. The PQ-learning method (Song et al. 2011) is also valid only under fixed alternatives but not under local alternatives. This method is non-conservative in Ex. 1–6, and is computationally the cheapest. However its coverage performance in Ex. A–C and the mean widths of CIs resulting from this method in all the examples are unknown to us at this point.

Note that the bias maps of Fig. 8.1 in Sect. 8.2 were created in a scenario where $\gamma_5 + \gamma_6 O_2 + \gamma_7 A_1 = 0$ with positive probability. As noted previously, the generative parameters γ_5, γ_6 and γ_7 correspond to the policy parameters ψ_{20}, ψ_{21}, and ψ_{22} of the analysis model, respectively. For all bias maps in the figure, $\gamma_1 = \gamma_2 = \gamma_4 = 0$ and $\gamma_3 = -0.5$; the first three plots (upper panel) explored the extent of bias in regions around the parameter setting given in Ex. 5 of Table 8.3, while the last three plots (lower panel) explore the extent of bias in regions around the parameter setting in

Ex. 6 of Table 8.3. More precisely, in the first three plots, $\delta_1 = 1, \delta_2 = 0$; and only one of $\psi_{20} (= \gamma_5)$, $\psi_{21} (= \gamma_6)$, or $\psi_{22} (= \gamma_7)$ was varied while the remaining were fixed (e.g. $(\psi_{21}, \psi_{22}) = (0.5, 0.5)$ fixed in the first plot, $(\psi_{20}, \psi_{22}) = (1.0, 0.5)$ fixed in the second plot, and $(\psi_{20}, \psi_{21}) = (1.0, 0.5)$ fixed in the third plot). Similarly, in the last three plots, $\delta_1 = \delta_2 = 0.1$; and only one of ψ_{20}, ψ_{21}, or ψ_{22} was varied while the remaining were fixed, e.g. $(\psi_{21}, \psi_{22}) = (0.5, 0.5)$ fixed in the first plot of the lower panel, $(\psi_{20}, \psi_{22}) = (0.25, 0.5)$ fixed in the second plot of the lower panel, and $(\psi_{20}, \psi_{21}) = (0.25, 0.5)$ fixed in the third plot of the lower panel.

8.9 Analysis of STAR*D Data: An Illustration

8.9.1 Background and Study Details

Selective serotonin reuptake inhibitors (SSRIs) are the most commonly prescribed class of antidepressants with simple dosing regimens and a preferable adverse effect profile in comparison to other types of antidepressants (Nelson 1997; Mason et al. 2000). Serotonin is a neurotransmitter in the human brain that regulates a variety of functions including mood. SSRIs affect the serotonin based brain circuits. Other classes of antidepressants may act on serotonin in concert with other neurotransmitter systems, or on entirely different neurotransmitter. While a meta-analysis of all efficacy trials submitted to the US Food and Drug Administration of four antidepressants for which full data sets were available found that pharmacological treatment of depression was no more effective than placebo for mild to moderate depression, other studies support the effectiveness of SSRIs and other antidepressants in primary care settings (Arroll et al. 2005, 2009). Few studies have examined treatment patterns, and in particular, few have studied best prescribing practices following treatment failure.

Sequenced Treatment Alternatives to Relieve Depression (STAR*D) was a multisite, multi-level randomized controlled trial designed to assess the comparative effectiveness of different treatment regimes for patients with major depressive disorder, and was introduced earlier in Chap. 2. See Sect. 2.4.2 for a detailed description of the study design along with a schematic of the treatment assignment algorithm. Here we will focus on levels 2, 2A, and 3 of the study only. For the purpose of the current analysis, we will classify the treatments into two categories: (i) treatment with an SSRI (alone or in combination): sertraline (SER), CIT + bupropion (BUP), CIT + buspirone (BUS), or CIT + cognitive psychotherapy (CT) or (ii) treatment with one or more non-SSRIs: venlafaxine (VEN), BUP, or CT alone. Only the patients assigned to CIT + CT or CT alone in level 2 were eligible, in the case of a non-satisfactory response, to move to a supplementary level of treatment (level 2A), to receive either VEN or BUP. Patients not responding satisfactorily at level 2 (and level 2A, if applicable) would continue to level 3. Treatment options at level 3 can again be classified into two categories, i.e. treatment with (i) SSRI: an augmentation of any SSRI-containing level 2 treatment with either lithium (Li) or thyroid hormone (THY), or (ii) non-SSRI: mirtazapine (MIRT) or nortriptyline (NTP), or an augmentation of any non-SSRI level 2 treatment with either Li or THY.

8.9.2 Analysis

Here we present the analysis originally conducted by Chakraborty et al. (2013). In this analysis, level 2A was considered a part of level 2. This implies that a patient who received an SSRI at level 2 but a non-SSRI at level 2A was considered a recipient of SSRI in the combined level 2 + 2A for the present analysis. Also, levels 2 (including 2A, if applicable) and 3 were treated as stages 1 and 2 respectively of the Q-learning framework (level 4 data were not considered in this analysis). As a feature of the trial design, the outcome data at stage 2 were available only for the non-remitters from stage 1; so Chakraborty et al. (2013) defined the overall primary outcome (Y) as the average $-$QIDS score over the stage(s) a patient was present in the study, i.e.

$$Y = R_1 \cdot Y_1 + (1 - R_1) \cdot \left(\frac{Y_1 + Y_2}{2}\right),$$

where Y_1 and Y_2 denote the $-$QIDS scores measured at the end of stages 1 and 2 respectively (the negative of QIDS score was taken to make higher values correspond to better outcomes), and $R_1 = 1$ if the subject achieved remission (QIDS ≤ 5) at the end of stage 1, and 0 otherwise.

Following Pineau et al. (2007), three covariates (tailoring variables) were included in this analysis: (i) QIDS-score measured at the start of the level (QIDS.start), (ii) the slope of the QIDS-score over the previous level (QIDS.slope), and (iii) preference. While QIDS.start and QIDS.slope are continuous variables, preference is a binary variable, coded 1 for preference to switch previous treatment and -1 for preference to augment previous treatment or no preference. Following the notation used earlier, let O_{1j} denote the QIDS.start at the jth stage, and O_{2j} denote the QIDS.slope at the jth stage, O_{3j} denote the preference at the jth stage, and A_j denote the treatment at the jth stage, for $j = 1, 2$. Treatment at each stage was coded 1 for SSRI and -1 for non-SSRI. The following models for the Q-functions were employed:

$$Q_2^{opt} = \beta_{02} + \beta_{12}O_{12} + \beta_{22}O_{22} + \beta_{32}O_{32} + \beta_{42}A_1 + \Big(\psi_{02} + \psi_{12}O_{12} + \psi_{22}O_{22}\Big)A_2,$$

$$Q_1^{opt} = \beta_{01} + \beta_{11}O_{11} + \beta_{21}O_{21} + \beta_{31}O_{31} + \Big(\psi_{01} + \psi_{11}O_{11} + \psi_{21}O_{21} + \psi_{31}O_{31}\Big)A_1.$$

To avoid singularity, a preference-by-treatment interaction was not included in the model for Q_2^{opt}; similarly no A_1A_2 interaction was included. According to the above models, the optimal DTR is given by the following two decision rules:

$$d_2^{opt}(H_2) = sign(\psi_{02} + \psi_{12}O_{12} + \psi_{22}O_{22}),$$

$$d_1^{opt}(H_1) = sign(\psi_{01} + \psi_{11}O_{11} + \psi_{21}O_{21} + \psi_{31}O_{31}).$$

One thousand two hundred and sixty patients were used at stage 1 (level 2); a small number (19) of patients were omitted altogether due to gross item missingness in the covariates. Of the 1,260 patients at stage 1, there were 792 who were non-remitters (QIDS > 5) who should have moved to stage 2 (level 3); however, only 324 patients were present at stage 2 while the rest dropped out. To adjust for this dropout, the model for Q_2^{opt} was fitted using inverse probability weighting where the probability of being present at stage 2 was estimated by logistic regression using $O_{11}, O_{21}, O_{31}, A_1, -Y_1, O_{22}, O_{11}A_1, O_{21}A_1$, and $O_{31}A_1$ as predictors.

Another complexity came up in the computation of the pseudo-outcome, $\max_{a_2} Q_2^{opt}$. Note that for $(792 - 324) = 468$ non-remitters who were absent from stage 2, covariates O_{12} (QIDS.start at stage 2) and O_{32} (preference at stage 2) were missing, rendering the computation of the pseudo-outcome impossible for them. For these patients, the value of O_{12} was imputed by the last observed QIDS score in the previous stage – a sensible strategy for a continuous, slowly changing variable like the QIDS score. On the other hand, the missing values of the binary variable O_{32} (preference at stage 2) were imputed using k nearest neighbor (k-NN) classification, where k was chosen via leave-one-out cross-validation. Following these imputations, Q-learning was implemented for this data; the estimates of the parameters of the Q-functions, along with their 95 % bootstrap CIs were computed. While only the usual bootstrap was used at stage 2, both the usual bootstrap and the adaptive m-out-of-n bootstrap procedure (with α chosen via double bootstrap) were employed at stage 1, to facilitate ready comparison.

8.9.3 Results

Results of the above analysis are presented in Table 8.6. In this analysis, m was chosen to be 1,059 in a data-driven way (using double bootstrap). At both stages, the coefficient of QIDS.start (β_{12} and β_{11}) and the coefficient of preference (β_{32} and β_{31}) were statistically significant. Additionally ψ_{31}, the coefficient of preference-by-treatment interaction at stage 1 was significantly different from 0; this fact is particularly interesting because it suggests that the decision rule at stage 1 should be individually tailored based on preference.

The estimated optimal DTR can be explicitly described in terms of the $\hat{\psi}$s: $\hat{d}_2^{opt}(H_2) = sign(-0.18 - 0.01O_{12} - 0.25O_{22})$, and $\hat{d}_1^{opt}(H_1) = sign(-0.73 + 0.01O_{11} + 0.01O_{21} - 0.67O_{31})$. That is, the estimated optimal DTR suggests treating a patient at stage 2 with an SSRI if $(-0.18 - 0.01 \times \text{QIDS.start}_2 - 0.25 \times \text{QIDS.slope}_2) > 0$, and with a non-SSRI otherwise. Similarly, it suggests treating a patient at stage 1 with an SSRI if $(-0.73 + 0.01 \times \text{QIDS.start}_1 + 0.01 \times \text{QIDS.slope}_1 - 0.67 \times \text{preference}_1) > 0$, and with a non-SSRI otherwise.

Table 8.6 Regression coefficients and their 95 % centered percentile bootstrap CIs (both the usual n-out-of-n and the novel m-out-of-n) in the analysis of STAR*D data (significant coefficients are in bold)

Parameter	Variable	Estimate	95 % CI (n-out-of-n)	95 % CI (m-out-of-n)
		Stage 2 ($n = 324$)		
β_{02}	Intercept$_2$	−1.66	(−3.70, 0.43)	–
β_{12}	QIDS.start$_2$	**−0.72**	(−0.87, −0.56)	–
β_{22}	QIDS.slope$_2$	0.79	(−0.32, 1.99)	–
β_{32}	Preference$_2$	**0.74**	(0.05, 1.50)	–
β_{42}	Treatment$_1$	0.26	(−0.38, 0.89)	–
ψ_{02}	Treatment$_2$	−0.18	(−2.15, 2.00)	–
ψ_{12}	Treatment$_2$ × QIDS.start$_2$	−0.01	(−0.18, 0.13)	–
ψ_{22}	Treatment$_2$ × QIDS.slope$_2$	−0.25	(−1.33, 0.94)	–
		Stage 1 ($n = 1,260$; $\hat{m} = 1,059$)		
β_{01}	Intercept$_1$	−0.47	(−1.64, 0.71)	(−1.82, 0.97)
β_{11}	QIDS.start$_1$	**−0.55**	(−0.63, −0.48)	(−0.65, −0.46)
β_{21}	QIDS.slope$_1$	0.12	(−0.36, 0.52)	(−0.41, 0.57)
β_{31}	Preference$_1$	**0.88**	(0.40, 1.40)	(0.35, 1.46)
ψ_{01}	Treatment$_1$	−0.73	(−1.84, 0.43)	(−1.91, 0.48)
ψ_{11}	Treatment$_1$ × QIDS.start$_1$	0.01	(−0.06, 0.09)	(−0.07, 0.09)
ψ_{21}	Treatment$_1$ × QIDS.slope$_1$	0.01	(−0.44, 0.46)	(−0.47, 0.49)
ψ_{31}	Treatment$_1$ × Preference$_1$	**−0.67**	(−1.17, −0.18)	(−1.29, −0.16)

However, these are just the "point estimates" of the optimal decision rules. A measure of confidence for these estimated decision rules can be formulated as follows. Note that the estimated difference in mean outcome at stage 2 corresponding to the two treatment options is given by

$$\begin{aligned} &Q_2^{opt}(H_2, 1; \hat{\beta}_2, \hat{\psi}_2) - Q_2^{opt}(H_2, -1; \hat{\beta}_2, \hat{\psi}_2) \\ &\quad = 2\big(-0.18 - 0.01 \times \text{QIDS.start}_2 - 0.25 \times \text{QIDS.slope}_2\big). \end{aligned}$$

Likewise, the estimated difference in mean pseudo-outcome at stage 1 corresponding to the two treatment options is given by

$$\begin{aligned} &Q_1^{opt}(H_1, 1; \hat{\beta}_1, \hat{\psi}_1) - Q_1^{opt}(H_1, -1; \hat{\beta}_1, \hat{\psi}_1) \\ &\quad = 2\big(-0.73 + 0.01 \times \text{QIDS.start}_1 + 0.01 \times \text{QIDS.slope}_1 - 0.67 \times \text{preference}_1\big). \end{aligned}$$

For any fixed values of QIDS.start, QIDS.slope, and preference, one can construct point-wise CIs for the above difference in mean outcome (or, pseudo-outcome) based on the CIs for the individual ψs, thus leading to a confidence band around the entire function. The mean difference function and its 95 % confidence band over the observed range of QIDS.start and QIDS.slope are plotted for stage 1 (separately for preference = "switch" and preference = "augment or no preference") and for stage 2 (patients with all preferences combined), and are presented in Fig. 8.3. Since the confidence bands in all three panels contain zero, there is insufficient evidence in the data to recommend a unique best treatment.

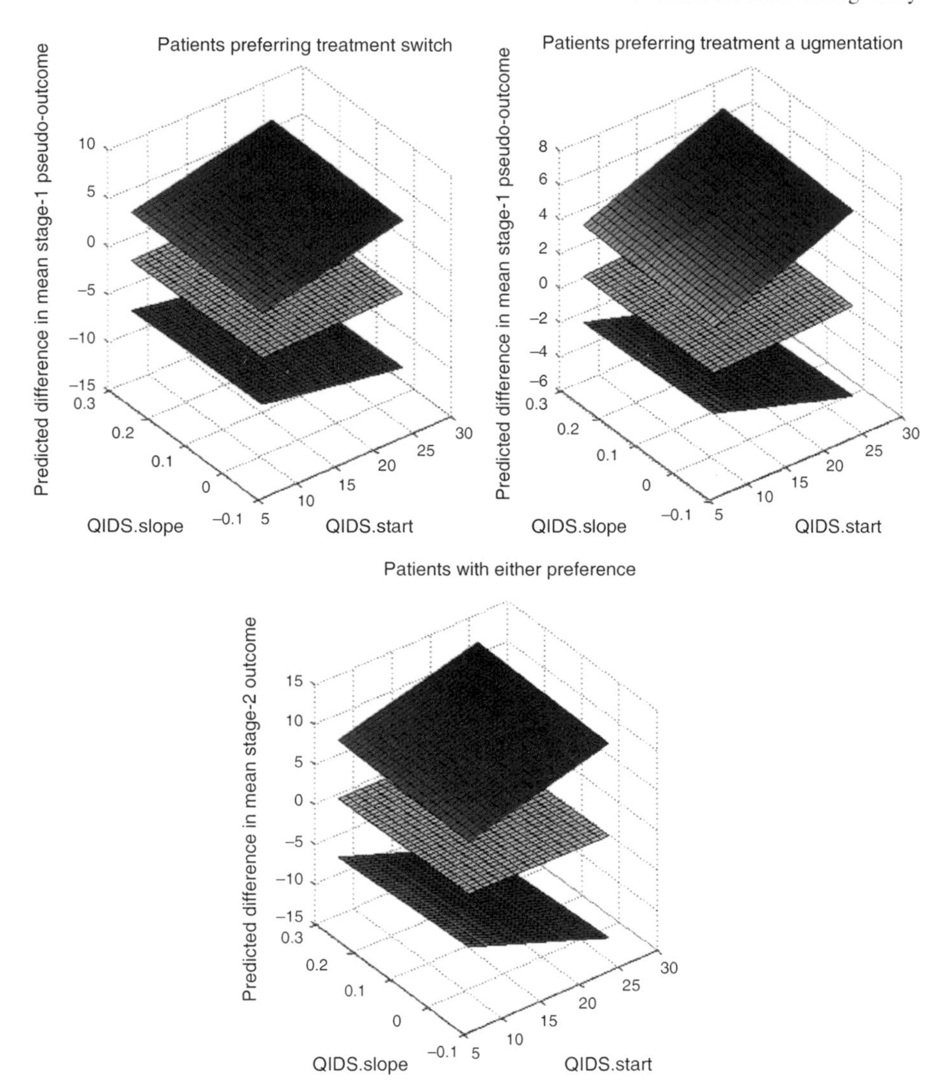

Fig. 8.3 Predicted difference in mean outcome and its 95 % confidence band for: (**a**) patients preferring treatment switch at stage 1; (**b**) patients either preferring treatment augmentation or without preference at stage 1; and (**c**) all patients at stage 2

8.10 Inference About the Value of an Estimated DTR

In Sect. 5.1, we discussed estimation of the *value* of an arbitrary DTR. Once a DTR $\hat{d}$ is estimated from the data (say, via Q-learning, G-estimation, etc.), a key quantity to assess its merit is its true value, $V^{\hat{d}}$. A point estimate of this quantity, say $\hat{V}^{\hat{d}}$, can be obtained, for example, by the IPTW formula (see Sect. 5.1). However it may be more interesting to construct a confidence interval for $V^{\hat{d}}$ and see if the confidence interval contains the optimal value V^{opt} (implying that the estimated DTR is not significantly different from the optimal DTR), or the value of some other pre-specified (not necessarily optimal) DTR. It turns out that the estimation of the value of an estimated DTR, or constructing a confidence interval for it, is a very difficult problem.

From Sect. 5.1, we can express the value of $\hat{d}$ by

$$V^{\hat{d}} = \int \Big(\prod_{j=1}^{K} \frac{\mathbb{I}[A_j = \hat{d}_j(H_j)]}{\pi_j(A_j|H_j)} \Big) Y dP_{\pi}, \tag{8.17}$$

where π is an embedded DTR in the study from which the data arose (e.g. the randomization probabilities in the study); see Sect. 5.1 for further details. Note that (8.17) can be alternatively expressed as

$$\begin{aligned} V^{\hat{d}} &= \int \Big\{ \prod_{j=1}^{K} \frac{1}{\pi_j(A_j|H_j)} Y \Big\} \Big(\prod_{j=1}^{K} \mathbb{I}[A_j = \hat{d}_j(H_j)] \Big) dP_{\pi} \\ &= \int c(O_1, A_1, \ldots, O_{K+1}; \pi) \Big(\prod_{j=1}^{K} \mathbb{I}[A_j = \hat{d}_j(H_j)] \Big) dP_{\pi} \end{aligned} \tag{8.18}$$

where

$$c(O_1, A_1, \ldots, O_{K+1}; \pi) = \Big\{ \prod_{j=1}^{K} \frac{1}{\pi_j(A_j|H_j)} Y \Big\}$$

is a function of the entire data trajectory and the embedded DTR π. Note that the form of the value function, as expressed in (8.18), is analogous to the test error (misclassification rate) of a classifier in a weighted (or, cost-sensitive) classification problem, where $c(O_1, A_1, \ldots, O_{K+1}; \pi)$ serves as the weight (or, cost) function. Zhao et al. (2012) vividly discussed this analogy in a single-stage decision problem; see also Sect. 5.3.

From this analogy, one can argue that the confidence intervals for the value function could be constructed in ways similar to those for confidence intervals for the test error of a learned classifier. Unfortunately, constructing valid confidence intervals for the test error in classification is an extremely difficult problem due to the inherent non-regularity (note the presence of non-smooth indicator functions in the definition of the value function); see Laber and Murphy (2011) for further details. Standard methods like normal approximation or the usual bootstrap fail in this problem. Laber and Murphy (2011) developed a method for constructing such confidence intervals by use of smooth data-dependent upper and lower bounds on the test error; this method is similar to the method described in Sect. 8.6 in the context of inference for Q-learning parameters. They proved that for linear classifiers, their proposed confidence interval automatically adapts to the non-smoothness of the test error, and is consistent under local alternatives. The method provided nominal coverage on a suite of test problems using a range of classification algorithms and sample sizes. While intuitively one can expect that this method could be successfully used for constructing confidence intervals for the value function, more research is needed to extend and fine-tune the procedure to the current setting.

8.11 Bayesian Estimation in Non-regular Settings

Robins (2004) considered the behavior of Bayesian estimators under exceptional laws, i.e. the situations where the data-generating distributions lead to non-regularity in frequentist approaches. He considered a prior distribution, $\pi(\psi)$, for the decision rule parameters that is absolutely continuous with respect to a Lebesgue measure and assigns positive mass over the area that includes the true (unknowable) parameter values. Robins (2004) showed that the posterior distribution of the decision rule parameters is non-normal, but that credible intervals based on the posterior distribution are well-defined under all data-generating distributions with probability 1. Furthermore, in many cases the frequentist confidence interval and the Bayesian credible interval based on the highest posterior density will coincide, even at exceptional laws, in very large samples. Robins noted:

> Nonetheless, in practice, if frequentist [confidence interval for ψ] includes exceptional laws (or laws very close to exceptional laws) and thus the set where the likelihood is relatively large contains an exceptional law, it is best not to use a normal approximation, but rather to use either Markov chain Monte Carlo or rejection sampling techniques to generate a sample $\psi^{(v)}, v = 1, \ldots, V$ [...] to construct highest posterior credible intervals, even if one had a prior mass of zero on the exceptional laws.

Following the estimation of the posterior density via direct calculation or, more likely, Markov Chain Monte Carlo, the Bayesian analyst must then formulate optimal decision rules. This can be done in a variety of manners, such as recommending treatment if the posterior median of $H_{j1}^T \psi_j$ is greater than some threshold or if the probability that the posterior mean of $H_{j1}^T \psi_j$ exceeds a threshold is greater than a half. Decisions based on either of these rules will coincide when the posterior is normally distributed, but may not in general (i.e. when laws are exceptional). Alternatively, both Arjas and Saarela (2010) and Zajonc (2012) considered a G-computation like approach, and choose as optimal the rule that maximizes the posterior predictive mean of the outcome.

8.12 Discussion

In this chapter, we have illustrated the problem of non-regularity that arises in the context of inference about the optimal "current" (stage j) treatment rule, when the optimal treatments at subsequent stages are non-unique for at least some non-null proportion of subjects in the population. We have discussed and illustrated the phenomenon using Q-learning as well as G-estimation.

As discussed by Chakraborty et al. (2010), the underlying non-regularity affects the analysis of optimal DTRs in at least two different ways: in some data-generating models it induces bias in the point estimates of the parameters indexing the optimal DTRs, and in other settings it causes lightness of tail of the asymptotic distribution but no bias. The coexistence of these two not-so-well-related issues makes this inference problem unique and challenging.

Non-regularity is an issue in the estimation of the optimal DTRs because it arises when there is no (or a very small) treatment effect at subsequent stages. This is exactly the setting that we are likely to face in many SMARTs in a variety of application areas, due to clinical equipoise (Freedman 1987). Thus we want estimators and inference tools to perform well particularly in non-regular settings. In the case of the hard-max estimator, unfortunately the point of non-differentiability coincides with the parameter value such that $\psi_2^T H_{21} = 0$ (non-unique optimal treatment at the subsequent stage), which causes non-regularity. The threshold estimators (both soft and hard), in some sense, redistribute the non-regularity from this "null point" to two different points symmetrically placed on either side of the null point (see Fig. 8.2). This is one reason why threshold estimators tend to work well in non-regular settings.

However, threshold estimators are still non-smooth, and hence cannot perform uniformly well throughout the parameter space (particularly in regular settings). Furthermore, due to their non-smoothness, the usual bootstrap procedure is still a theoretically invalid inference procedure. Song et al. (2011) extended the idea of thresholding into penalized regression in the Q-learning steps which led to the PQ-learning estimators. Asymptotic CIs for PQ-learning estimators are constructed via analytical formulae, making the procedure computationally cheap. While threshold methods focused primarily on bias correction, PQ-learning was perhaps a more comprehensive attack on the root of the problem.

A different class of methods emerged from the works of Laber et al. (2011) and Chakraborty et al. (2013). These methods do not disturb the original Q-learning (hard-max) estimators, but employ more sophisticated versions of the ordinary bootstrap to mimic the non-regular asymptotic distributions of the estimators. The adaptive method of Laber et al. (2011) is computationally and conceptually complex, while the m-out-of-n bootstrap method is simpler and thus may be more attractive to practitioners. Another computationally expensive method is the double bootstrap, which performs well in conjunction with the original estimator. Yet another method to construct CIs in non-regular settings is the *score method* due to Robins (2004); except for the work of Moodie and Richardson (2010), this approach has not been thoroughly investigated in simulations, likely due to its computational burden.

As discussed by Chakraborty et al. (2013), their adaptive m-out-of-n resampling scheme is conceptually very similar to the *subsampling* method without replacement. In particular, a subsample size of $\tilde{m} = \hat{m}/2$ would enjoy similar asymptotic theory to the adaptive m-out-of-n bootstrap and hence provide consistent confidence sets (see, for example, Politis et al. 1999). One possible advantage of the adaptive m-out-of-n scheme over an adaptive subsampling scheme is that in a regular setting, the m-out-of-n procedure reduces to the familiar n-out-of-n bootstrap which may be more familiar to applied quantitative researchers. Many of the inference tools discussed in this chapter can be extended to involve more stages and more treatment options at each stage; see, for example, Laber et al. (2011) and Song et al. (2011). Aside from notational complications, extending the adaptive m-out-of-n procedure should also be straightforward.

Finally, we touched on the problems of inference for the value of an estimated DTR, discussing the work of Laber and Murphy (2011), and Bayesian estimation. These are very interesting yet very difficult problems, and little has yet appeared in the literature. More targeted research is warranted.

Chapter 9
Additional Considerations and Final Thoughts

The statistical study of DTRs and associated methods of estimation is a young and growing field. As such, there are many topics which are only beginning to be explored. In this chapter, we point to some new developments and areas of research in the field.

9.1 Variable Selection

In estimating optimal adaptive treatment strategies, the variables used to tailor treatment to patient characteristics are typically hand-picked by experts who seek to use a minimum set of variables routinely available in clinical practice. However, studies often use a large set of easy-to-measure covariates (e.g., multiple surveys of mental health status and functioning) from which a smaller subset of variables must be selected for any practical implementation of treatment tailoring. It may therefore be desirable to be able to select tailoring variables with which to index the class of regimes using automated or data-adaptive procedures. It has been noted that prediction methods such as boosting could aid in selecting variables to adapt treatments (LeBlanc and Kooperberg 2010); many such methods can be applied with ease, particularly to the regression-based approaches to estimating optimal DTRs, however their ability to select variables for strong *interactions* with treatment rather than simply strong predictive power may require special care and further study.

Recall the distinction between *predictive* variables (used to increase precision of estimates) and *prescriptive* variables (used to adapt treatment strategies to patients), i.e. tailoring variables (Gunter et al. 2007). In the Q-learning notation, predictive variables correspond to the H_{j0} terms in the Q-function associated with parameters β, while the prescriptive or tailoring variables are those contained in H_{j1}, associated with parameters ψ. Tailoring variables must *qualitatively* interact with the treatment, meaning that the choice of optimal treatment varies for different values of such variables. The usefulness of a prescriptive variable can be characterized by

B. Chakraborty and E.E.M. Moodie, *Statistical Methods for Dynamic Treatment Regimes*, 169
Statistics for Biology and Health 76, DOI 10.1007/978-1-4614-7428-9_9,

the magnitude of the interaction and the proportion of the population for whom the optimal action changes given the knowledge of the variable (Gunter et al. 2007).

We will focus the discussion in this section on the randomized trial setting, so that variable selection is strictly for the purposes of optimal treatment tailoring, rather than elimination of bias due to confounding. Further, we will restrict attention to the one-stage setting, as to date there have been no studies on the use of variable selection for dynamic treatment regimes in the multi-stage setting.

9.1.1 Penalized Regression

Lu et al. (2013) proposed an adaptation of the lasso which penalizes only interaction terms. Specifically, they consider the loss function

$$L_n(\psi,\beta,\alpha) = \mathbb{P}_n[Y_i - \phi(O_i;\beta) - \psi^T O_i(A_i - \pi(O_i))]^2 \qquad (9.1)$$

where the covariate vector O_i is augmented by a column of 1s and has total length $p+1$, $\pi(o) = P(A=1|O=o;\alpha)$ is the propensity score for a binary treatment A and $\phi(O)$ is an arbitrary function. Lu et al. (2013) noted that the estimating function found by taking the derivative of the loss function $L_n(\psi,\beta,\alpha)$ with respect to ψ corresponds to an A-learning method of estimation, and is therefore robust to mis-specification of the conditional mean model $\phi(O;\beta)$ for the response Y in the sense that the estimator requires correct specification of either the propensity score or the mean model $\phi(O;\beta)$. The decision (or treatment interaction) parameters ψ are then shrunk using an adaptive lasso which penalizes parameters with a weight inversely proportional to their estimated value, solving

$$\min_{\psi} L_n(\psi,\hat{\beta},\hat{\alpha}) + \lambda_n \sum_{j=1}^{p+1} |\hat{\psi}_j|^{-1}|\psi_j|$$

where $\hat{\psi},\hat{\beta}$ are solutions to Eq. (9.1), $\hat{\alpha}$ is a consistent estimate of the propensity score model parameters, and λ_n is a tuning parameter that may be selected using cross-validation or some form of Bayesian Information Criterion (BIC). By penalizing the interaction parameters with the inverse of their estimated values, important interactions (i.e. those estimated to have large coefficients) will receive little penalty, while those with small estimates will be highly penalized.

Lu et al. (2013) showed that under standard regularity conditions, the estimators of the parameters ψ resulting from the penalized regression will be asymptotically normal and the set of selected treatment-covariate interactions will equal the set of treatment-interaction which are truly non-zero. The properties of the penalized estimator in multi-stage or non-regular settings were not examined. The estimator was compared to the unpenalized estimator $\hat{\psi}$ that results from solving Eq. (9.1) in low and high dimensional problems (10 and 50 variables, respectively). Using a linear working model for $\phi(O_i;\beta)$, the penalized estimator selected the truly non-zero interaction terms with very high probability in samples of size 100 or larger. In high dimensional settings, the penalized estimator increased the selection of the correct treatment choice relative to the unpenalized estimator by 7–8 %; in low dimensional settings, the improvement was more modest (2–3 %).

9.1.2 Variable Ranking by Qualitative Interactions

As proposed by Gunter et al. (2007, 2011b), the *S-score* for a (univariate) variable O is defined as:

$$S_O = \mathbb{P}_n \left\{ \max_{a \in \mathscr{A}} \mathbb{P}_n \left[Y | A = a, O \right] - \max_{a \in \mathscr{A}} \mathbb{P}_n \left[Y | A = a \right] \right\}.$$

The S-score of a variable O captures the expected increase in the response that is observed by adapting treatment based on the value of that variable. S-scores combine two characteristics of a useful tailoring variable: the interaction of the variable with the treatment and the proportion of the population exhibiting variability in its value. A high S-score for a variable is indicative of a strong qualitative interaction between the variable and the treatment, as well as a high proportion of patients for whom the optimal action would change if the value of the variable were taken into consideration. Thus, S-scores may be used to rank variables and select those that have the highest scores. The performance of the S-score ranking method was found to be superior to the standard lasso (Tibshirani 1996) in terms of consistent selection of a small number of variables from a large set of covariates of interest.

In the real-data implementation of the S-score ranking performed by Gunter et al. (2007), each variable was evaluated separately, without taking into account potential correlation between variables. Two variables that are highly correlated may have similar S-scores (Biernot and Moodie 2010) but may not both be necessary for decision making. The S-score may be modified in a straight-forward fashion to examine the usefulness of sets of variables, O' given the use of others, O, by considering, for example,

$$S_{O'|O} = \mathbb{P}_n \left\{ \max_{a \in \mathscr{A}} \mathbb{P}_n \left[Y | A = a, O, O' \right] - \max_{a \in \mathscr{A}} \mathbb{P}_n \left[Y | A = a, O \right] \right\}.$$

Thus, the S-score approach could be used to select the variable, O, with the highest score, then select a second variable, O', with the highest S-score given the use of O as a prescriptive variable, and so on.

For $i = 1, \ldots, n$ subjects and $j = 1, \ldots, p$ possible tailoring variables, Gunter et al. (2007, 2011b) proposed an alternative score, also based on both the strength of interaction as measured by

$$D_j = \max_{1 \leq i \leq n} (\mathbb{P}_n[Y|O_j = o_{ij}, A = 1] - \mathbb{P}_n[Y|O_j = o_{ij}, A = 0])$$
$$- \min_{1 \leq i \leq n} (\mathbb{P}_n[Y|O_j = o_{ij}, A = 1] - \mathbb{P}_n[Y|O_j = o_{ij}, A = 0])$$

and the proportion of the population for whom the optimal decision differs if a variable is used for tailoring, captured by

$$P_j = \mathbb{P}_n \mathbb{I}\left[\operatorname{argmax}_a \mathbb{P}_n[Y|O_j = o_{ij}, A = a] \neq a^*\right]$$

where $a^* = \operatorname{argmax}_a \mathbb{P}_n[Y|A = a]$ is the optimal decision in the absence of tailoring. These values are combined to form another means of ranking the importance of tailoring variables, called the U-score:

$$U_j = \left(\frac{D_j - \min_{1 \leq k \leq p} D_k}{\max_{1 \leq k \leq p} D_k - \min_{1 \leq k \leq p} D_k}\right)\left(\frac{P_j - \min_{1 \leq k \leq p} P_k}{\max_{1 \leq k \leq p} P_k - \min_{1 \leq k \leq p} P_k}\right).$$

Gunter et al. (2007, 2011b) suggested the use of the S- and U-scores in combination with lasso:

1. Select variables that are predictive of the outcome Y from among the variables in (H_{10}, AH_{11}), using cross-validation or the BIC to select the penalty parameter.
2. Rank each variable O_j using the S- or U-score, retaining the predictive variables selected in step (1) to reduce the variability in the estimated mean response. Choose the M most highly-ranked variables, where M is the cardinality of the variables in H_{11} for which the S- or U-score is non-zero.
3. Create nested subsets of variables.

   (a) Let H_{11}^* be the top M variables found in step (2), and let H_{10}^* denote the union of the predictive variables chosen in step (1) and H_{11}^*. Let M^* denote the cardinality of (H_{10}^*, H_{11}^*).
   (b) Run a weighted lasso where all main effect and interaction variables chosen in step (1) only have weight 1, and all interaction variables chosen in step (2) are given a weight $0 < w \leq 1$ which is a non-decreasing function of the U- or S-score. This downweights the importance of the prescriptive variables, which are favored by lasso.
   (c) Create M^* nested subsets based on the order of entry of the M^* variables in the weighted lasso.

4. Choose from among the subsets based on the highest expected response, or alternatively, the highest adjusted gain in the outcome relative to not using any tailoring variables.

The variable selection approaches based on the S- and U-scores were found to perform well in simulation, leading to variable choices that provided higher expected outcomes than lasso alone (Gunter et al. 2007, 2011b).

9.1.3 Stepwise Selection

Gunter et al. (2011a) suggested that the qualitative ranking of the previous section is complex and difficult to interpret, and instead proposed the use of a stepwise procedure, using the expected response conditional on treatment A and covariates O, as the criterion on which to select or omit tailoring variables.

The suggested approach begins by fitting a regression model for the response Y as a function of treatment only, and estimating the mean response to the overall ("un-tailored") optimal treatment; denote this by $\hat{V}_0^*$. Next, let $\mathscr{C}$ contain the treatment variable as well as all variables which are known to be important predictors of the response. Fit a regression model for the response Y as a function of treatment and all variables in $\mathscr{C}$ and estimate the mean response to the overall (un-tailored) optimal treatment when the predictors in $\mathscr{C}$ are included in the model; denote this by $\hat{V}_C^*$. A key quantity that will be used to decide variable inclusion or exclusion is the *adjusted value* of the model. For $\mathscr{C}$, the adjusted value is $AV_C = (\hat{V}_C^* - \hat{V}_0^*)/|\mathscr{C}|$ where $|\mathscr{C}|$ is the rank of the model matrix used in the estimation of the response conditional on the variables in $\mathscr{C}$.

Letting $\mathscr{E}$ denote all eligible variables, both predictive variables and treatment-covariate interaction terms, not included in $\mathscr{C}$. The procedure is then carried out by performing forward selection and backwards elimination at each step.

Forward selection: For each variable $e \in \mathscr{E}$,

1. Estimate the predictive model using all the variables in $\mathscr{C}$ plus the variable e.
2. Optimize the estimated predictive model over the treatment actions to obtain the optimal mean response, $\hat{V}_E^*$, and calculate the adjusted value, $AV_e = (\hat{V}_e^* - \hat{V}_0^*)/|\mathscr{C} + e|$.
3. Retain the covariate e^* which results in the largest value of AV_e.

Backward elimination: For each variable $c \in \mathscr{C}$,

1. Estimate the predictive model using all the variables in $\mathscr{C}$ except the variable c.
2. Optimize the estimated predictive model over the treatment actions to obtain the optimal mean response, $\hat{V}_{-c}^*$, and calculate the adjusted value, $AV_{-c} = (\hat{V}_{-c}^* - \hat{V}_0^*)/|\mathscr{C} - c|$.
3. Let c^* be the covariate which results in the largest value of AV_{-c}.

If each of AV_C, AV_{e^*}, and AV_{-c^*} are negative, the stepwise procedure is complete and no further variable selection is required. If $AV_{e^*} > \max\{AV_C, AV_{-c^*}\}$, e^* is included in $\mathscr{C}$ and AV_C is set to AV_{e^*}; otherwise, if $AV_{-c^*} > \max\{AV_C, AV_{e^*}\}$, remove c from $\mathscr{C}$ and AV_C is set to AV_{-c^*}. Gunter et al. (2011a) suggested that all covariate main effects should be retained in a model in which a treatment-covariate interaction is present, and to group covariates relating to a single characteristic (e.g. dummy variables indicating covariate level for categorical variables).

In simulation, the stepwise method was found to have higher specificity but lower sensitivity than the qualitative interaction ranking approach of the previous section (Gunter et al. 2011a). That is, the stepwise procedure was less likely to falsely include variables which did not qualitatively interact with treatment, at the cost of being less able to identify variables which did. However, the stepwise procedure is rather easier to implement and can be applied to different outcome types such as binary or count data.

Gunter et al. (2011c) used a similar, but more complex, method to perform variable selection while controlling the number of falsely significant findings by using bootstrap sampling and permutation thresholding in combination. The bootstrap procedure is used as a form of voting algorithm to ensure selection of variables that modify treatment in a single direction, while the permutation algorithm is used to maintain a family-wise error rate across the tests of significance for the coefficients associated with the tailoring variables.

9.2 Model Checking via Residual Diagnostics

There has been relatively little work on the topic of model checking for estimating optimal DTRs. The regret-regression approach of Henderson et al. (2010) is one of the first in which the issues of model checking and diagnostics were specifically addressed. Because regret-regression uses ordinary least squares for estimation of the model parameters, standard tools for regression model checking and diagnostics can be employed. In particular, Henderson et al. (2010) showed that residual plots can be used to diagnose model mis-specification. In fact, these standard approaches can and should be used whenever a regression-based approach to estimating DTR parameters, such as Q-learning or A-learning as implemented by Almirall et al. (2010), is taken.

Consider the following small example using Q-learning: data are generated such that $O_{11} \sim N(0,1)$ and $O_{21} \sim N(-0.5_0 + 0.5O_{11}, 1)$, treatment is randomly assigned at each stage with probability 1/2, and the binary tailoring variables are generated via

$$P[O_{12} = 1] = P[O_{12} = -1] = 1/2,$$
$$P[O_{22} = 1|O_{12}, A_1] = 1 - P[O_{22} = -1|O_{12}, A_1] = \text{expit}(0.1O_{12} + 0.1A_1).$$

Thus the state variables are $O_1 = (O_{11}, O_{12})$ and $O_2 = (O_{21}, O_{22})$. Then for $\varepsilon \sim N(0,1)$,

$$Y = 0.5O_{11} - 0.5A_1 + 0.5O_{12}A_1 + 0.5O_{21} + A_2 + 1.4O_{22}A_2 + A_1A_2 + \varepsilon.$$

We fit three models. The first is correctly specified, the second omits the single predictive variable, O_{j1}, from the model for the Q-function at each stage, and the third omits the interaction A_jO_{j2} from the Q-function model. As observed in Fig. 9.1, residuals from the OLS fit at each stage of the Q-learning algorithm can be used to detect the omission of important predictors of the response, but may not be sufficiently sensitive to detect the omission of important tailoring variables from the Q-function model.

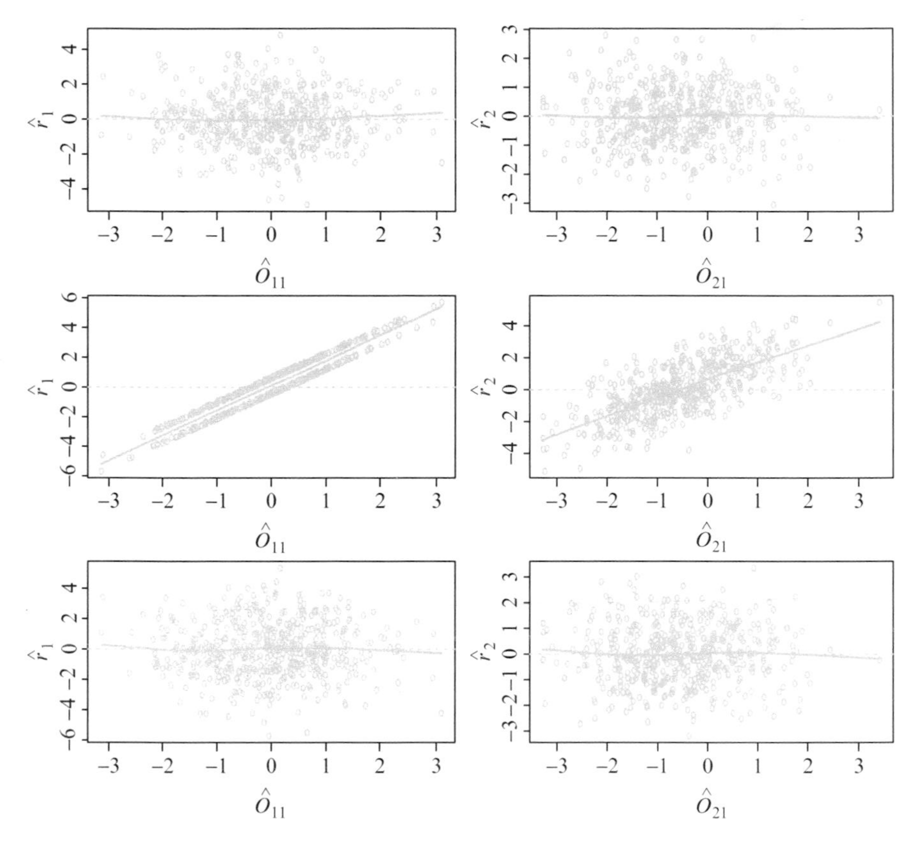

Fig. 9.1 Residual diagnostic plots for Q-learning using a simulated data set with n = 500. The first and second columns show plots for residuals at the first and second stages, respectively. The first row corresponds to a correctly specified Q-function model. In the second and third rows, Q-function models at each stage are mis-specified by the omission, respectively, of a predictive variable and an interaction with a tailoring variable

It is also possible to generalize the ideas of model-checking in regression to G-estimation, producing a type of residual that can be used to construct residual diagnostic plots. Recall that doubly-robust G-estimation can be based on the estimating function:

$$U = \sum_{j=0}^{K-1} U_j = \sum_{j=0}^{K-1} \left\{G_{\text{mod},j}(\psi) - E[G_{\text{mod},j}(\psi)|H_j]\right\}\left\{S_j(A_j) - E[S_j(A_j)|H_j]\right\}$$

where

$$G_{\text{mod},j}(\psi) \equiv G_{\text{mod},j}(\psi)(H_K, A_K, \psi_j) = Y - \gamma_j(H_j, A_j; \psi_j) + \sum_{m=j+1}^{K-1} \mu_m(H_m, A_m; \psi_m),$$

for $S_j(A_j)$ an analyst-specified function of H_j and A_j. In general, due to high dimensionality of the covariate space, estimation is made more tractable when parametric models are specified for:

1. The blip function $\gamma_j(h_j, a_j; \psi_j)$;
2. The expected potential outcome $E[G_{\text{mod},j}(\psi)|H_j; \varsigma_j]$;
3. The treatment model $E[A_j|H_j; \alpha_j]$, required for $E[S_j(A_j)|H_j; \alpha_j]$.

The first of these provides estimates of the decision rule parameters while the other two are considered nuisance models. Although some model mis-specification is permitted in the doubly-robust framework, there are efficiency gains when both models (2) and (3) are correct (Moodie et al. 2007).

Rich et al. (2010) note that, letting G_{ij} be $G_{\text{mod},j}(\psi)$ for subject i at stage j,

$$\begin{aligned}
G_{ij} - E[G_{ij}|H_j; \varsigma_j(\psi_j)] &= \left\{Y_i - \gamma_j(H_j, A_j; \psi_j)) + \sum_{m=j+1}^{K-1} \mu_m(H_m, A_m; \psi_m)\right\} - E[G_{ij}|H_j; \varsigma_j(\psi_j)] \\
&= Y_i - \left\{E[G_{ij}|H_j; \varsigma_j(\psi_j)] - \sum_{m=j+1}^{K-1} \mu_m(H_m, A_m; \psi_m) + \gamma_j(H_j, A_j; \psi_j))\right\}
\end{aligned}$$

has mean zero conditional on history H_j, so that a fitted value for Y_i is given by

$$\hat{Y}_{ij}(\psi) = \left\{E[G_{ij}|H_j; \varsigma_j(\psi_j)] - \sum_{m=j+1}^{K-1} \mu_m(H_m, A_m; \psi_m) + \gamma_j(H_j, A_j; \psi_j))\right\}.$$

The residual for the ith individual at the jth stage is then defined to be

$$r_{ij}(\psi) = Y_i - \left\{E[G_{ij}|H_j; \varsigma_j(\psi_j)] - \sum_{m=j+1}^{K-1} \mu_m(H_m, A_m; \psi_m) + \gamma_j(H_j, A_j; \psi_j))\right\}.$$

To use the residual for model-checking purposes, estimates $\hat{\psi}$ and $\hat{\varsigma}_j(\hat{\psi}_j)$ must be substituted for the unknown parameters. The residuals r_{ij} can be used to verify the models $E[G_{ij}|H_j; \varsigma_j(\psi_j)]$ and $\gamma(h_j, a_j; \psi_j)$, diagnosing underspecification (that is, the omission of a variable) and checking the assumptions regarding the functional form in which covariates were included in the models.

Rich et al. (2010) considered a two-stage simulation, and examined plots of the first- and second-stage residuals against covariates and fitted values. The residual plots were able to detect incorrectly-specified models in a variety of settings, and appeared able to distinguish at which stage the model was mis-specified. While patterns in residual plots provide a useful indicator of problems with model specification, they do not necessarily indicate in *which* model a problem occurs, i.e. whether the problem is in the specification of the blip function or the expected counterfactual model.

Consider the following example, where data are generated as follows:

$$O_1 \sim N(0, 140)$$
$$O_2 \sim N(50 + 1.25O_1, 120)$$

$A_j = 1$ with probability p_j and $A_j = -1$ with probability $1 - p_j$ for $j = 1, 2$

$$Y \sim N(300 + 1.6O_1 + 1.2O_2, 300) - \mu_1(H_1, A_1; \psi_1) - \mu_2(H_2, A_2; \psi_2)$$

where $p_1 = \text{expit}(0.1 - 0.003O_1)$, $p_2 = \text{expit}(0.5 - 0.004O_2)$, and the regret functions $\mu_1(O_j, A_1; \psi_1)$, $\mu_2(H_2, A_2; \psi_2)$ are based on the linear blip functions

$$\gamma_1(O_1, A_1; \psi_1) = (170 - 3.4O_1)\mathbb{I}[A_1 = 1]$$
$$\gamma_2(H_2, A_2; \psi_2) = (420 - 2.8O_2)\mathbb{I}[A_1 = 1].$$

In Fig. 9.2, we plot the residuals for four different models, three of which have mis-specified components, from a single data set of size 500. The first and second models mis-specified the form of $E[G_{ij}|H_j; \varsigma_j(\psi_j)]$, the expected counterfactual model, at stage one and two, respectively. The third model correctly specified the expected counterfactual models, but omitted O_1 and O_2 from the blip models at both stages. The fourth model was correctly specified. In the first, second, and fourth rows, the stage(s) where no models are mis-specified provide residual plots with no systematic patterns. However, if the expected counterfactual model (row 1 and 2) or the blip models (row 3) are mis-specified at one or both stages, obvious trends appear in the residual plots. As noted by Rich et al. (2010), mis-specification of the expected counterfactual model and the blip function result in similar patterns in the residual plots; it is therefore not possible to determine which model is incorrect simply by inspection of residual plots.

9.3 Discussion and Concluding Remarks

In this book, we have attempted to provide an introduction to the key findings in the statistical literature of dynamic treatment regimes. In Chaps. 1 and 2, we introduced the motivation for seeking evidence-based decision rules for treating chronic conditions, and outlined the key features of the structures of longitudinal data which are used to make inference about optimal treatment policies: observational follow-up studies and sequential multiple-assignment randomized trials. In the third chapter, we delved more deeply into the mathematics of the decision making problem and the reinforcement learning perspective. We also introduced Q-learning in Chap. 3, which is increasingly finding favor in the scientific community for the ease with which it can be implemented. Chapter 4 presented several semi-parametric methods arising from the causal inference literature: G-estimation and

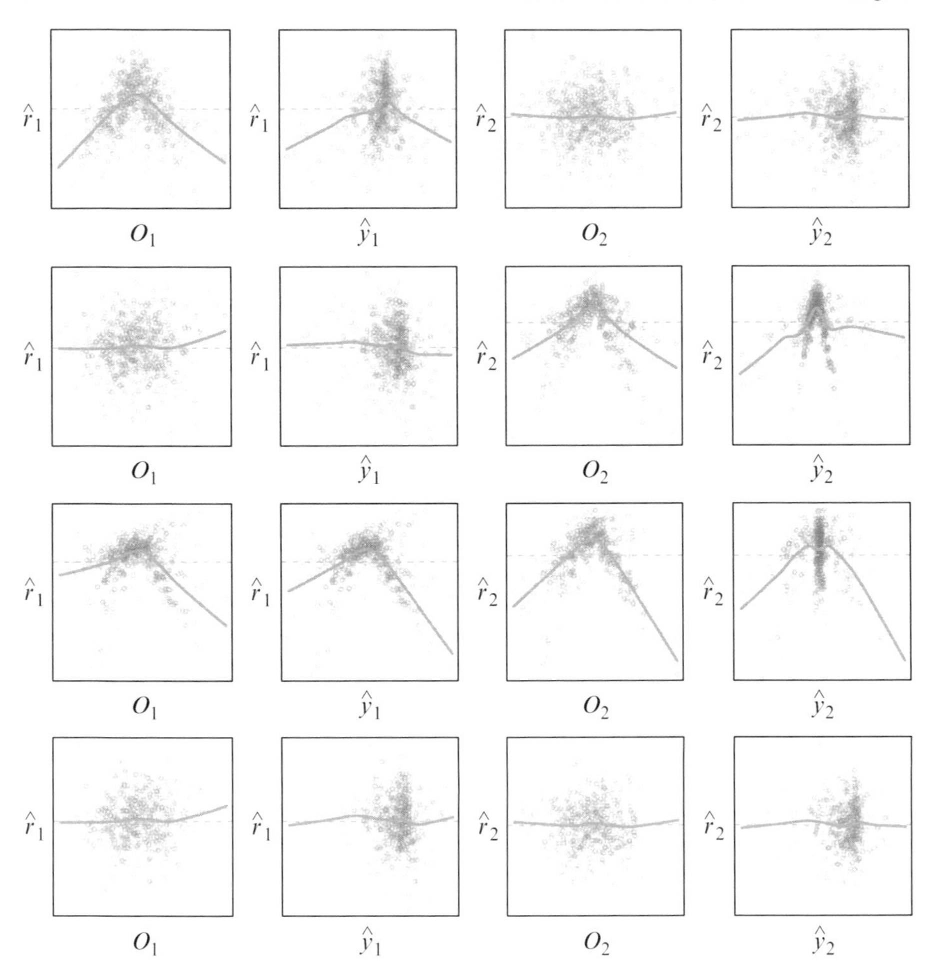

Fig. 9.2 Residual diagnostic plots for G-estimation using simulated data set with n = 500. The first two columns show plots for residuals and the first stage ($j = 1$), the last two for residuals at the second stage ($j = 2$). Specifically, the columns plot: (1) first stage residuals vs. O_1, (2) residuals vs. fitted values at the first stage, (3) second stage residuals vs. O_2, and (4) residuals vs. fitted values at the second stage. Rows correspond model choices: (1) $E[G_{\text{mod},1}(\psi)|O_1;\varsigma_1(\psi_1)]$ mis-specified, (2) $E[G_{\text{mod},2}(\psi)|H_2;\varsigma_2(\psi_2)]$ mis-specified, (3) $\gamma_1(O_1,A_1;\psi_1)$ and $\gamma_2(H_2,A_2;\psi_2)$ mis-specified, and (4) all models correctly specified. The solid grey curve indicates a loess smooth through the points

the regret-based methods including A-learning and regret-regression; where connections exist between methods, they were demonstrated. In Chap. 5, we turned our attention to methods that model regimes directly, including inverse probability weighting, marginal structural models, and classification-based approaches.

Our survey of estimation methods continued in Chap. 6, where the likelihood-based method of G-computation was demonstrated in both the frequentist and Bayesian contexts. In Chap. 7, we turned our attention to estimating DTRs for alternative outcome types, including outcomes that are compound measures or multi-component in nature, as well as time-to-event and discrete valued. A range of methods have been applied in these settings, from Q-learning to marginal structural models to a likelihood-based approach.

Chapter 8 focused on improving estimation and inference, which presents a particular challenge in the dynamic treatment regime setting due to non-regularity of the estimators under certain underlying longitudinal data distributions, including those in which treatment has no effect. Three methods of bias reduction are considered: hard- and soft-thresholding, and penalized Q-learning. We then presented three bootstrap-based approaches to constructing confidence intervals which yield greatly improved coverage over any naively constructed interval at and near points in the parameter space that cause non-regularity of the estimators.

Finally, in this chapter, we have brought together a collection of topics that are at the forefront of research activity in dynamic regimes. The first two sections considered practical problems in implementing optimal DTR estimation: variable selection and model checking. In Sect. 9.1, we presented proposed approaches to the selection of tailoring variables, which differs from the usual problem of variable selection in that the analyst is seeking to find variables which qualitatively interact with treatment rather than those which are good predictors of the outcome. In the following section, we demonstrated the use of residual plots to assess model specification in Q-learning and G-estimation. As a summary of current or ongoing work, it is likely that this chapter is incomplete since the study of dynamic treatment regimes is, as a field, so active and is attracting new researchers from a diversity of backgrounds. The refinement and application of estimation techniques and the need to provide reliable measures of goodness-of-fit will continue to provide inspiration for many researchers in the coming years.

With the anticipated popularity of SMARTs in clinical and behavioral research, we foresee an inevitable complexity in the near future. Note that many interventions, either due to their very nature or due to logistical feasibility, need to be administered in group settings, requiring the design and analysis of cluster-randomized SMARTs. Some such complex trials are currently being considered. At the design level, cluster randomization would imply increased sample size requirements due to intra-class correlation, as expected. At the analysis level, on the other hand, it would open up several questions, e.g. how to incorporate random effects models or generalized estimating equations (GEE) methods into the framework of estimation techniques like Q-learning or G-estimation, whether the correlation would enhance the phenomenon of non-regularity in inference, and so on. These are areas of active current research.

While much of the personalized medicine literature is occupied by the use of patients' genetic information in personalizing treatments, the use of genetic information in the dynamic regime context, as of now, is surprisingly limited. Thus we envision this as a critically important research direction in the near future. This being one of the most natural next steps, methodologists will have to carefully investigate how best to handle the associated high dimensionality.

In today's health care, there seems to be an increasing trend in the use of sophisticated mobile devices (e.g. smart phones, actigraph units containing accelerometers, etc.) to remotely monitor patients' chronic health conditions and to act on the fly, when needed. According to the reinforcement learning literature, this is an instance of *online* decision making in a possibly *infinite horizon* setting involving many stages of intervention. Development of statistically sound estimation and inference techniques for such a setting seems to be another very important future research direction.

The call to personalize medicine is growing more urgent, and reaching beyond the walls of academia. Even in popular literature (see, e.g. Topol 2012), it has been declared that

> This is a new era of medicine, in which each person can be near fully defined at the individual level, instead of how we practice medicine at the population level, with [...] use of the same medication and dosage for a diagnosis rather than for a patient.

While it is true that high dimensional data, even genome scans, are increasingly available to the average "consumer" of medicine, there remains the need to adequately and appropriately evaluate any new, tailored approach to treatment. It is that evaluation, by statistical means, that has proven theoretically, computationally, and practically challenging and has driven many of the methodological innovations described in this text.

The study of estimation and inference for dynamic treatment regimes is still relatively young, and constantly evolving. Many inferential problems, including inference about the optimal value function, remain incompletely addressed. A further key challenge is the dissemination of the statistical results into the medical and public health spheres, so that the methods being developed are not used in 'toy' examples, but are deployed in routine use for the evidence-based improvement of treatment of chronic illnesses. While observational data can help drive hypotheses and suggest good regimes to explore, increasing the use of SMARTs in clinical research will be required to better understand and evaluate the sequential treatment decisions that are routinely taken in the care of chronic illnesses.

Glossary

Action From the reinforcement learning literature: a treatment or exposure.

Action-value function See *Q-function*.

Acute care model A treatment paradigm which focuses on intensive short-term care for an episode of illness or trauma, often in a hospital setting.

Adaptive treatment strategy See *Dynamic treatment regime*.

Berkson's bias See *Collider-stratification bias*.

Blip function A function describing the expected difference in outcome when receiving a treatment regime d_j^* instead of the observed treatment a_j at stage j and subsequently receiving the regime d instead of the observed treatments, given covariate history h_j:

$$\gamma_j(h_j, a_j) = E[Y(\overline{a}_j, \underline{d}_{j+1}) - Y(\overline{a}_{j-1}, d_j^*, \underline{d}_{j+1}) | H_j = h_j].$$

A common choice for d_j^* is no treatment (or placebo, standard of care); this is often called the reference function. The regime d is typically chosen to be the optimal treatment regime. The blip function can be formulated as a difference of Q-functions, $\gamma_j(h_j, a_j) = Q_j^d(h_j, a_j) - Q_j^d(h_j, d_j^*)$.

Chronic care model A treatment (or prevention) paradigm for chronic illness based on the principle that effective care requires teams of providers with resources at the community and health services levels who interact with an engaged and informed patient. The six key elements of a chronic care model are health care organization, community resources, self-management support, delivery system design, decision support, and a clinical information system.

B. Chakraborty and E.E.M. Moodie, *Statistical Methods for Dynamic Treatment Regimes*, Statistics for Biology and Health 76, DOI 10.1007/978-1-4614-7428-9,

Collider-stratification bias Bias that arises due to the selection of the sample or conditioning of an analysis model on a covariate that is a common effect of the treatment of interest (or a variable which causes treatment) and the outcome (or one of its causes).

Confounding The bias that occurs when the treatment and the outcome have a common cause that is not appropriately accounted for in an analysis.

Counterfactual outcome The outcome that would have been observed if individual i had received treatment a where a is not the treatment actually received. Often used interchangeably with the term potential outcome.

Dynamic treatment regime A set of rules for determining effective treatments for individuals based on personal characteristics such as treatment and covariate history.

G-computation An estimation procedure that models the dependence of covariates on the history, then simulates from these models the outcome that would have been observed had exposures been fixed by intervention.

G-estimation An estimation procedure typically coupled with structural nested models that aims to simulate nested randomized-controlled trials at each stage of treatment within strata of treatment and covariate history.

Marginal structural model A model for the mean counterfactual outcome which conditions on treatment (and sometimes also baseline covariates) only, but does not include any post-baseline covariates.

Non-regular estimator An estimator whose asymptotic distribution does not converge uniformly over the parameter space. In the context of the estimation of optimal dynamic treatment regimes, this typically occurs due to non-differentiability of the estimating function with respect to a parameter that indexes a decision rule.

Policy From the reinforcement learning literature: a dynamic treatment regime.

Policy search methods In the reinforcement learning literature, a class of methods which finds the optimal regime directly by estimating the value or marginal mean outcome under each candidate regime within a pre-specified class and then selects as optimal the regimes that maximize the estimated value.

Potential outcome The outcome that would be observed if individual i were to receive treatment a, where here treatment may indicate a single- or multi-component intervention that is either static or dynamic.

Propensity score For a binary-valued treatment, it is the conditional probability of receiving treatment given covariates.

Q-function The total expected future reward, starting from stage j with covariate history h_j, taking an action a_j, and following the treatment policy d thereafter. Thus,

$$Q_j^d(h_j,a_j) = E[Y_j(H_j,A_j,O_{j+1}) + V_{j+1}^d(H_{j+1})|H_j = h_j,A_j = a_j].$$

Note that if a_j follows policy d, then the Q-function equals the value function.

Regret A blip function where both the reference regime d_j^* and d are taken to the optimal treatment regime. It is the expected difference in the outcome among participants with history h_j that would be observed had the participants taken the optimal treatment from stage j onwards instead of taking the observed treatment regime a_j and subsequently followed the optimal regime:

$$\mu_j(h_j,a_j) = E[Y(\bar{a}_{j-1},\underline{d}_j^{opt}) - Y(\bar{a}_j,\underline{d}_{j+1}^{opt})|H_j = h_j].$$

The regret can be expressed as a difference of optimal Q-functions, $\mu_j(h_j,a_j) = Q_j^{opt}(h_j,a_j) - Q_j^{opt}(h_j,d_j)$ or as a function of optimal blip functions: $\mu_j(h_j,a_j) = \max_{a_j}\gamma_j(h_j,a_j) - \gamma_j(h_j,a_j)$. Alternatively, the difference of regrets can be taken to find the corresponding blip function, $\gamma_j(h_j,a_j) = \mu_j(h_j,d_j^*) - \mu_j(h_j,a_j)$. The negative of the regret is called the *advantage function*.

Reward From the reinforcement learning literature: an outcome which may be observed at the end of the study following the final stage of treatment, or at intermediate stages after each stage-specific treatment.

Selection bias See *Collider-stratification bias*.

Sequential multiple assignment randomized trial A randomized experimental design developed specifically for building time-varying adaptive interventions, whereby participants may require more than one stage of treatment, and are randomized to one of a set of possible treatments at each stage.

State From the reinforcement learning literature: the values of the covariates of an individual at a particular time, e.g. at the beginning of a stage.

Static treatment regime A treatment regimen which does not change in response to patient characteristics.

Structural nested mean model A model, or sequence of models (one per stage), that parameterizes only the effect treatment (and any interactions between the treatment and covariates) on the outcome. Any covariates that are purely predictive, and do not act as treatment effect modifiers, are not included in the model.

Tailoring variable A personal characteristic, either fixed or time-varying, used to adapt treatment to an individual. Also called a *prescriptive variable*.

Utility See *Reward*.

Value function The total expected future reward, starting with a particular covariate history, and following the given treatment regime actions thereafter. The stage-j value function for history h_j with respect to a regime d is

$$\begin{aligned} V_j^d(h_j) &= E_d\Big[\sum_{k=j}^{K} Y_k(H_k, A_k, O_{k+1})\Big| H_j = h_j\Big] \\ &= E_d\Big[Y_j(H_j, A_j, O_{j+1}) + V_{j+1}^d(H_{j+1})\Big| H_j = h_j\Big], \quad 1 \leq j \leq K. \end{aligned}$$

The value function, or simply value, represents the expected future reward starting at stage j with history h_j and thereafter choosing treatments according to the policy d.

References

Abbring, J. J., & Heckman, J. J. (2007). Econometric evaluation of social programs, part III: Distributional treatment effects, dynamic treatment effects, dynamic discrete choice, and general equilibrium policy evaluation. In J. J. Heckman & E. E. Leamer (Eds.), *Handbook of econometrics* (Vol. 6, Part B). Amsterdam: Elsevier.

Almirall, D., Ten Have, T., & Murphy, S. A. (2010). Structural nested mean models for assessing time-varying effect moderation. *Biometrics, 66*, 131–139.

Almirall, D., Compton, S. N., Gunlicks-Stoessel, M., Duan, N., & Murphy, S. A. (2012a). Designing a pilot sequential multiple assignment randomized trial for developing an adaptive treatment strategy. *Statistics in Medicine, 31*, 1887–1902.

Almirall, D., Lizotte, D., & Murphy, S. A. (2012b). SMART design issues and the consideration of opposing outcomes, Discussion of "Evaluation of Viable Dynamic Treatment Regimes in a Sequentially Randomized Trial of Advanced Prostate Cancer" by Wang et al. *Journal of the American Statistical Association, 107*, 509–512.

Anderson, J. W., Johnstone, B. M., & Remley, D. T. (1999). Breast-feeding and cognitive development: A meta-analysis. *American Journal of Clinical Nutrition, 70*, 525–535.

Andrews, D. W. K. (2000). Inconsistency of the bootstrap when a parameter is on the boundary of the parameter space. *Econometrica, 68*, 399–405.

Angrist, J. D., Imbens, G. W., & Rubin, D. B. (1996). Identification of causal effects using instrumental variables. *Journal of the American Statistical Association, 91*, 444–455.

Arjas, E. (2012). Causal inference from observational data: A Bayesian predictive approach. In C. Berzuini, A. P. Dawid, & L. Bernardinelli (Eds.), *Causality: Statistical perspectives and applications* (pp. 71–84). Chichester, West Sussex, United Kindom.

Arjas, E., & Andreev, A. (2000). Predictive inference, causal reasoning, and model assessment in nonparametric Bayesian analysis: A case study. *Lifetime Data Analysis, 6*, 187–205.

B. Chakraborty and E.E.M. Moodie, *Statistical Methods for Dynamic Treatment Regimes*, Statistics for Biology and Health 76, DOI 10.1007/978-1-4614-7428-9,

Arjas, E., & Parner, J. (2004). Causal reasoning from longitudinal data. *Scandinavian Journal of Statistics, 31*, 171–187.

Arjas, E., & Saarela, O. (2010). Optimal dynamic regimes: Presenting a case for predictive inference. *The International Journal of Biostatistics, 6*.

Arroll, B., MacGillivray, S., Ogston, S., Reid, I., Sullivan, F., Williams, B., & Crombie, I. (2005). Efficacy and tolerability of tricyclic antidepressants and ssris compared with placebo for treatment of depression in primary care: A meta-analysis. *Annals of Family Medicine, 3*, 449–456.

Arroll, B., Elley, C. R., Fishman, T., Goodyear-Smith, F. A., Kenealy, T., Blashki, G., Kerse, N., & MacGillivray, S. (2009). Antidepressants versus placebo for depression in primary care. *Cochrane Database of Systematic Reviews, 3*, CD007954.

Auyeung, S. F., Long, Q., Royster, E. B., Murthy, S., McNutt, M. D., Lawson, D., Miller, A., Manatunga, A., & Musselman, D. L. (2009). Sequential multiple-assignment randomized trial design of neurobehavioral treatment for patients with metastatic malignant melanoma undergoing high-dose interferon-alpha therapy. *Clinical Trials, 6*, 480–490.

Banerjee, A., & Tsiatis, A. A. (2006). Adaptive two-stage designs in phase II clinical trials. *Statistics in Medicine, 25*, 3382–3395.

Bellman, R. E. (1957). *Dynamic programming*. Princeton: Princeton University Press.

Bembom, O., & Van der Laan, M. J. (2007). Statistical methods for analyzing sequentially randomized trials. *Journal of the National Cancer Institute, 99*, 1577–1582.

Berger, R. L. (1996). More powerful tests from confidence interval p values. *American Statistician, 50*, 314–318.

Berger, R. L., & Boos, D. D. (1994). P values maximized over a confidence set for the nuisance parameter. *Journal of the American Statistical Association, 89*, 1012–1016.

Berkson, J. (1946). Limitations of the application of fourfold tables to hospital data. *Biometrics Bulletin, 2*, 47–53.

Berry, D. A. (2001). Adaptive clinical trials and Bayesian statistics in drug development (with discussion). *Biopharmaceutical Report, 9*, 1–11.

Berry, D. A. (2004). Bayesian statistics and the efficiency and ethics of clinical trials. *Statistical Science, 19*, 175–187.

Berry, D. A., Mueller, P., Grieve, A. P., Smith, M., Parke, T., Blazek, R., Mitchard, N., & Krams, M. (2001). Adaptive Bayesian designs for dose-ranging drug trials. In Gatsonis, C., Kass, R.E., Carlin, B., Carriquiry, A. Gelman, A. Verdinelli, I., and West, M. (Eds.), *Case studies in Bayesian statistics* (Vol. V, pp. 99–181). New York: Springer.

Bertsekas, D. P., & Tsitsiklis, J. (1996). *Neuro-dynamic programming*. Belmont: Athena Scientific.

Berzuini, C., Dawid, A. P., & Didelez, V. (2012). Assessing dynamic treatment strategies. In C. Berzuini, A. P. Dawid, & L. Bernardinelli (Eds.), *Causality: Statistical perspectives and applications* (pp. 85–100). Chichester, West Sussex, United Kindom.

Bickel, P. J., & Sakov, A. (2008). On the choice of m in the m out of n bootstrap and confidence bounds for extrema. *Statistica Sinica, 18*, 967–985.

Bickel, P. J., Klaassen, C. A. J., Ritov, Y., & Wellner, J. A. (1993). *Efficient and adaptive estimation for semiparametric models*. Baltimore: Johns Hopkins University Press.

Bickel, P. J., Gotze, F., & Zwet, W. V. (1997). Resampling fewer than n observations: Gains, losses and remedies for losses. *Statistica Sinica, 7*, 1–31.

Biernot, P., & Moodie, E. E. M. (2010). A comparison of variable selection approaches for dynamic treatment regimes. *The International Journal of Biostatistics, 6*.

Bodnar, L. M., Davidian, M., Siega-Riz, A. M., & Tsiatis, A. A. (2004). Marginal structural models for analyzing causal effects of time-dependent treatments: An application in perinatal epidemiology. *American Journal of Epidemiology, 159*, 926–934.

Box, G. E. P., Hunter, W. G., & Hunter, J. S. (1978). *Statistics for experimenters: An introduction to design, data analysis, and model building*. New York: Wiley.

Breiman, L. (1995). Better subset regression using the nonnegative garrote. *Technometrics, 37*, 373–384.

Breiman, L. (1996). Bagging predictors. *Machine Learning, 24*, 123–140.

Brotman, R. M., Klebanoff, M. A., Nansel, T. R., Andrews, W. W., Schwebke, J. R., Zhang, J., Yu, K. F., Zenilman, J. M., & Scharfstein, D. O. (2008). A longitudinal study of vaginal douching and bacterial vaginosis – A marginal structural modeling analysis. *American Journal of Epidemiology, 168*, 188–196.

Buhlmann, P., & Yu, B. (2002). Analyzing bagging. *Annals of Statistics, 30*, 927–961.

Cain, L. E., Robins, J. M., Lanoy, E., Logan, R., Costagliola, D., & Hernán, M. A. (2010). When to start treatment? A systematic approach to the comparison of dynamic regimes using observational data. *The International Journal of Biostatistics, 6*.

Carlin, B. P., Kadane, J. B., & Gelfand, A. E. (1998). Approaches for optimal sequential decision analysis in clinical trials. *Biometrics, 54*, 964–975.

Chakraborty, B. (2009). *A study of non-regularity in dynamic treatment regimes and some design considerations for multicomponent interventions* (Dissertation, University of Michigan, 2009).

Chakraborty, B. (2011). Dynamic treatment regimes for managing chronic health conditions: A statistical perspective. *American Journal of Public Health, 101*, 40–45.

Chakraborty, B., & Moodie, E. E. M. (2013). Estimating optimal dynamic treatment regimes with shared decision rules across stages: An extension of Q-learning (under revision).

Chakraborty, B., Collins, L. M., Strecher, V. J., & Murphy, S. A. (2009). Developing multicomponent interventions using fractional factorial designs. *Statistics in Medicine, 28*, 2687–2708.

Chakraborty, B., Murphy, S. A., & Strecher, V. (2010). Inference for non-regular parameters in optimal dynamic treatment regimes. *Statistical Methods in Medical Research, 19*, 317–343.

Chakraborty, B., Laber, E. B., & Zhao, Y. (2013). Inference for optimal dynamic treatment regimes using an adaptive *m*-out-of-*n* bootstrap scheme. *Biometrics*, (in press).

Chapman, G. B., & Sonnenberg, F. B. (2000). *Decision making in health care: Theory, psychology, and applications*. Cambridge, UK: Cambridge University Press.

Chen, Y. K. (2011). *Dose finding by the continual reassessment method*. Boca Raton: Chapman & Hall/CRC.

Chen, M.-H., Muller, P., Sun, D., & Ye, K. (Eds.). (2010). *Frontiers of statistical decision making and Bayesian analysis: In Honor of James O. Berger*. New York: Springer.

Cheung, K. Y., Lee, S. M. S., & Young, G. A. (2005). Iterating the *m* out of *n* bootstrap in nonregular smooth function models. *Statistica Sinica, 15*, 945–967.

Chow, S. C., & Chang, M. (2008). Adaptive design methods in clinical trials – A review. *Orphanet Journal of Rare Diseases, 3*.

Clemen, R. T., & Reilly, T. (2001). *Making hard decisions*. Pacific Grove: Duxbury.

Coffey, C. S., Levin, B., Clark, C., Timmerman, C., Wittes, J., Gilbert, P., & Harris, S. (2012). Overview, hurdles, and future work in adaptive designs: Perspectives from an NIH-funded workshop. *Clinical Trials, 9*, 671–680.

Cohen, J. (1988). *Statistical power for the behavioral sciences* (2nd ed.). Hillsdale: Erlbaum.

Cole, S. R., & Frangakis, C. (2009). The consistency statement in causal inference: A definition or an assumption? *Epidemiology, 20*, 3–5.

Cole, S. A., & Hernán, M. A. (2008). Constructing inverse probability weights for marginal structural models. *American Journal of Epidemiology, 168*, 656–664.

Collins, L. M., Murphy, S. A., & Bierman, K. (2004). A conceptual framework for adaptive preventive interventions. *Prevention Science, 5*, 185–196.

Collins, L. M., Murphy, S. A., Nair, V. N., & Strecher, V. J. (2005). A strategy for optimizing and evaluating behavioral interventions. *Annals of Behavioral Medicine, 30*, 65–73.

Collins, L. M., Chakraborty, B., Murphy, S. A., & Strecher, V. J. (2009). Comparison of a phased experimental approach and a single randomized clinical trial for developing multicomponent behavioral interventions. *Clinical Trials, 6*, 5–15.

Cortes, C., & Vapnik, V. (1995). Support-vector networks. *Machine Learning, 20*, 273–297.

Cotton, C. A., & Heagerty, P. J. (2011). A data augmentation method for estimating the causal effect of adherence to treatment regimens targeting control of an intermediate measure. *Statistics in Bioscience, 3*, 28–44.

Cox, D. R. (1958). *Planning of experiments*. New York: Wiley.

Cox, D. R., & Oaks, D. (1984). *Analysis of survival data*. Boca Raton, Florida: Chapman & Hall/CRC.

D'Agostino, R. B., Jr. (1998). Tutorial in biostatistics: Propensity score methods for bias reduction in the comparison of a treatment to a non-randomized control group. *Statistics in Medicine, 17*, 2265–2281.

Daniel, R. M., De Stavola, B. L., & Cousens, S. N. (2011). gformula: Estimating causal effects in the presence of time-varying confounding or mediation using the g-computation formula. *The Stata Journal, 11*, 479–517.

Daniel, R. M., Cousens, S. N., De Stavola, B. L., Kenwood, M. G., & Sterne, J. A. C. (2013). Methods for dealing with time-dependent confounding. *Statistics in Medicine, 32,* 1584–1618.

Davison, A. C., & Hinkley, D. V. (1997). *Bootstrap methods and their application.* Cambridge, UK: Cambridge University Press.

Dawid, A. P., & Didelez, V. (2010). Identifying the consequences of dynamic treatment strategies: A decision-theoretic overview. *Statistics Surveys, 4*, 184–231.

Dawson, R., & Lavori, P. W. (2010). Sample size calculations for evaluating treatment policies in multi-stage designs. *Clinical Trials, 7*, 643–652.

Dawson, R., & Lavori, P. W. (2012). Efficient design and inference for multistage randomized trials of individualized treatment policies. *Biostatistics, 13*, 142–152.

Dehejia, R. H. (2005). Program evaluation as a decision problem. *Journal of Econometrics, 125*, 141–173.

Diggle, P. J., Heagerty, P., Liang, K.-Y., Zeger, S. L. (2002). *Analysis of longitudinal data* (2nd ed.). Oxford: Oxford University Press.

Donoho, D. L., & Johnstone, I. M. (1994). Ideal spatial adaptation by wavelet shrinkage. *Biometrika, 81*, 425–455.

Dragalin, V. (2006). Adaptive designs: Terminology and classification. *Drug Information Journal, 40*, 425–435.

Efron, B. (1979). Bootstrap methods: Another look at the jackknife. *Annals of Statistics, 7*, 1–26.

Efron, B., & Tibshirani, R. (1993). *An introduction to the bootstrap* (Vol. 57). London: Chapman & Hall/CRC.

Ernst, D., Geurts, P., & Wehenkel, L. (2005). Tree-based batch mode reinforcement learning. *Journal of Machine Learning Research, 6*, 503–556.

Ernst, D., Stan, G. B., Goncalves, J., & Wehenkel, L. (2006). Clinical data based optimal STI strategies for HIV: A reinforcement learning approach. In *Proceedings of the machine learning conference of Belgium and The Netherlands (Benelearn)*, Ghent (pp. 65–72).

Ertefaie, A., Asgharian, M., & Stephens, D. A. (2012). Estimation of average treatment effects using penalization (submitted).

Fan, J., & Li, R. (2001). Variable selection via nonconcave penalized likelihood and its oracle properties. *Journal of the American Statistical Association, 96*, 1348–1360.

Fava, M., Rush, A. J., Trivedi, M. H., Nierenberg, A. A., Thase, M. E., Sackeim, H. A., Quitkin, F. M., Wisniewski, S., Lavori, P. W., Rosenbaum, J. F., & Kupfer, D. J. (2003). Background and rationale for the Sequenced Treatment Alternatives to Relieve Depression (STAR*D) study. *Psychiatric Clinics of North America, 26*, 457–494.

Feng, W., & Wahed, A. S. (2009). Sample size for two-stage studies with maintenance therapy. *Statistics in Medicine, 28*, 2028–2041.

Ferguson, T. S. (1996). *A course in large sample theory*. London: Chapman & Hall/CRC.

Figueiredo, M., & Nowak, R. (2001). Wavelet-based image estimation: An empirical Bayes approach using Jeffreys' noninformative prior. *IEEE Transactions on Image Processing, 10*, 1322–1331.

Freedman, B. (1987). Equipoise and the ethics of clinical research. *The New England Journal of Medicine, 317*, 141–145.

French, S. (1986). *Decision theory: An introduction to the mathematics of rationality*. Chichester: Ellis Horwood.

Gail, M. H., & Benichou, J. (Eds.). (2000). *Encyclopedia of epidemiologic methods*. Chichester/New York: Wiley.

Gao, H. (1998). Wavelet shrinkage denoising using the nonnegative garrote. *Journal of Computational and Graphical Statistics, 7*, 469–488.

Geurts, P., Ernst, D., & Wehenkel, L. (2006). Extremely randomized trees. *Machine Learning, 11*, 3–42.

Greenland, S. (2003). Quantifying biases in causal models: Classical confounding vs collider-stratification bias. *Epidemiology, 14*, 300–306.

Greenland, S., Pearl, J., & Robins, J. M. (1999). Causal diagrams for epidemiologic research. *Epidemiology, 10*, 37–48.

Guez, A., Vincent, R., Avoli, M., & Pineau, J. (2008). Adaptive treatment of epilepsy via batch-mode reinforcement learning. In *Proceedings of the innovative applications of artificial intelligence (IAAI)*, Chicago.

Gunter, L., Zhu, J., & Murphy, S. A. (2007). Variable selection for optimal decision making. In *Proceedings of the 11th conference on artificial intelligence in medicine*, Amsterdam.

Gunter, L., Chernick, M., & Sun, J. (2011a). A simple method for variable selection in regression with respect to treatment selection. *Pakistan Journal of Statistics and Operation Research, VII*, 363–380.

Gunter, L., Zhu, J., & Murphy, S. A. (2011b). Variable selection for qualitative interactions. *Statistical Methodology, 8*, 42–55.

Gunter, L., Zhu, J., & Murphy, S. A. (2011c). Variable selection for qualitative interactions in personalized medicine while controlling the family-wise error rate. *Journal of Biopharmaceutical Statistics, 21*, 1063–1078.

Hall, P., Horowitz, J., & Jing, B. (1995). On blocking rules for the bootstrap with dependent data. *Biometrika, 82*, 561–574.

Hastie, T., Tibshirani, R., & Friedman, J. (2009). *The elements of statistical learning: Data mining, inference, and prediction* (2nd ed.). New York: Springer.

Henderson, R., Ansell, P., & Alshibani, D. (2010). Regret-regression for optimal dynamic treatment regimes. *Biometrics, 66*, 1192–1201.

Henmi, M., & Eguchi, S. (2004). A paradox concerning nuisance parameters and projected estimating functions. *Biometrika, 91*, 929–941.

Hernán, M. A., & Robins, J. M. (2013). *Causal inference*. Chapman & Hall/CRC (in revision).

Hernán, M. A., & Taubman, S. L. (2008). Does obesity shorten life? The importance of well-defined interventions to answer causal questions. *International Journal of Obesity, 32*, S8–S14.

Hernán, M. A., Brumback, B., & Robins, J. M. (2000). Marginal structural models to estimate the causal effect of zidovudine on the survival of HIV-positive men. *Epidemiology, 11*, 561–570.

Hernán, M. A., Hernández-Díaz, S., & Robins, J. M. (2004). A structural approach to selection bias. *Epidemiology, 15*, 615–625.

Hernán, M. A., Cole, S. J., Margolick, J., Cohen, M., & Robins, J. M. (2005). Structural accelerated failure time models for survival analysis in studies with time-varying treatments. *Pharmacoepidemiology and Drug Safety, 14*, 477–491.

Hernán, M. A., Lanoy, E., Costagliola, D., & Robins, J. M. (2006). Comparison of dynamic treatment regimes via inverse probability weighting. *Basic & Clinical Pharmacology & Toxicology, 98*, 237–242.

Hirano, K., & Porter, J. (2009). Asymptotics for statistical treatment rules. *Econometrica, 77*, 1683–1701.

Holland, P. (1986). Statistics and causal inference. *Journal of the American Statistical Association, 81*, 945–970.

Huang, F., & Lee, M.-J. (2010). Dynamic treatment effect analysis of TV effects on child cognitive development. *Journal of Applied Econometrics, 25*, 392–419.

Huang, X., & Ning, J. (2012). Analysis of multi-stage treatments for recurrent diseases. *Statistics in Medicine, 31*, 2805–2821.

Huber, P. (1964). Robust estimation of a location parameter. *Annals of Mathematical Statistics, 53*, 73–101.

Joffe, M. M. (2000). Confounding by indication: The case of calcium channel blockers. *Pharamcoepidemiology and Drug Safety, 9*, 37–41.

Joffe, M. M., & Brensinger, C. (2003). Weighting in instrumental variables and G-estimation. *Statistics in Medicine, 22*, 1285–1303.

Jones, H. (2010). *Reinforcement-based treatment for pregnant drug abusers (home ii)*. Bethesda: National Institutes of Health. http://clinicaltrials.gov/ct2/show/NCT01177982?term=jones+pregnant&rank=9.

Kaelbling, L. P., Littman, M. L., & Moore, A. (1996). Reinforcement learning: A survey. *The Journal of Artificial Intelligence Research, 4*, 237–385.

Kakade, S. M. (2003). *On the sample complexity of reinforcement learning* (Dissertation, University College London).

Kasari, C. (2009). *Developmental and augmented intervention for facilitating expressive language (ccnia)*. Bethesda: National Institutes of Health. http://clinicaltrials.gov/ct2/show/NCT01013545?term=kasari&rank=5.

Kaslow, R. A., Ostrow, D. G., Detels, R., Phair, J. P., Polk, B. F., & Rinaldo, C. R. (1987). The Multicenter AIDS Cohort Study: Rationale, organization, and selected characteristics of the participants. *American Journal of Epidemiology, 126*, 310–318.

Kearns, M., Mansour, Y., & Ng, A.Y. (2000). *Approximate planning in large POMDPs via reusable trajectories* (Vol. 12). MIT.

Kramer, M. S., Chalmers, B., Hodnett, E. D., Sevkovskaya, Z., Dzikovich, I., Shapiro, S., Collet, J., Vanilovich, I., Mezen, I., Ducruet, T., Shishko, G., Zubovich, V., Mknuik, D., Gluchanina, E., Dombrovsky, V., Ustinovitch, A., Ko, T., Bogdanovich, N., Ovchinikova, L., & Helsing, E. (2001). Promotion of

Breastfeeding Intervention Trial (PROBIT): A randomized trial in the Republic of Belarus. *Journal of the American Medical Association, 285*, 413–420.

Kramer, M. S., Aboud, F., Miranova, E., Vanilovich, I., Platt, R., Matush, L., Igumnov, S., Fombonne, E., Bogdanovich, N., Ducruet, T., Collet, J., Chalmers, B., Hodnett, E., Davidovsky, S., Skugarevsky, O., Trofimovich, O., Kozlova, L., & Shapiro, S. (2008). Breastfeeding and child cognitive development: New evidence from a large randomized trial. *Archives of General Psychiatry, 65*, 578–584.

Laber, E. B., & Murphy, S. A. (2011). Adaptive confidence intervals for the test error in classification. *Journal of the American Statistical Association, 106*, 904–913.

Laber, E. B., Qian, M., Lizotte, D., & Murphy, S. A. (2011). Statistical inference in dynamic treatment regimes. arXiv:1006.5831v2 [stat.ME].

Lavori, P. W., & Dawson, R. (2000). A design for testing clinical strategies: Biased adaptive within-subject randomization. *Journal of the Royal Statistical Society, Series A, 163*, 29–38.

Lavori, P. W., & Dawson, R. (2004). Dynamic treatment regimes: Practical design considerations. *Clinical Trials, 1*, 9–20.

Lavori, P. W., & Dawson, R. (2008). Adaptive treatment strategies in chronic disease. *Annual Review of Medicine, 59*, 443–453.

Lavori, P. W., Rush, A. J., Wisniewski, S. R., Alpert, J., Fava, M., Kupfer, D. J., Nierenberg, A., Quitkin, F. M., Sackeim, H. M., Thase, M. E., & Trivedi, M. (2001). Strengthening clinical effectiveness trials: Equipoise-stratified randomization. *Biological Psychiatry, 48*, 605–614.

LeBlanc, M., & Kooperberg, C. (2010). Boosting predictions of treatment success. *Proceedings of the National Academy of Sciences, 107*, 13559–13560.

Lee, S. M. S. (1999). On a class of *m* out of *n* bootstrap confidence intervals. *Journal of the Royal Statistical Society, Series B, 61*, 901–911.

Lee, M.-J., & Huang, F. (2012). Finding dynamic treatment effects under anticipation: The effects of spanking on behaviour. *Journal of the Royal Statistical Society, Series A, 175*, 535–567.

Leeb, H., & Pötscher, B. M. (2005). Model selection and inference: Facts and fiction. *Econometric Theory, 21*, 21–59.

Lei, H., Nahum-Shani, I., Lynch, K., Oslin, D., & Murphy, S. A. (2012). A SMART design for building individualized treatment sequences. *The Annual Review of Psychology, 8*, 21–48.

Levin, B., Thompson, J. L. P., Chakraborty, R. B., Levy, G., MacArthur, R., & Haley, E. C. (2011). Statistical aspects of the TNK-S2B trial of tenecteplase versus alteplase in acute ischemic stroke: An efficient, dose-adaptive, seamless phase II/III design. *Clinical Trials, 8*, 398–407.

Li, Z., & Murphy, S. A. (2011). Sampe size formulae for two-stage randomized trials with survival outcomes. *Biometrika, 98*, 503–518.

Lieberman, J. A., Stroup, T. S., McEvoy, J. P., Swartz, M. S., Rosenheck, R. A., Perkins, D. O., Keefe, R. S. E., Davis, S., Davis, C. E., Lebowitz, B. D., & Severe, J. (2005). Effectiveness of antipsychotic drugs in patients with chronic schozophrenia. *New England Journal of Medicine, 353*, 1209–1223.

Lindley, D. V. (1985). *Making decisions* (2nd ed.). New York: Wiley.

Lindley, D. V. (2002). Seeing and doing: The concept of causation. *International Statistical Review, 70*, 191–214.

Little, R. J. A., & Rubin, D. B. (2002). *Statistical analysis with missing data* (2nd ed.). New York: Wiley.

Lizotte, D., Bowling, M., & Murphy, S. A. (2010). Efficient reinforcement learning with multiple reward functions for randomized clinical trial analysis. In *Twenty-seventh international conference on machine learning (ICML)*, Haifa (pp. 695–702). Omnipress.

Lu, W., Zhang, H. H., & Zeng, D. (2013). Variable selection for optimal treatment decision. *Statistical Methods in Medical Research* (in press). doi:10.1177/0962280211428383.

Lunceford, J. K., Davidian, M., & Tsiatis, A. A. (2002). Estimation of survival distributions of treatment policies in two-stage randomization designs in clinical trials. *Biometrics, 58*, 48–57.

Lusted, L. B. (1968). *Introduction to medical decision making*. Springfield: Thomas.

Manski, C. F. (2000). Identification problems and decisions under ambiguity: Empirical analysis of treatment response and normative analysis of treatment choice. *Journal of Econometrics, 95*, 415–442.

Manski, C. F. (2002). Treatment choice under ambiguity induced by inferential problems. *Journal of Statistical Planning and Inference, 105*, 67–82.

Manski, C. F. (2004). Statistical treatment rules for heterogeneous populations. *Econometica, 72*, 1221–1246.

Mark, S. D., & Robins, J. M. (1993). Estimating the causal effect of smoking cessation in the presence of confounding factors using a rank preserving structural failure time model. *Statistics in Medicine, 12*, 1605–1628.

Mason, J., Freemantle, N., & Eccles, M. (2000). Fatal toxicity associated with antidepressant use in primary care. *British Journal of General Practice, 50*, 366–370.

McEvoy, J. P., Lieberman, J. A., Stroup, T. S., Davis, S., Meltzer, H. Y., Rosenheck, R. A., Swartz, M. S., Perkins, D. O., Keefe, R. S. E., Davis, C. E., Severe, J., & Hsiao, J. K. (2006). Effectiveness of clozapine versus olanzapine, quetiapine and risperidone in patients with chronic schizophrenia who did not respond to prior atypical antipsychotic treatment. *American Journal of Psychiatry, 163*, 600–610.

Moodie, E. E. M. (2009a). A note on the variance of doubly-robust G-estimates. *Biometrika, 96*, 998–1004.

Moodie, E. E. M. (2009b). Risk factor adjustment in marginal structural model estimation of optimal treatment regimes. *Biometrical Journal, 51*, 774–788.

Moodie, E. E. M., & Richardson, T. S. (2010). Estimating optimal dynamic regimes: Correcting bias under the null. *Scandinavian Journal of Statistics, 37*, 126–146.

Moodie, E. E. M., Richardson, T. S., & Stephens, D. A. (2007). Demystifying optimal dynamic treatment regimes. *Biometrics, 63*, 447–455.

Moodie, E. E. M., Platt, R. W., & Kramer, M. S. (2009). Estimating response-maximized decision rules with applications to breastfeeding. *Journal of the American Statistical Association, 104*, 155–165.

Moodie, E. E. M., Chakraborty, B., & Kramer, M. S. (2012). Q-learning for estimating optimal dynamic treatment rules from observational data. *Canadian Journal of Statistics, 40*, 629–645.

Moodie, E. E. M., Dean, N., & Sun, Y. R. (2013). Q-learning: Flexible learning about useful utilities. *Statistics in Biosciences*, (in press).

Mortimer, K. M., Neugebauer, R., Van der Laan, M. J., & Tager, I. B. (2005). An application of model-fitting procedures for marginal structural models. *American Journal of Epidemiology, 162*, 382–388.

Murphy, S. A. (2003). Optimal dynamic treatment regimes (with Discussion). *Journal of the Royal Statistical Society, Series B, 65*, 331–366.

Murphy, S. A. (2005a). An experimental design for the development of adaptive treatment strategies. *Statistics in Medicine, 24*, 1455–1481.

Murphy, S. A. (2005b). A generalization error for Q-learning. *Journal of Machine Learning Research, 6*, 1073–1097.

Murphy, S. A., & Bingham, D. (2009). Screening experiments for developing dynamic treatment regimes. *Journal of the American Statistical Association, 184*, 391–408.

Murphy, S. A., Van der Laan, M. J., Robins, J. M., & CPPRG (2001). Marginal mean models for dynamic regimes. *Journal of the American Statistical Association, 96*, 1410–1423.

Murphy, S. A., Lynch, K. G., Oslin, D., Mckay, J. R., & TenHave, T. (2007a). Developing adaptive treatment strategies in substance abuse research. *Drug and Alcohol Dependence, 88*, s24–s30.

Murphy, S. A., Oslin, D., Rush, A. J., & Zhu, J. (2007b). Methodological challenges in constructing effective treatment sequences for chronic psychiatric disorders. *Neuropsychopharmacology, 32*, 257–262.

Nahum-Shani, I., Qian, M., Almiral, D., Pelham, W., Gnagy, B., Fabiano, G., Waxmonsky, J., Yu, J., & Murphy, S. A. (2012a). Experimental design and primary data analysis methods for comparing adaptive interventions. *Psychological Methods, 17*, 457–477.

Nahum-Shani, I., Qian, M., Almiral, D., Pelham, W., Gnagy, B., Fabiano, G., Waxmonsky, J., Yu, J., & Murphy, S. (2012b). Q-learning: A data analysis method for constructing adaptive interventions. *Psychological Methods, 17*, 478–494.

Nankervis, J. C. (2005). Computational algorithms for double bootstrap confidence intervals. *Computational Statistics & Data Analysis, 49*, 461–475.

Nelson, J. C. (1997). Safety and tolerability of the new antidepressants. *Journal of Clinical Psychiatry, 58*(Suppl. 6), 26–31.

Neugebauer, R., & Van der Laan, M. J. (2005). Why prefer double robust estimators in causal inference? *Journal of Statistical Planning and Inference, 129*, 405–426.

Neugebauer, R., & Van der Laan, M. J. (2006). G-computation estimation for causal inference with complex longitudinal data. *Computational Statistics & Data Analysis, 51*, 1676–1697.

Neugebauer, R., Silverberg, M. J., & Van der Laan, M. J. (2010). *Observational study and individualized antiretroviral therapy initiation rules for reducing cancer incidence in HIV-infected patients* (Technical report). U.C. Berkeley Division of Biostatistics Working Paper Series.

Newey, W. K., & McFadden, D. (1994). Large sample estimation and hypothesis testing. In R. F. Engle & D. L. McFadden (Eds.), *Handbook of econometrics* (Vol. IV, pp. 2113–2245). Amsterdam/Oxford: Elsevier Science.

Neyman, J. (1923). On the application of probability theory to agricultural experiments. Essay in principles. Section 9 (translation published in 1990). *Statistical Science, 5*, 472–480.

Ng, A., & Jordan, M. (2000). PEGASUS: A policy search method for large MDPs and POMDPs.

Oetting, A. I., Levy, J. A., Weiss, R. D., & Murphy, S. A. (2011). Statistical methodology for a SMART design in the development of adaptive treatment strategies. In: P. E. Shrout, K. M. Keyes, & K. Ornstein (Eds.) *Causality and Psychopathology: Finding the Determinants of Disorders and their Cures* (pp. 179–205). Arlington: American Psychiatric Publishing.

Olshen, R. A. (1973). The conditional level of the F-test. *Journal of the American Statistical Association, 68*, 692–698.

Orellana, L., Rotnitzky, A., & Robins, J. M. (2010a). Dynamic regime marginal structural mean models for estimation of optimal dynamic treatment regimes, part I: Main content. *The International Journal of Biostatistics, 6.*

Orellana, L., Rotnitzky, A., & Robins, J. M. (2010b). Dynamic regime marginal structural mean models for estimation of optimal dynamic treatment regimes, part II: Proofs and additional results. *The International Journal of Biostatistics, 6.*

Ormoneit, D., & Sen, S. (2002). Kernel-based reinforcement learning. *Machine Learning, 49*, 161–178.

Oslin, D. (2005). *Managing alcoholism in people who do not respond to naltrexone (ExTENd)*. Bethesda: National Institutes of Health. http://clinicaltrials.gov/ct2/show/NCT00115037?term=oslin&rank=8.

Pampallona, S., & Tsiatis, A. A. (1994). Group sequential designs for one and two sided hypothesis testing with provision for early stopping in favour of the null hypothesis. *Journal of Statistical Planning and Inference, 42*, 19–35.

Parmigiani, G. (2002). *Modeling in medical decision making: A Bayesian approach*. New York: Wiley.

Pearl, J. (2009). *Causality* (2nd ed.). New York: Cambridge University Press.

Petersen, M. L., Deeks, S. G., & Van der Laan, M. J. (2007). Individualized treatment rules: Generating candidate clinical trials. *Statistics in Medicine, 26*, 4578–4601.

Petersen, M. L., Porter, K. E., Gruber, S., Wang, Y., & Van der Laan, M. J. (2012). Diagnosing and responding to violations in the positivity assumption. *Statistical Methods in Medical Research, 21*, 31–54.

Partnership for Solutions (2004). *Chronic conditions: Making the case for ongoing care: September 2004 update*. Baltimore: Partnership for Solutions, Johns Hopkins University.

Pineau, J., Bellernare, M. G., Rush, A. J., Ghizaru, A., & Murphy, S. A. (2007). Constructing evidence-based treatment strategies using methods from computer science. *Drug and Alcohol Dependence, 88*, S52–S60.

Pliskin, J. S., Shepard, D., & Weinstein, M. C. (1980). Utility functions for life years and health status: Theory, assessment, and application. *Operations Research, 28*, 206–224.

Pocock, S. J. (1977). Group sequential methods in the design and analysis of clinical trials. *Biometrika, 64*, 191–199.

Politis, D. N., Romano, J. P., & Wolf, M. (1999). *Subsampling*. New York: Springer.

Pötscher, B. M. (2007). Confidence sets based on sparse estimators are necessarily large. Arxiv preprint arXiv:0711.1036.

Pötscher, B. M., & Schneider, U. (2008). *Confidence sets based on penalized maximum likelihood estimators*. Mpra paper, University Library of Munich, Germany.

Qian, M., & Murphy, S. A. (2011). Performance guarantees for individualized treatment rules. *Annals of Statistics, 39*, 1180–1210.

Rich, B., Moodie, E. E. M., Stephens, D. A., & Platt, R. W. (2010). Model checking with residuals for g-estimation of optimal dynamic treatment regimes. *The International Journal of Biostatistics, 6*.

Rich, B., Moodie, E. E. M., and Stephens, D.A. (2013) Adaptive individualized dosing in pharmacological studies: Generating candidate dynamic dosing strategies for warfarin treatment. (submitted).

Robins, J. M. (1986). A new approach to causal inference in mortality studies with sustained exposure periods – Application to control of the healthy worker survivor effect. *Mathematical Modelling, 7*, 1393–1512.

Robins, J. M. (1994). Correcting for non-compliance in randomized trials using structural nested mean models. *Communications in Statistics, 23*, 2379–2412.

Robins, J. M. (1997). Causal inference from complex longitudinal data. In M. Berkane (Ed.), *Latent variable modeling and applications to causality: Lecture notes in statistics* (pp. 69–117). New York: Springer.

Robins J. M. (1999a). Marginal structural models versus structural nested models as tools for causal inference. In: M. E. Halloran & D. Berry (Eds.) *Statistical models in epidemiology: The environment and clinical trials. IMA, 116*, NY: Springer-Verlag, pp. 95–134.

Robins, J. M. (1999b). Association, causation, and marginal structural models. *Synthese, 121*, 151–179.

Robins, J. M. (2004). Optimal structural nested models for optimal sequential decisions. In D. Y. Lin & P. Heagerty (Eds.), *Proceedings of the second Seattle symposium on biostatistics* (pp. 189–326). New York: Springer.

Robins, J. M., & Hernán, M. A. (2009). Estimation of the causal effects of time-varying exposures. In G. Fitzmaurice, M. Davidian, G. Verbeke, & G. Molenberghs (Eds.), *Longitudinal data analysis*. Boca Raton: Chapman & Hall/CRC.

Robins, J. M., & Wasserman, L. (1997). Estimation of effects of sequential treatments by reparameterizing directed acyclic graphs. In D. Geiger & P. Shenoy (Eds.), *Proceedings of the thirteenth conference on uncertainty in artificial intelligence* (pp. 409–430). Providence.

Robins, J. M., Hernán, M. A., & Brumback, B. (2000). Marginal structural models and causal inference in epidemiology. *Epidemiology, 11*, 550–560.

Robins, J. M., Orellana, L., & Rotnitzky, A. (2008). Estimation and extrapolation of optimal treatment and testing strategies. *Statistics in Medicine, 27*, 4678–4721.

Rosenbaum, P. R. (1991). Discussing hidden bias in observational studies. *Annals of Internal Medicine, 115*, 901–905.

Rosenbaum, P. R., & Rubin, D. B. (1983). The central role of the propensity score in observational studies for causal effects. *Biometrika, 70*, 41–55.

Rosenbaum, P. R., & Rubin, D. B. (1984). Reducing bias in observational studies using subclassification on the propensity score. *Journal of the American Statistical Association, 79*, 516–524.

Rosenbaum, P. R., & Rubin, D. B. (1985). Constructing a control group using multivariate matched sampling methods that incorporate the propensity score. *The American Statistician, 39*, 33–38.

Rosthøj, S., Fullwood, C., Henderson, R., & Stewart, S. (2006). Estimation of optimal dynamic anticoagulation regimes from observational data: A regret-based approach. *Statistics in Medicine, 25*, 4197–4215.

Rubin, D. B. (1974). Estimating causal effects of treatments in randomized and nonrandomized studies. *Journal of Educational Psychology, 66*, 688–701.

Rubin, D. B. (1980). Discussion of "randomized analysis of experimental data: The Fisher randomization test" by D. Basu. *Journal of the American Statistical Association, 75*, 591–593.

Rubin, D. B., & Shenker, N. (1991). Multiple imputation in health-case data bases: An overview and some applications. *Statistics in Medicine, 10*, 585–598.

Rubin, D. B., & van der Laan, M. J. (2012). Statistical issues and limitations in personalized medicine research with clinical trials. *International Journal of Biostatistics, 8*.

Rush, A. J., Fava, M., Wisniewski, S. R., Lavori, P. W., Trivedi, M. H., Sackeim, H. A., Thase, M. E., Nierenberg, A. A., Quitkin, F. M., Kashner, T. M., Kupfer, D. J., Rosenbaum, J. F., Alpert, J., Stewart, J. W., McGrath, P. J., Biggs, M. M., Shores-Wilson, K., Lebowitz, B. D., Ritz, L., & Niederehe, G. (2004). Sequenced treatment alternatives to relieve depression (STAR*D): Rationale and design. *Controlled Clinical Trials, 25*, 119–142.

Saarela, O., Moodie, E. E. M., Stephens, D. A., & Klein, M. B. (2013a). On Bayesian estimation of marginal structural models (submitted).

Saarela, O., Stephens, D. A., & Moodie, E. E. M. (2013b). The role of exchangeability in causal inference (submitted).

Schneider, L. S., Tariot, P. N., Lyketsos, C. G., Dagerman, K. S., Davis, K. L., & Davis, S. (2001). National Institute of Mental Health Clinical Antipsychotic Trials of Intervention Effectiveness (CATIE): Alzheimer disease trial methodology. *American Journal of Geriatric Psychiatry, 9*, 346–360.

Schulte, P. J., Tsiatis, A. A., Laber, E. B., & Davidian, M. (2012). Q- and A-learning methods for estimating optimal dynamic treatment regimes. arXiv, 1202.4177v1.

Sekhon, J. S. (2011). Multivariate and propensity score matching software with automated balance optimization: The matching package for R. *Journal of Statistical Software, 42*, 1–52.

Shao, J. (1994). Bootstrap sample size in nonregular cases. *Proceedings of the American Mathematical Society, 122*, 1251–1262.

Shao, J., & Sitter, R. R. (1996). Bootstrap for imputed survey data. *Journal of the American Statistical Association, 91*, 1278–1288.

Shepherd, B. E., Jenkins, C. A., Rebeiro, P. F., Stinnette, S. E., Bebawy, S. S., McGowan, C. C., Hulgan, T., & Sterling, T. R. (2010). Estimating the optimal CD4 count for HIV-infected persons to start antiretroviral therapy. *Epidemiology, 21*, 698–705.

Shivaswamy, P., Chu, W., & Jansche, M. (2007). A support vector approach to censored targets. In *Proceedings of the seventh IEEE international conference on data mining*, Omaha (pp. 655–660).

Shortreed, S. M., & Moodie, E. E. M. (2012). Estimating the optimal dynamic antipsychotic treatment regime: Evidence from the sequential-multiple assignment randomized CATIE Schizophrenia Study. *Journal of the Royal Statistical Society, Series B, 61*, 577–599.

Shortreed, S. M., Laber, E., & Murphy, S. A. (2010). *Imputation methods for the clinical antipsychotic trials of intervention and effectiveness study* (Technical report SOCS-TR-2010.8). School of Computer Science, McGill University.

Shortreed, S. M., Laber, E., Lizotte, D. J., Stroup, T. S., Pineau, J., & Murphy, S. A. (2011). Informing sequential clinical decision-making through reinforcement learning: An empirical study. *Machine Learning, 84*, 109–136.

Sjölander, A., Nyrén, O., Bellocco, R., & Evans, M. (2011). Comparing different strategies for timing of dialysis initiation through inverse probability weighting. *American Journal of Epidemiology, 174*, 1204–1210.

Song, R., Wang, W., Zeng, D., & Kosorok, M. R. (2011). Penalized Q-learning for dynamic treatment regimes arXiv:1108.5338v1 [stat.ME].

Sox, H. C., Blatt, M. A., Higgins, M. C., & Marton, K. I. (1988). *Medical decision making*. Boston: Butterworth-Heinemann.

Sterne, J. A. C., May, M., Costagliola, D., de Wolf, F., Phillips, A. N., Harris, R., Funk, M. J., Geskus, R. B., Gill, J., Dabis, F., Miró, J. M., Justice, A. C., Ledergerber, B., Fätkenheuer, G., Hogg, R. S., D'Arminio Monforte, A., Saag, M., Smith, C., Staszewski, S., Egger, M., Cole, S. R., & The When To Start Consortium (2009). Timing of initiation of antiretroviral therapy in AIDS-free HIV-1-infected patients: A collaborative analysis of 18 HIV cohort studies. *Lancet, 373*, 1352–1363.

Stewart, C. E., Fielder, A. R., Stephens, D. A., & Moseley, M. J. (2002). Design of the Monitored Occlusion Treatment of Amblyopia Study (MOTAS). *British Journal of Ophthalmology, 86*, 915–919.

Stewart, C. E., Moseley, M. J., Stephens, D. A., & Fielder, A. R. (2004). Treatment dose-response in amblyopia therapy: The Monitored Occlusion Treatment of Amblyopia Study (MOTAS). *Investigations in Ophthalmology and Visual Science, 45*, 3048–3054.

Stone, R. M., Berg, D. T., George, S. L., Dodge, R. K., Paciucci, P. A., Schulman, P., Lee, E. J., Moore, J. O., Powell, B. L., & Schiffer, C. A. (1995). Granulocyte macrophage colony-stimulating factor after initial chemotherapy for elderly patients with primary acute myelogenous leukemia. *The New England Journal of Medicine, 332*, 1671–1677.

Strecher, V., McClure, J., Alexander, G., Chakraborty, B., Nair, V., Konkel, J., Greene, S., Collins, L., Carlier, C., Wiese, C., Little, R., Pomerleau, C., & Pomerleau, O. (2008). Web-based smoking cessation components and tailoring depth: Results of a randomized trial. *American Journal of Preventive Medicine, 34*, 373–381.

Stroup, T. S., McEvoy, J. P., Swartz, M. S., Byerly, M. J., Glick, I. D., Canive, J. M., McGee, M., Simpson, G. M., Stevens, M. D., & Lieberman, J. A. (2003). The National Institute of Mental Health Clinical Antipschotic Trials of Intervention Effectiveness (CATIE) project: Schizophrenia trial design and protocol deveplopment. *Schizophrenia Bulletin, 29*, 15–31.

Stroup, T. S., Lieberman, J. A., McEvoy, J. P., Davis, S. M., Meltzer, H. Y., Rosenheck, R. A., Swartz, M. S., Perkins, D. O., Keefe, R. S. E., Davis, C. E., Severe, J., & Hsiao, J. K. (2006). Effectiveness of olanzapine, quetiapine, risperidone, and ziprasidone in patients with chronic schizophrenia folllowing discontinuation of a previous atypical antipsychotic. *American Journal of Psychiatry, 163*, 611–622.

Sturmer, T., Schneeweiss, S., Brookhart, M. A., Rothman, K. J., Avorn, J., & Glynn, R. J. (2005). Analytic strategies to adjust confounding using exposure propensity scores and disease risk scores: Nonsteroidal antiinflammatory drugs and short-term mortality in the elderly. *American Journal of Epidemiology, 161*, 891–898.

Sutton, R. S., & Barto, A. G. (1998). *Reinforcement learning: An introduction*. Cambridge, MA: MIT.

Swartz, M. S., Perkins, D. O., Stroup, T. S., McEvoy, J. P., Nieri, J. M., & Haal, D. D. (2003). Assessing clinical and functional outcomes in the Clinical Antipsychotic Trials of Intervention Effectiveness (CATIE) schizophrenia trial. *Schizophrenia Bulletin, 29*, 33–43.

Taubman, S. L., Robins, J. M., Mittleman, M. A., & Hernán, M. A. (2009). Intervening on risk factors for coronary heart disease: An application of the parametric g-formula. *International Journal of Epidemiology, 38*, 1599–1611.

Thall, P. F., & Wathen, J. K. (2005). Covariate-adjusted adaptive randomization in a sarcoma trial with multi-stage treatments. *Statistics in Medicine, 24*, 1947–1964.

Thall, P. F., Millikan, R. E., & Sung, H. G. (2000). Evaluating multiple treatment courses in clinical trials. *Statistics in Medicine, 30*, 1011–1128.

Thall, P. F., Sung, H. G., & Estey, E. H. (2002). Selecting therapeutic strategies based on efficacy and death in multicourse clinical trials. *Journal of the American Statistical Association, 97*, 29–39.

Thall, P. F., Wooten, L. H., Logothetis, C. J., Millikan, R. E., & Tannir, N. M. (2007a). Bayesian and frequentist two-stage treatment strategies based on sequential failure times subject to interval censoring. *Statistics in Medicine, 26*, 4687–4702.

Thall, P. F., Logothetis, C., Pagliaro, L. C., Wen, S., Brown, M. A., Williams, D., & Millikan, R. E. (2007b). Adaptive therapy for androgen-independent prostate cancer: A randomized selection trial of four regimens. *Journal of the National Cancer Institute, 99*, 1613–1622.

Tibshirani, R. (1996). Regression shrinkage and selection via the lasso. *Journal of the Royal Statistical Society, Series B, 58*, 267–288.

Topol, E. (2012). *Creative destruction of medicine: How the digital revolution and personalized medicine will create better health care*. New York: Basic Books.

Torrance, G. W. (1986). Measurement of health state utilities for economic appraisal. *Journal of Health Economics, 5*, 1–30.

Tsiatis, A. A. (2006). *Semiparametric theory and missing data*. New York: Springer.

Van der Laan, M. J., & Petersen, M. L. (2007a). Causal effect models for realistic individualized treatment and intention to treat rules. *The International Journal of Biostatistics, 3*.

Van der Laan, M. J., & Petersen, M. L. (2007b). Statistical learning of origin-specific statically optimal individualized treatment rules. *The International Journal of Biostatistics, 3*.

Van der Laan, M. J., & Robins, J. M. (2003). *Unified methods for censored longitudinal data and causality*. New York: Springer.

Van der Laan, M. J., & Rubin, D. (2006). Targeted maximum likelihood learning. *The International Journal of Biostatistics, 2*.

Van der Vaart, A. W. (1998). *Asymptotic statistics*. Cambridge, UK: Cambridge University Press.

Vansteelandt, S., & Goetghebeur, E. (2003). Causal inference with generalized structural mean models. *Journal of the Royal Statistical Society, Series B, 65*, 817–835.

Vapnik, V. (1995). *The nature of statistical learning theory*. New York: Springer.

Vogt, W. P. (1993). *Dictionary of statistics and methodology: A nontechnical guide for the social sciences*. Newbury Park: Sage Publications.

Wagner, E. H., Austin, B. T., Davis, C., Hindmarsh, M., Schaefer, J., & Bonomi, A. (2001). Improving chronic illness care: Translating evidence into action. *Health Affairs, 20*, 64–78.

Wahed, A. S., & Tsiatis, A. A. (2004). Optimal estimator for the survival distribution and related quantities for treatment policies in two-stage randomized designs in clinical trials. *Biometrics, 60*, 124–133.

Wahed, A. S., & Tsiatis, A. A. (2006). Semiparametric efficient estimation of survival distributions in two-stage randomisation designs in clinical trials with censored data. *Biometrika, 93*, 163–177.

Wald, A. (1949). *Statistical decision functions*. New York: Wiley.

Wang, Y., Petersen, M. L., Bangsberg, D., & Van der Laan, M. J. (2006). *Diagnosing bias in the inverse probability of treatment weighted estimator resulting from violation of experimental treatment assignment*. UC Berkeley Division of Biostatistics Working Paper Series.

Wang, L., Rotnitzky, A., Lin, X., Millikan, R. E., & Thall, P. F. (2012). Evaluation of viable dynamic treatment regimes in a sequentially randomized trial of advanced prostate cancer. *Journal of the American Statistical Association, 107*, 493–508.

Wathen, J. K., & Thall, P. F. (2008). Bayesian adaptive model selection for optimizing group sequential clinical trials. *Statistics in Medicine, 27*, 5586–5604.

Watkins, C. J. C. H. (1989). *Learning from delayed rewards* (Dissertation, Cambridge University).

Weinstein, M. C., Feinberg, H., Elstein, A. S., Frazier, H. S., Neuhauser, D., Neutra, R. R., & McNeil, B. J. (1980). *Clinical decision analysis*. Philadelphia: Saunders.

Westreich, D., Cole, S. R., Young, J. G., Palella, F., Tien, P. C., Kingsley, L., Gange, S. J., & Hernán, M. A. (2012). The parametric g-formula to estimate the effect of highly active antiretroviral therapy on incident AIDS or death. *Statistics in Medicine, 31*, 2000–2009.

WHO (1997). *The World Health Report 1997: Conquering suffering, enriching humanity*. Geneva: The World Health Organization.

Wood, S. N. (2006). *Generalized additive models: An introduction with R*. Boca Raton: Chapman & Hall/CRC.

Wood, S. N. (2011). Fast stable restricted maximum likelihood and marginal likelihood estimation of semiparametric generalized linear models. *Journal of the Royal Statistical Society, Series B, 73*, 3–36.

Xiao, Y., Abrahamowicz, M., Moodie, E. E. M., Weber, R., and Young, J. (2013) Flexible marginal structural models for estimating cumulative effect of time-dependent treatment on the hazard: Reassessing the cardiovascular risks of didanosine treatment in the Swiss HIV Cohort. (In revision.)

Young, J. G., Cain, L. E., Robins, J. M., O'Reilly, E. J., & Hernán, M. A. (2011). Comparative effectiveness of dynamic treatment regimes: An application of the parametric G-formula. *Statistics in Biosciences, 1*, 119–143.

Zajonc, T. (2012). Bayesian inference for dynamic treatment regimes: Mobility, equity, and efficiency in student tracking. *Journal of the American Statistical Association, 107*, 80–92.

Zhang, T. (2004). Statistical behavior and consistency of classification methods based on convex risk minimization. *Annals of Statistics, 32*, 56–85.

Zhang, B., Tsiatis, A. A., Davidian, M., Zhang, M., & Laber, E. B. (2012a). Estimating optimal treatment regimes from a classification perspective. *Stat, 1*, 103–114.

Zhang, B., Tsiatis, A. A., Laber, E. B., & Davidian, M. (2012b). A robust method for estimating optimal treatment regimes. *Biometrics*, 68, 1010–1018.

Zhao, Y., Kosorok, M. R., & Zeng, D. (2009). Reinforcement learning design for cancer clinical trials. *Statistics in Medicine, 28*, 3294–3315.

Zhao, Y., Zeng, D., Socinski, M. A., & Kosorok, M. R. (2011). Reinforcement learning strategies for clinical trials in nonsmall cell lung cancer. *Biometrics, 67*, 1422–1433.

Zhao, Y., Zeng, D., Rush, A. J., & Kosorok, M. R. (2012). Estimating individual treatment rules using outcome weighted learning. *Journal of the American Statistical Association, 107*, 1106–1118.

Zou, H. (2006). The adaptive lasso and its oracle properties. *Journal of the American Statistical Association, 101*, 1418–1429.

Index

B. Chakraborty and E.E.M. Moodie, *Statistical Methods for Dynamic Treatment Regimes*,
Statistics for Biology and Health 76, DOI 10.1007/978-1-4614-7428-9,